Methods in Neurosciences

Volume 18

Lipid Metabolism in Signaling Systems

Methods in Neurosciences

Editor-in-Chief
P. Michael Conn

Methods in Neurosciences

Volume 18
Lipid Metabolism in Signaling Systems

Edited by
John N. Fain
Department of Biochemistry
University of Tennessee
Center for Health Science
Memphis, Tennessee

ACADEMIC PRESS, INC.
A Division of Harcourt Brace & Company
San Diego   New York   Boston   London   Sydney   Tokyo   Toronto

Front cover photograph: Rat embryo fibroblasts (REF52 cells) were grown on glass coverslips. Soluble proteins were extracted with Triton X-100. The remaining insoluble components (cytoskeletons) were fixed in formaldehyde and stained with α-protein kinase C specific antibody M6. Preparations were then stained with fluorescein-conjugated goat anti-mouse antibody and photographed under a fluorescence microscope using a 60X objective. In these cells, α-PKC is concentrated in sites of cell–substratum attachment known as focal contacts. Courtesy of Drs. Susan Jaken and Sussanah L. Hyatt, W. Alton Jones Cell Science Center Incorporated, Lake Placid, New York.

This book is printed on acid-free paper. ∞

Academic Press, Inc.
525 B Street, Suite 1900, San Diego, California 92101-4495

United Kingdom Edition published by
Academic Press Limited
24–28 Oval Road, London NW1 7DX

International Standard Serial Number: 1043-9471

International Standard Book Number: 0-12-185285-7

PRINTED IN THE UNITED STATES OF AMERICA
93 94 95 96 97 98   E B   9 8 7 6 5 4 3 2 1

Table of Contents

Section V Inositol Phosphate Receptors and Their Regulation

Contributors to Volume 18

Article numbers are in parentheses following the names of contributors. Affiliations listed are current.

JOHN C. ANTHES (3), Schering-Plough Research Institute, Kenilworth, New Jersey 07033

ELAINE S. G. BARDES (15), Section of Cell Growth, Department of Biochemistry, Duke University Medical Center, Durham, North Carolina 27710

ROBERT M. BELL (15), Section of Cell Growth, Department of Biochemistry, Duke University Medical Center, Durham, North Carolina 27710

M. MOTASIM BILLAH (3), Schering–Plough Research Institute, Kenilworth, New Jersey 07033

JOHN BLOOMENTHAL (15), Section of Cell Growth, Department of Biochemistry, Duke University Medical Center, Durham, North Carolina 27710

ROY A. BORCHARDT (15), Section of Cell Growth, Department of Biochemistry, Duke University Medical Center, Durham, North Carolina 27710

URS BRODBECK (1), Department of Neurochemistry, Institute of Biochemistry and Molecular Biology, University of Bern, CH-3012 Bern, Switzerland

LEWIS C. CANTLEY (12), Division of Signal Transduction, Department of Medicine, Beth Israel Hospital, Boston, Massachusetts 02115

VERED CHALIFA (2), Department of Hormone Research, The Weizmann Institute of Science, Rehovot 76100, Israel

R. A. JOHN CHALLISS (21), Department of Pharmacology and Therapeutics, University of Leicester, Leicester LE1 9HN, United Kingdom

ENRIQUE CLARO (5), Departamento de Bioquímica y Biología Molecular, Universidad Autónoma de Barcelona, E-08193 Bellaterra, Barcelona, Spain

MICHAL DANIN (2), Department of Hormone Research, The Weizmann Institute of Science, Rehovot 76100, Israel

JOHN F. DIXON (28), Department of Pharmacology, University of Wisconsin Medical School, Madison, Wisconsin 53706

JOSEPH EICHBERG (10), Department of Biochemical and Biophysical Sciences, University of Houston, Houston, Texas 77204

CHRISTOPHE ERNEUX (26), Institut de Recherche Interdisciplinaire (IRIBHN), Université Libre de Bruxelles, B-1070 Brussels, Belgium

JOHN N. FAIN (4, 5), Department of Biochemistry, University of Tennessee, Center for Health Science, Memphis, Tennessee 38163

DAVID FRITH (16), Max-Delbrück-Laboratorium, Max-Planck-Gesellschaft, D-50829 Köln, Germany

ABDALLAH GHALAYINI (10), Department of Ophthamology, Baylor College of Medicine, Houston, Texas 77030

AMIYA K. HAJRA (18), Mental Health Research Institute and Department of Biological Chemistry, University of Michigan, Ann Arbor, Michigan 48104

MASATO HIRATA (25), Department of Biochemistry, Faculty of Dentistry, Kyushu University, Fukuoka 812, Japan

MARIUS C. HOENER (1), Department of Neurochemistry, Institute of Biochemistry and Molecular Biology, University of Bern, CH-3012 Bern, Switzerland

ARIANE HÖER (27), Institut für Pharmakologie, Freie Universität Berlin, D-14195 Berlin, Germany

LOWELL E. HOKIN (28), Department of Pharmacology, University of Wisconsin Medical School, Madison, Wisconsin 53706

FONG-FU HSU (19), Department of Medicine, Washington University School of Medicine, St. Louis, Missouri 63110

FREESIA L. HUANG (14), Section on Metabolic Regulation, Endocrinology and Reproduction Research Branch, NICHHD, National Institutes of Health, Bethesda, Maryland 20892

KUO-PING HUANG (14), Section on Metabolic Regulation, Endocrinology and Reproduction Research Branch, NICHHD, National Institutes of Health, Bethesda, Maryland 20892

SUSAN JAKEN (17), W. Alton Jones Cell Science Center, Lake Placid, New York 12946

DEOK-YOUNG JHON (7), Section on Signal Transduction, Laboratory of Biochemistry, NHLBI, National Institutes of Health, Bethesda, Maryland 20892

TAKASHI KANEMATSU (25), Department of Biochemistry, Faculty of Dentistry, Kyushu University, Fukuoka 812, Japan

DAVID R. KAPLAN (12), Eukaryotic Signal Transduction Group, Molecular Mechanisms of Carcinogenesis Laboratory, ABL-Basic Research Program, National Cancer Institute, Frederick Cancer Research and Development Center, Frederick, Maryland 21702

RYUICHI KATO (20), Department of Pharmacology, Keio University School of Medicine, Tokyo 160, Japan

KAREN LEACH (17), Department of Cell Biology, The Upjohn Company, Kalamazoo, Michigan 49001

CHANG-WON LEE (8), Section on Signal Transduction, Laboratory of Biochemistry, NHLBI, National Institutes of Health, Bethesda, Maryland 20892

CHUNGHEE LEE (18), Molecular Pathophysiology Branch, NIDDK, National Institutes of Health, Bethesda, Maryland 20892

KWEON-HAENG LEE (8), Section on Signal Transduction, Laboratory of Biochemistry, NHLBI, National Institutes of Health, Bethesda, Maryland 20892

MORDECHAI LISCOVITCH (2), Department of Hormone Research, The Weizmann Institute of Science, Rehovot 76100, Israel

MAREK LIYANAGE (16), Max-Delbrück-Laboratorium, Max-Planck-Gesellschaft, D-50829 Köln, Germany

SILVIA LLAHI (4), Department of Biochemistry, University of Tennessee, Center for Health Science, Memphis, Tennessee 38163

GREGORY A. MIGNERY (22), Department of Physiology, Stritch School of Medicine, Loyola University Medical Center, Maywood, Illinois 60153

HEIDI MÖHN (2), Department of Hormone Research, The Weizmann Institute of Science, Rehovot 76100, Israel

STEFAN R. NAHORSKI (21, 23), Department of Pharmacology and Therapeutics, University of Leicester, Leicester LE1 9HN, United Kingdom

TOSHIO NAKAKI (20), Department of Pharmacology, Keio University School of Medicine, Tokyo 160, Japan

ECKARD OBERDISSE (27), Institut für Pharmakologie, Freie Universität Berlin, D-14195 Berlin, Germany

KEN-ICHI OSADA (14), Section of Metabolic Regulation, Endocrinology and Reproduction Research Branch, NICHHD, National Institutes of Health, Bethesda, Maryland 20892

DONGEUN PARK (7), Section on Signal Transduction, Laboratory of Biochemistry, NHLBI, National Institutes of Health, Bethesda, Maryland 20892

LATHAKUMARI PARTHASARATHY (13), Department of Biochemistry, University of Madras, Madras 600025, India

RANGANATHAN PARTHASARATHY (13), Molecular Neuroscience Laboratory, VA Medical Center, Memphis, Tennessee 38104

FERNANDO PICATOSTE (5), Departamento de Bioquímica y Biología Molecular, Universidad Autónoma de Barcelona, E-08193 Bellaterra, Barcelona, Spain

ANDREW F. G. QUEST (15), Section of Cell Growth, Department of Biochemistry, Duke University Medical Center, Durham, North Carolina 27710

GEORG REISER (24), Physiologisch-chemisches Institut, Universität Tübingen, 72076 Tübingen, Germany

SUE GOO RHEE (7, 8), Section on Signal Transduction, Laboratory of Biochemistry, NHLBI, National Institutes of Health, Bethesda, Maryland 20892

LEONA J. RUBIN (19), Department of Veterinary Biomedical Sciences, College of Veterinary Medicine, University of Missouri, Columbia, Missouri 65211

NOBUYUKI SASAKAWA (20), Department of Pharmacology, Keio University School of Medicine, Tokyo 160, Japan

UTA-SUSANNE SCHMIDT (2), Department of Hormone Research, The Weizmann Institute of Science, Rehovot 76100, Israel

WILLIAM R. SHERMAN (19), Department of Psychiatry, Washington University School of Medicine, St. Louis, Missouri 63110

FWU-SHAN SHEU (14), Section on Metabolic Regulation, Endocrinology and Reproduction Research Branch, NICHHD, National Institutes of Health, Bethesda, Maryland 20892

ALAN V. SMRCKA (9), Department of Pharmacology, University of Texas, Southwestern Medical Center, Dallas, Texas 75235

STEPHEN P. SOLTOFF (12), Division of Signal Transduction, Department of Medicine, Beth Israel Hospital, Boston, Massachusetts 02115

SILVIA STABEL (16), Max-Delbrück-Laboratorium, Max-Planck-Gesellschaft, D-50829 Köln, Germany

PAUL C. STERNWEIS (9), Department of Pharmacology, University of Texas, Southwestern Medical Center, Dallas, Texas 75235

THOMAS C. SÜDHOF (22), Howard Hughes Medical Institute and Department of Molecular Genetics, University of Texas, Southwestern Medical Center, Dallas, Texas 75235

KAZUNAGA TAKAZAWA (26), Third Department of Internal Medicine, University of Yamanashi Medical School, Yamanashi 409-38, Japan

TADAOMI TAKENAWA (11), Department of Molecular Oncology, Institute of Medical Science, University of Tokyo, Tokyo 108, Japan

ROBERT E. VADNAL (13), Molecular Neuroscience Laboratory, VA Medical Center, Memphis, Tennessee 38104

BENOÎT VERJANS (26), Institut de Recherche Interdisciplinaire (IRIBHN), Université Libre de Bruxelles, B-1070 Brussels, Belgium

MICHAEL A. WALLACE (6), Department of Biochemistry, University of Tennessee, Center for Health Science, Memphis, Tennessee 38163

PENG WANG (3), Schering-Plough Research Institute, Kenilworth, New Jersey 07033

RICHARD J. H. WOJCIKIEWICZ (23), Department of Pharmacology and Therapeutics, University of Leicester, Leicester LE1 9HN, United Kingdom

AKIO YAMAKAWA (11), Department of Biosignal Research, Tokyo Metropolitan Institute of Gerontology, Tokyo 173, Japan

Preface

In the past few years there has been an enormous expansion of knowledge among neuroscience investigators concerning the role of phospholipid breakdown products. There is abundant evidence that phosphoinositide breakdown is involved in the mode of signal transduction for many neurotransmitters and emerging evidence for the importance of the breakdown of other cellular phospholipids in the regulation of neuronal function.

It has been less than ten years since many investigators thought that the effects of neurotransmitters on phosphoinositide breakdown were secondary to elevations in intracellular calcium. There is ample evidence that breakdown of neuronal phosphoinositides can be activated simply by an increase in intracellular calcium, but this results primarily in the accumulation of inositol mono- and bisphosphates. However, there is direct activation of phosphoinositide breakdown involving receptors with seven transmembrane spanning regions, unique guanine nucleotide-binding (G) proteins, and a phosphoinositide-specific phospholipase C. It was also recently demonstrated that in the presence of a muscarinic cholinergic agonist along with its receptor, a G_q protein and a phosphoinositidase C isozyme, there is enhanced breakdown of phosphatidylinositol 4,5-bisphosphate to inositol 1,4,5-trisphosphate and diacyglycerol.

Ligand-activated breakdown of phosphatidylinositol 4,5-bisphosphate to inositol 1,4,5-trisphosphate also results in the conversion of this compound to inositol 1,3,4,5-tetrakisphosphate. The inositol 1,4,5-trisphosphate interacts with a calcium channel in the endoplasmic reticulum, resulting in the release of intracellular stores of calcium to the cytosol. The role of inositol 1,3,4,5-tetrakisphosphate remains to be elucidated, but there is a specific receptor for this messenger in the cerebellum and in other areas of the brain, and it may be involved in the regulation of calcium entry into cells. The diacylglycerol released during phosphoinositide breakdown in the plasma membrane activates membrane-bound protein kinase C. There are other sources of diacylglycerol, especially during continued stimulation, including ligand-activated breakdown of phosphatidylcholine and other membrane phospholipids by phospholipases of the C and D category.

This volume emphasizes new techniques and presents methods which will be of use to investigators in the field. For example, it is no longer necessary or even desirable to measure phosphoinositide breakdown in cells by exposing them to tritiated inositol and then measuring the accumulation of inositol monophosphates over prolonged incubation periods in the presence of lithium. There are now easy procedures for the determination of inositol 1,4,5-trisphosphate mass within seconds after the addition of neurotransmitters.

I am grateful to the contributors for their willingness to prepare chapters for this volume and for doing so in a timely manner.

JOHN N. FAIN

Methods in Neurosciences

Section I

Phospholipases Involved in Signaling Systems

[1] Phosphatidylinositol Glycan-Anchor-Specific Phospholipase D from Mammalian Brain

Marius C. Hoener and Urs Brodbeck

Introduction

A steadily increasing number of proteins are known to be anchored to membranes via a covalently linked phosphatidylinositol glycan (PIG) moiety (1) consisting of phosphatidylinositol to which a nonacetylated glucosamine and three mannose residues are attached. The linkage to the carboxyl group of the C-terminal amino acid is brought about by an ethanolamine–phosphate residue (Fig. 1). Although this core structure appears to be highly conserved in evolution, variability exists in attached sugar and ethanolamine residues as well as in the hydrophobic part of the anchor.

In brain several PIG-anchored proteins exist that display widely different functions (2) (Table I; 3–23). This special type of membrane anchoring is thought to be a possible targeting signal in the sorting of apically located surface proteins of polarized cells (6, 24–26). It was shown that PIG-anchored proteins and glycans are enriched up to 10-fold in the apical surface, presumably through sorting in the trans-Golgi network. As shown by Lemansky et al. (27), PIG anchorage may function to prolong the cell-surface half-life of proteins whose function does not require internalization. It has been suggested by Rothberg et al. (28) that certain PIG-anchored receptors can undergo a novel, clathrin-independent form of endocytosis and recycling. PIG-linked proteins are attractive candidates for mediating the dynamic remodeling of membranes that occur during nerve fiber outgrowth, synaptogenesis, and particularly in myelination by allowing for a stable but potentially fluid adhesion between the plasma membranes of apposed cells. In addition, the increased mobility of PIG-anchored proteins within the membrane may promote adhesion by facilitating the recruitment of these proteins into membrane domains engaged in adhesion.

Furthermore, the PIG-anchor could provide a unique mechanism for the regulated release of PIG-anchored proteins and glycolipids at the cell surface by serving as a substrate for PIG-specific phospholipases. PIG-specific phospholipase D (PIG–PLD) was found in serum (29–32), in the islets of Langerhans (33), in mast cells (34), in bovine brain (35), and in different neurons (36). The primary structure of PIG–PLD was deduced from a full-length

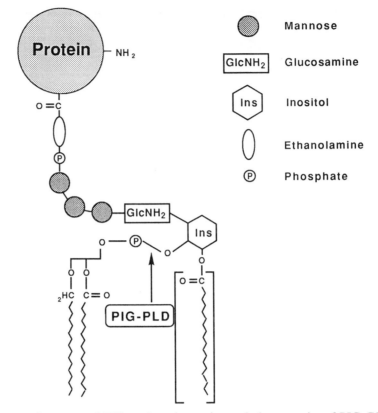

FIG. 1   Structure of PIG-anchored proteins and cleavage site of PIG–PLD.

cDNA construct from bovine liver (37). Recently a PIG–PLD-specific cDNA was found in calf brain (B. Stadelmann, personal communication). A brain PIG-specific phospholipase C (PIG–PLC) was found by Fouchier *et al.* (38).

Assay Methods

PIG–PLD is assayed as described previously by Hoener and Brodbeck (39) using the purified membrane form of acetylcholinesterase from bovine erythrocytes as substrate (Fig. 2). Erythrocyte acetylcholinesterase is membrane bound through covalently linked PIG, and its conversion from the amphiphilic membrane form to soluble acetylcholinesterase serves as measure for anchor-degrading activity. If purified acetylcholinesterase is not available, the

TABLE I   Phosphatidylinositol Glycan-Anchored Proteins in the Nervous System

Function	Examples	Source	Refs.
Hydrolytic enzymes	Acetylcholinesterase	Insect brain	3
	5'-Nucleotidase	Bovine brain	4
Mammalian antigens	Thy-1	Mammalian brain	5–7
Cell–cell interaction	Heparan sulfate proteoglycan	Schwann cells	8, 9
	Neural cell adhesion molecule (N-CAM$_{120}$)	Mammalian and chicken brain	10, 11
	Axon-associated cell adhesion molecules TAG-1 and axonin-1	Rat and chicken brain	12, 13
	Neuronal cell recognition molecules F3 and F11 (gp130)	Mouse and chicken brain	14–16
	T-cadherin (gp90)	Chicken brain	16
	Opiate-binding protein cell adhesion molecule	Bovine brain	17
	Fasciclin, chaoptin	*Drosophila* nervous system	18, 19
Miscellaneous	Scrapie prion protein	Hamster brain	20
	Ciliary neurotrophic factor receptor	Chicken brain	21
	Oligodendrocyte–myelin protein	Human brain	22
	Sgp-1, Sgp-2	Squid neural tissues	23

commercially available enzyme from Boehringer Mannheim (Mannheim, Germany) is also suitable (Cat. No. 1143 026). This preparation contains acetylcholinesterase essentially in membrane-bound form, and consequently the rate of conversion by PIG–PLD is lower than with purified acetylcholinesterase.

To assay PIG–PLD, samples are placed in a 1-ml tube and adjusted to 21 μl with 20 mM Tris (pH 7.4). To this, 4 μl of substrate solution containing 0.60 pmol (0.24 IU) of the membrane form of acetylcholinesterase in 10 mM Tris (pH 7.4), 144 mM NaCl, 6 mM CaCl$_2$, and 0.1% (w/v) Triton X-100 is added and incubated at 37°C for varying lengths of time. The product of the reaction, namely, soluble acetylcholinesterase, is separated from the substrate by phase separation in Triton X-114 (40) as follows. The incubation mixture is put on ice, and 0.4 ml of an ice-cold solution of 4% (w/v) Triton X-114 in 10 mM Tris (pH 7.4), 144 mM NaCl is added. Phase separation is carried out by incubation at 37°C for 5 min, and product formation is assessed by measuring soluble acetylcholinesterase in the aqueous phase by the method of Ellman *et al.* (41) in standard microtiter plates. The assay solution contains 1 mM acetylthiocholine iodide and 0.25 mM 5,5'-dithiobis(2-nitro-

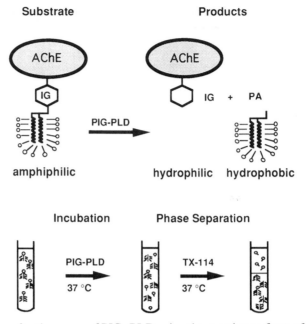

FIG. 2   Scheme for the assay of PIG–PLD using the membrane form of acetylcholinesterase (AChE) from bovine erythrocytes as substrate. IG, Inositol glycan; PA, phosphatidic acid; TX-114, Triton X-114.

benzoic acid) in 100 mM sodium phosphate buffer (pH 7.4) containing 0.1% (w/v) Triton X-100. The change in absorbance is read at 405 nm by a Molecular Devices (Menlo Park, CA) V_{max} kinetic microplate reader interfaced to a Hewlett Packard (Palo Alto, CA) Vectra computer, and rates are calculated using the Softmax version 2.01d program. Alternatively, any standard spectrophotometer may be used without, however, the convenience of the large sample throughput of the microplate reader.

PIG–PLD activity is calculated as the percentage of soluble acetylcholinesterase in the aqueous phase in relation to total conversion. Conversion of 100% of the membrane form of acetylcholinesterase to the soluble form is obtained by adding excess amounts of PIG–PLD to a given sample. PIG–PLD activity is expressed either as arbitrary units or as units where 1 unit equals 1 nmol of mf-AChE converted per minute at 37°C.

As shown for the serum enzyme, the activity of PIG–PLD is strongly influenced by the concentration of Triton X-100 in the assay (39). The substrate for PIG–PLD is an amphiphilic molecule that must be kept in solution by a micellar concentration of a detergent. At detergent concentrations above the critical micellar concentration (CMC), however, PIG–PLD becomes increasingly inhibited, and the highest activity is obtained with detergent concentrations just around the CMC. Similar results are obtained with PIG–PLD from bovine brain. The following detergents were tested and found to inhibit significantly the bovine brain enzyme above their CMC: Various Tweens, Tritons, Nonidet P-40 (NP-40), sodium cholate and deoxycholate, Brij, Span 20, and Sarcomega 12. So far no detergent has been found that does not interfere with the assay above its CMC.

Protein is determined with the BCA reagent kit (Pierce Chemicals, Rockford, IL) as described by Sørensen and Brodbeck (42) with bovine serum albumin (BSA) as standard.

Purification of Phosphoinositol Glycan-Specific Phospholipase D from Bovine and Human Brain

Whole fresh brain is carefully freed from meninges and blood vessels and extensively washed with 10 mM Tris (pH 7.4), 144 mM NaCl. Then the brain is cut into little slices, which are bathed for 5 hr with three changes of the buffer as described before. Slices (1030 g) are homogenized with 3090 ml of 20 mM Tris buffer (pH 7.4) and centrifuged at 4°C at 25,000 g for 1 hr. The resulting pellet (800 ml) is homogenized with 1600 ml Tris buffer and centrifuged under the same conditions.

The combined supernatants are applied to a DEAE-cellulose DE-53 Whatman Biosystems (Maidstone, Kent, England) column (4 × 20 cm) equilibrated with 20 mM Tris (pH 7.4). The column is washed with 400 ml equilibrating buffer followed by 800 ml buffer containing 50 mM NaCl. PIG–PLD activity is eluted by 2000 ml of a gradient from 50 to 250 mM NaCl. The flow rate is kept at 150 ml/hr. The human brain enzyme elutes between 420 and 1000 ml in a relatively sharp peak together with the first of three protein peaks, and the bovine brain enzyme elutes between 420 and 1520 ml in a broad peak of activity.

Fractions containing PIG–PLD activity are pooled and to them is added NaCl to a final concentration of 400 mM. The solution is applied to an octyl-Sepharose column (4 × 12 cm) equilibrated with 20 mM Tris (pH 7.4) containing 400 mM NaCl. The column is first washed with equilibrating buffer until the absorbance at 280 nm reaches baseline and then with 450 ml of 5 mM Tris (pH 7.4). PIG–PLD is eluted with 1200 ml of 3 mM Tris (pH 7.4) containing 0.15% reduced Triton X-100.

NaCl is added to the pooled PIG–PLD fractions to a final concentration of 400 mM, and the enzyme is applied to a concanavalin A (con A)–Sepharose column (4 × 3 cm) equilibrated with 20 mM Tris (pH 7.4) containing 400 mM NaCl, 1 mM CaCl$_2$, 1 mM MgCl$_2$, and 1 mM MnCl$_2$. The column is

TABLE II   Purification of Phosphoinositol Glycan-Specific Phospholipase D from Bovine and Human Brain

Purification step	Volume (ml)	Total protein (mg)	Total activity[a] (units)	Yield (%)	Purification (-fold)
Bovine brain homogenate	4070	81,520	—	—	1
Supernatant	5030	12,680	1370	100	6.4
DEAE-cellulose DE-53	1100	4336	960	70	13
Octyl-Sepharose Cl-4B	930	553	790	58	85
Concanavalin A–Sepharose	460	53	590	43	662
Human brain homogenate	4100	82,820	—	—	1
Supernatant	5100	13,910	1290	100	6.0
DEAE-cellulose DE-53	580	1065	730	57	44
Octyl-Sepharose Cl-4B	930	170	450	35	170
Concanavalin A–Sepharose	540	16	300	23	1204

[a] 1 unit equals 1 nmol of mf-AChE converted per minute at 37°C.

washed with 400 ml of equilibrating buffer, and PIG–PLD is eluted with 1000 ml of buffer containing 0.5 M methyl-α-D-mannopyranoside. Fractions with PIG–PLD activity are collected, concentrated to 10 ml using an Amicon (Danvers, MA) 52 stirred cell equipped with a PM50 Diaflow ultrafiltration membrane, and dialyzed against 20 mM Tris (pH 7.4).

After these steps a 660-fold purification resulted for bovine brain and a 1200-fold purification for human brain (Table II). The recovery of purified enzyme compared to the supernatant is 43% for the bovine brain and 23% for the human brain. Bovine and human brain supernatants have comparable amounts of PIG–PLD activity, but the specific activity is about 100 times less than that of PIG–PLD in human serum and about 1000 times less than that of the bovine serum enzyme (for comparison see Ref. 39, in which 1 μmol/min equals 1 unit in Table II in the present report).

Density Gradient Centrifugation

PIG–PLD from bovine and human brain (50 μl in 20 mM Tris, pH 7.4) is layered on top of a 11.0-ml linear sucrose density gradient in buffer (10 mM Tris, pH 7.4, 144 mM NaCl, without and with 0.1% Triton X-100). The gradients are centrifuged at 4°C and 195,000 g_{av} for 15 hr in a Centrikon/ 2070 centrifuge (Kontron, Zürich, Switzerland) equipped with a TST 4114 rotor. The gradients are emptied from the bottom with a glass capillary by means of a peristaltic pump. Fractions of about 0.35 ml are collected in microplates and assayed for PIG–PLD activity under standard assay conditions.

Cell Fractionation in Isotonic Sucrose

Cell fractionation of human brain in isotonic sucrose is done as described by Aronson and Touster (43), and enzyme activities of subcellular organelles are measured as described by Storrie and Madden (44).

Postnatal Quantification of Enzyme in Rat Brain

Rat brains at 2, 10, 17, 24, and 35 days after birth (0.1 g) are homogenized in 0.3 ml of 20 mM Tris (pH 7.4) with a syringe and centrifuged for 15 min in an Eppendorf centrifuge at maximal speed. PIG–PLD activity and protein are measured in the supernatants without further purification.

Characterization of Phosphoinositol Glycan-Specific Phospholipase D

PIG–PLD from serum is quite well characterized (31, 32, 39). It is an amphiphilic, nonspherical glycoprotein of about 110 kDa that binds to high-density lipoprotein particles. It is inhibited by EDTA, EGTA, o-phenanthroline, p-chloromercuribenzene sulfonate, $HgCl_2$, bicarbonate (45), lipids (46), and detergents (39). Ca^{2+} and Zn^{2+}, but not Mg^{2+}, stimulate PIG–PLD activity. In these aspects PIG–PLD from brain resembles the enzyme from serum. The K_m value with acetylcholinesterase as the substrate for PIG–PLD is around 50 nM for both the brain and serum enzyme. There is, however, a significant difference in the behavior of the two enzymes on ion-exchange chromatography with DEAE-cellulose. PIG–PLD from bovine brain elutes in a buffer of 20 mM Tris (pH 7.4) between 60 and 250 mM NaCl, whereas the enzyme from serum elutes at higher NaCl concentrations. Similarly, the enzyme from human brain enzyme elutes in a sharp peak between 60 and 110 mM NaCl, whereas that from human serum PIG–PLD also elutes at higher concentrations. In that respect the brain enzyme resembles one of the isoenzymes described in bovine liver (47).

As shown by density gradient centrifugation, PIG–PLD from bovine brain is an amphiphilic protein that in the absence of detergents forms higher molecular weight aggregates in the range of 5.9 to 9.4 S (Fig. 3). The human brain enzyme, on the other hand, seems to be nonamphiphilic, as it does not aggregate in the absence of detergent. Its sedimentation coefficient is about 6.7 S regardless of the absence or presence of 0.1% Triton X-100 in the density gradient. Subcellular distribution studies of PIG–PLD reveal that the majority of enzyme activity is contained in the 100,000 g supernatant fraction, whereas the microsomal, mitochondrial

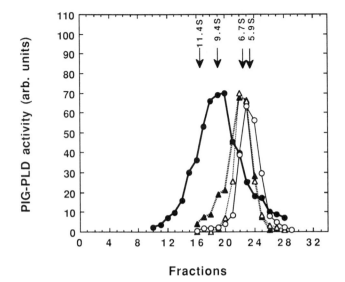

Fractions

FIG. 3 Sedimentation analysis of PIG–PLD from bovine and human brain. Sucrose density gradient centrifugation was carried out in the absence of Triton X-100 (filled symbols) or in the presence of 0.1% Triton X-100 (open symbols) with enzyme from bovine brain (circles) and human brain (triangles). PIG–PLD activity was assayed under standard assay conditions. Numbers above the arrows give sedimentation values of peak fractions in relation to the position of catalase (11.4 S).

TABLE III   Intracellular Distribution of Phosphoinositol Glycan-Specific Phospholipase D and Marker Enzymes in Human Brain

	Cell fraction				
Enzyme	Final supernatant (%)	Microsomal fraction (%)	Mitochondrial plus lysosomal fraction (%)	Nuclear fraction (%)	Recovery (%)
PIG–PLD	76.1	2.1	3.8	4.6	86.6
Alkaline phosphatase	27.0	42.3	6.3	22.9	98.5
α-Glucosidase	0.8	62.3	21.9	11.7	96.7
β-Galactosidase	3.8	6.8	63.8	28.5	102.9
Cytochrome-c oxidase	0	1.0	83.5	5.7	90.2
Total protein	50.7	18.9	20.4	8.5	98.5

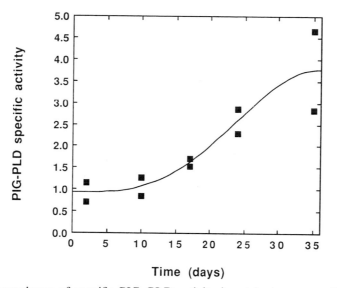

Fɪɢ. 4 Dependence of specific PIG–PLD activity in rat brain on age. Rat brains (two each of the chosen ages) were measured for PIG–PLD activity and protein. Specific PIG–PLD activity was calculated as arbitrary units of PIG–PLD activity per milligram of protein.

plus lysosomal, and nuclear fractions contain between 2 and 5% of the activity (Table III).

The cleavage specificity of anchor-degrading activity in the subcellular fractions has been determined using radioactive 3-trifluoromethyl-3-(*m*-[^{125}I]iodophenyl)diazirine-labeled acetylcholinesterase as substrate. The anchor-degrading activity assayed in all subcellular fractions could be assigned to a phospholipase D (for assay conditions, see Ref. 35). Our finding is in contrast to that of Fouchier *et al.* (38), who presented evidence for the presence in brain of a PIG–PLC. The cleavage of the PIG anchor by such an enzyme would lead to the formation of alkylacylglycerol rather than phosphatidic acid. As shown for PIG anchor-degrading activity in bovine liver, the hydrophobic cleavage product of acetylcholinesterase in the absence of phosphatase inhibitors is exclusively alkylacylglycerol (45). In the presence of such inhibitors, however, mainly phosphatidic acid is recovered, which clearly shows that in liver alkylacylglycerol is formed through the combined effects of PIG–PLD and a phosphatase (47). It is thus reasonable to assume that in brain alkylacylglycerol is formed through the combination of the two activities, too. PIG–PLD activity could also be assayed in rat brain; as shown in Fig. 4, the specific activity of the enzyme increases about 3- to 4-fold within 35 days postnatally.

References

1. G. A. M. Cross, *Annu. Rev. Cell Biol.* **6,** 1 (1990).
2. C. L. Rosen, M. P. Lisanti, and J. L. Salzer, *J. Cell Biol.* **117,** 617 (1992).
3. D. Fournier, J. B. Bergé, M. L. Cardoso de Almeida, and C. Bordier, *J. Neurochem.* **50,** 1158 (1988).
4. M. Vogel, H. Kowalewski, H. Zimmermann, N. M. Hooper, and A. J. Turner, *Biochem. J.* **284,** 621 (1992).
5. S. W. Homans, M. A. J. Ferguson, R. A. Dwek, T. W. Rademacher, R. Anand, and R. F. Williams, *Nature (London)* **333,** 269 (1988).
6. S. K. Powell, B. A. Cunningham, G. M. Edelman, and E. Rodriguez-Boulan, *Nature (London)* **353,** 76 (1991).
7. N. K. Mahanthappa and P. H. Patterson, *Dev. Biol.* **150,** 47 (1992).
8. D. J. Carey and R. C. Stahl, *J. Cell Biol.* **111,** 2053 (1990).
9. M. Yanagishita and V. C. Hascall, *J. Biol. Chem.* **267,** 9451 (1992).
10. H.-T. He, J. Barbet, J.-C. Chaix, and C. Goridis, *EMBO J.* **5,** 2489 (1986).
11. H. J. Gower, C. H. Barton, V. L. Elson, J. Thompson, S. E. Moore, G. Dickson, and F. S. Walsh, *Cell (Cambridge, Mass.)* **55,** 955 (1988).
12. A. J. Furley, S. B. Morton, D. Manalo, D. Karagogeos, J. Dodd, and T. M. Jessell, *Cell (Cambridge, Mass.)* **61,** 517 (1990).
13. R. A. Zuelling, C. Rader, A. Schroeder, M. B. Kalousek, F. von Bohlen und Halbach, T. Osterwalder, C. Inan, E. T. Stoeckli, H.-U. Affolter, A. Fritz, E. Hafen, and P. Sonderegger, *Eur. J. Biochem.* **204,** 453 (1992).
14. G. Gennarini, G. Cibelli, G. Rougon, M. Mattei, and C. Goridis, *J. Cell Biol.* **109,** 775 (1989).
15. J. M. Wolff, T. Brümmendorf, and F. G. Rathjen, *Biochem. Biophys. Res. Commun.* **161,** 931 (1989).
16. D. J. Moss and C. A. White, *Eur. J. Cell Biol.* **57,** 59 (1992).
17. P. R. Schofield, K. C. McFarland, J. S. Hayflick, J. N. Wilcox, T. M. Cho, S. Roy, N. M. Lee, H. H. Loh, and P. H. Seeburg, *EMBO J.* **8,** 489 (1989).
18. M. Hortsch and C. S. Goodman, *J. Biol. Chem.* **265,** 15104 (1990).
19. D. E. Krantz and S. L. Zipursky, *EMBO J.* **9,** 1969 (1990).
20. N. Stahl and S. B. Prusiner, *FASEB J.* **5,** 2799 (1991).
21. S. Davis, T. H. Aldrich, D. M. Valenzuela, V. Wong, M. E. Furth, S. P. Squinto, and G. D. Yancopoulos, *Science* **253,** 59 (1991).
22. D. D. Mikol and K. S. Stefansson, *J. Cell Biol.* **106,** 1273 (1988).
23. A. F. Williams, A. G. D. Tse, and J. Gagnon, *Immunogenetics* **27,** 265 (1988).
24. M. P. Lisanti and E. Rodriguez-Boulan, *Trends Biochem. Sci.* **15,** 113 (1990).
25. T. L. Dotti, R. G. Parton, and K. Simons, *Nature (London)* **349,** 158 (1991).
26. D. A. Brown and J. K. Rose, *Cell (Cambridge, Mass.)* **68,** 533 (1992).
27. P. Lemansky, S. H. Fatemi, B. Gorican, S. Meyale, R. Rossero, and A. M. Tartakoff, *J. Cell Biol.* **110,** 1525 (1990).
28. K. G. Rothberg, Y. Ying, J. F. Kolhouse, B. A. Kamen, and R. G. W. Anderson, *J. Cell Biol.* **110,** 637 (1990).
29. M. A. Davitz, D. Hereld, S. Shak, J. Krakow, P. T. Englund, and V. Nussenzweig, *Science* **238,** 81 (1987).

30. M. G. Low and A. R. S. Prasad, *Proc. Natl. Acad. Sci. U.S.A.* **85,** 980 (1988).
31. M. A. Davitz, J. Hom, and S. Schenkman, *J. Biol. Chem.* **264,** 13760 (1989).
32. K. S. Huang, S. Li, W. J. Fung, J. D. Hulmes, L. Reik, Y. C. E. Pan, and M. G. Low, *J. Biol. Chem.* **265,** 17738 (1990).
33. C. N. Metz, Y. Zhang, Y. Guo, T. C. Tsang, J. P. Kochan, N. Altszuler, and M. A. Davitz, *J. Biol. Chem.* **266,** 17733 (1991).
34. C. N. Metz, P. Thomas, and M. A. Davitz, *Am. J. Pathol.* **140,** 1275 (1992).
35. M. C. Hoener, S. Stieger, and U. Brodbeck, *Eur. J. Biochem.* **190,** 593 (1990).
36. A. M. Sesko and M. G. Low, *FASEB J.* **5,** A839 (1991).
37. B. J. Scallon, W. J. C. Fung, T. C. Tsang, S. Li, H. Kado-Fong, K. S. Huang, and J. P. Kochan, *Science* **252,** 446 (1991).
38. F. Fouchier, T. Baltz, and G. Rougon, *Biochem. J.* **269,** 321 (1990).
39. M. C. Hoener and U. Brodbeck, *Eur. J. Biochem.* **206,** 747 (1992).
40. C. Bordier, *J. Biol. Chem.* **256,** 1604 (1981).
41. G. L. Ellman, D. K. Courtney, V. Andres, and R. M. Featherstone, *Biochem. Pharmacol.* **7,** 88 (1961).
42. K. Sørensen and U. Brodbeck, *Experientia* **42,** 161 (1986).
43. N. N. Aronson, Jr., and O. Touster, *in* "Methods in Enzymology" (S. Fleischer and L. Packer, eds.), Vol. 31, p. 90. Academic Press, New York, 1974.
44. B. Storrie and E. A. Madden, *in* "Methods in Enzymology" (M. P. Deutscher, ed.), Vol. 182, p. 203. Academic Press, San Diego, 1990.
45. S. Stieger, S. Diem, A. Jakob, and U. Brodbeck, *Eur. J. Biochem.* **197,** 67 (1991).
46. M. G. Low and K. S. Huang, *Biochem. J.* **279,** 483 (1991).
47. M. Heller, S. Bieri, and U. Brodbeck, *Biochim. Biophys. Acta* **1109,** 109 (1992).

[2] Rat Brain Membrane-Bound Phospholipase D

Michal Danin, Vered Chalifa, Heidi Möhn,
Uta-Susanne Schmidt, and Mordechai Liscovitch

Introduction

Phospholipase D (EC 3.1.4.4; PLD) is a phosphodiesterase that attacks the distal phosphodiester bond in phospholipids, for example, phosphatidylcholine (PC), producing phosphatidic acid (PA) and releasing the free polar head group, for example, choline (Fig. 1). PLD also catalyzes a unique transphosphatidylation reaction, which, in the presence of primary alcohols, yields a phosphatidyl alcohol (Fig. 1).

Mammalian phospholipase D activity was unequivocally first observed by Saito and Kanfer in rat brain tissue (1). In a series of studies, this brain membrane-bound PLD activity was further characterized and distinguished from a related phospholipid base-exchange activity by its acidic pH optimum, its independence of Ca^{2+}, and its activation by free fatty acids *in vitro* (2). Insight into the possible role of mammalian PLD was gained as numerous studies have demonstrated the activation of PLD by a variety of receptor agonists in many cell types (see Ref. 3 for review). These results raise the hypothesis that signal-dependent formation of PA, by PLD-catalyzed hydrolysis of phospholipids, may represent a novel and ubiquitous signal transduction pathway in mammalian cells. However, the cellular PLD(s) that operates in stimulated cells is rather poorly defined in molecular terms. Studies with intact cells, labeled with different phospholipid polar head groups, suggested that PLDs which hydrolyze PC, phosphatidylethanolamine, and phosphatidylinositol are activated during signaling. In accordance with these findings, various forms of soluble and membrane-bound PLD activities have been characterized using *in vitro* assays (4–6).

We have been studying a neutral-active PLD found in rat brain synaptic plasma membranes that utilizes PC as a substrate (5, 7, 8). In this chapter we describe methods for the solubilization of this activity from brain membranes and its assay using a fluorescent substrate, namely, 1-palmitoyl-2-[6-*N*-(7-nitrobenzo-2-oxa-1,3-diazol-4-yl)amino]caproylphosphatidylcholine (C_6-NBD-PC).

Methods in Neurosciences, Volume 18

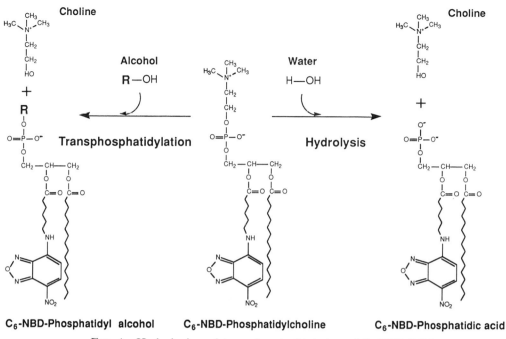

FIG. 1   Hydrolysis and transphosphatidylation of C_6-NBD-PC by PLD.

Materials

1-Palmitoyl-2-[6-*N*-(7-nitrobenzo-2-oxa-1,3-diazol-4-yl)amino]caproylphosphatidylcholine (C_6-NBD-PC) and C_6-NBD-PA are purchased from Avanti Polar Lipids (Alabaster, AL). Sodium oleate is obtained from Sigma (St. Louis, MO). Cholic acid obtained from Fluka (Buchs, Switzerland) is further purified by crystallization according to Kagawa and Racker (9), dissolved in water by neutralization with NaOH, and further diluted to give a final concentration of 20% (w/v) cholic acid. Thin-layer chromatography (TLC) plates (LK6) are obtained from Whatman (Maidstone, UK). All other chemicals and solvents are of analytical or higher grade.

Preparation of Rat Brain Membranes

Reagents

Sucrose solution: 0.25 *M* sucrose; 10 m*M* HEPES, pH 7.2; 1 m*M* EDTA
Hypotonic buffer: 10 m*M* HEPES, pH 7.2; 1 m*M* EDTA
4 *M* NaCl, 10 m*M* HEPES, pH 7.2
HEPES, pH 7.2, 50 m*M*

Procedure

Usually, 12 Wistar-derived male rats (60 days old) are used for preparation of 600–900 mg of brain membrane protein. Fewer rats may be used if so desired, and the volumes are accordingly reduced. During the membrane preparation, all the solutions and instruments must be kept at 4°C. Vortexing is avoided whenever possible.

1. Whole brains are removed from decapitated rats, then transferred to a beaker containing sucrose solution. The brains are minced using a razor blade and homogenized in 9 volumes per weight of sucrose solution using a tight motor-driven Teflon–glass homogenizer (6 strokes, 500 rpm).
2. Nuclei and cell debris are removed from the homogenate by centrifugation (1000 g, 10 min) and collection of the supernatant. The pellet is further washed by resuspension in sucrose solution and centrifugation. The two supernatants are pooled and then ultracentrifuged (60 min, 100,000 g). The clear supernatant is removed by suction and discarded.
3. To remove cytosolic proteins that are trapped within the membrane vesicles, the 100,000 g pellet is treated with hypotonic buffer as follows. Several milliliters of buffer is added to the pellet, which is then suspended with the aid of a glass rod. The suspension is transferred to a homogenization tube, and hypotonic buffer is added to a final volume of 50 ml. Several strokes with a Telfon pestle is sufficient to make the suspension homogeneous. An additional 100 ml of hypotonic buffer is mixed with the suspension, which is then incubated at 4°C for 30 min.
4. To remove peripheral membrane proteins, 50 ml of 4 M NaCl, 10 mM Na–HEPES (pH 7.2) is added to the membrane suspension (final NaCl concentration is 1 M), followed by incubation at 4°C for 30 min.
5. The suspension is finally ultracentrifuged at 100,000 g for 60 min, the supernatant removed by suction, and the pellet suspended with a small volume of 50 mM Na–HEPES, pH 7.2, as above. The membrane suspension is divided into aliquots, frozen immediately in liquid nitrogen, and stored at or below −70°C. Protein concentration in the membranes is determined according to the modified Lowry assay (10), and is usually 20–30 mg/ml.

Solubilization of Brain Membrane Phospholipase D Activity with Sodium Cholate

Reagents

Rat brain membranes, prepared as above

2× Solubilization buffer: 1.6% cholate, 0.3 M NaCl, and 0.1 M Na–HEPES, pH 7.2

Procedure

The required amount of total brain membranes is diluted with water to 10 mg/ml and mixed with 2× solubilization buffer to give the following final concentrations: 0.8% cholate, 150 mM NaCl, 50 mM Na–HEPES, pH 7.2, and 5 mg/ml membrane protein. (Brain membranes may be solubilized with 1% cholate, given essentially similar results.) The mixture is incubated at 4°C for 15 min and mixed by vortexing every 5 min. It is then centrifuged for 90 min at 100,000 g, and the supernatant is carefully collected with a pipette. This supernatant contains around 2.5 mg/ml protein as determined by the modified Lowry assay (10), and it may be either used directly for measuring PLD activity or immediately frozen in liquid nitrogen and stored at −130°C.

Assay of Solubilized Brain Membrane Phospholipase D Using C$_6$-NBD-PC as Substrate

Reagents

> Solubilized brain-membrane PLD, approximately 2.5 mg protein/ml in 0.8% cholate, 150 mM NaCl, and 50 mM Na–HEPES, pH 7.2
> C$_6$-NBD-PC, 0.5 mg/ml in chloroform/methanol (19 : 1, v/v)
> Na–HEPES/1-propanol: 0.6 M 1-propanol, 0.2 M Na–HEPES buffer, pH 7.2
> Sodium oleate, 4.8 mM (dissolved in warm water)
> Termination mixture: chloroform/methanol/9 N HCl (1 : 1 : 0.006, v/v)
> Silica gel TLC plates, sprayed with 1% potassium oxalate and activated by heating at 115°C for 60 min
> TLC solvent mixture: upper phase of ethyl acetate/2,2,4-trimethylpentane/acetic acid/water (65 : 10 : 15 : 50, v/v)
> Methanol

Procedure

Prior to the assay, an appropriate volume of C$_6$-NBD-PC stock (0.5 mg/ml) is dried under a stream of nitrogen, redissolved in water, and combined with one-half volume of sodium oleate to give a solution of 0.4 mM C$_6$-NBD-PC/ 1.6 mM sodium oleate. The solubilized brain membranes are diluted 2-fold with water. When PLD-catalyzed transphosphatidylation is measured, a solution of 600 mM 1-propanol in Na–HEPES buffer is freshly prepared and kept on ice to minimize evaporation.

A standard reaction mixture (120 μl) contains 0.1 mM C$_6$-NBD-PC, 0.4 mM sodium oleate, 50 mM Na–HEPES (pH 7.2), 0.1% cholate, 150 mM

1-propanol (optional), and around 37.5 μg solubilized membrane protein.*
Thirty microliters of Na–HEPES or Na–HEPES/1-propanol mixture, 30 μl
of C_6-NBD-PC/sodium oleate mixture, 30 μl of water or additive, and, finally,
30 μl of diluted solubilized membranes are added to each tube. Incubation
is carried out for 5 min at 37°C. The reaction is stopped by the addition of
2 ml of termination mixture. Phase separation is accomplished by the addition
of 1 ml water, mixing, and centrifugation (2000 rpm, 10 min). The lower,
lipid-containing chloroform phase (900 μl) is collected, dried by centrifugation under vacuum, and redissolved in 25 μl chloroform/methanol (1 : 1, v/v).

Samples are spotted on activated Whatman LK6 TLC plates. Plates are
developed in the TLC solvent mixture and dried at room temperature. To
visualize the fluorescent C_6-NBD-lipid spots, plates are illuminated with a
long-wavelength ultraviolet table at 365 nm (Vilber Lourmat, TF-20L, Marne
la Vallée, France), and fluorescent spots are marked. The illuminated plate
may be photographed with a Polaroid MP-3 Land camera (see Fig. 2). The
silica from the relevant C_6-NBD-PA or C_6-NBD-phosphatidylpropanol (C_6-
NBD-PPr) bands are subsequently scraped into disposable glass tubes. C_6-
NBD-phospholipids are extracted by mixing the silica with 0.6 ml methanol,
spinning down (1 min, 3000 rpm), and collecting 0.4 ml of the supernatant
into a 10 $\times$ 75 mm disposable glass tube (Kimble). The procedure is repeated
with additional 0.5 ml methanol, and 0.5 ml of the resulting supernatant is
combined with the first one.

NBD-phospholipids are quantified by measuring the fluorescence of the
methanol extracts in a Perkin-Elmer (Norwalk, CT) LS-5B luminescence
spectrometer (excitation and emmission at 468 and 520 nm, respectively),
the 10 $\times$ 75 mm glass tubes being used as disposable cuvettes. The relative
fluorescence units are converted (after subtracting the zero time or zero
protein control) to picomoles of phospholipids using a fluorescence standard
curve of C_6-NBD-PA (the mean slope is 1.39 fluorescence units/pmol). The
values presented are not corrected for recovery of C_6-NBD-PA and thus
likely represent an underestimation of the true PLD activity.

Properties of Cholate-Solubilized Phospholipase D Activity

C_6-NBD-PC is a fluorescent PC analog that can serve as a substrate to brain
PLD. Figure 2 shows a TLC separation of NBD-lipids produced in the course

---

* In the course of these studies we noted that the stimulatory effect of Mg^{2+} on PLD activity
(Ref. 5) is no longer observed following solubilization. Thus, Mg^{2+} ions are omitted from the
standard assay mix although they were present in some of the experiments, as indicated in
the figure legends.

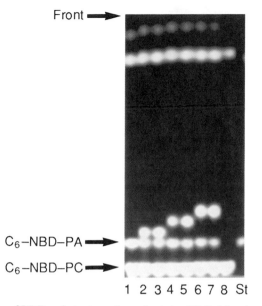

FIG. 2   Separation of PLD substrate and products by TLC. Membranes were solubilized with 1% cholate. Approximately 30 μg protein/tube was incubated for 5 min with 0.1 mM C$_6$-NBD-PC, 0.4 mM sodium oleate, 1.0 mM MgCl$_2$ and in the presence of ethanol (lanes 2, 3), 1-propanol (lanes 4, 5), or 1-butanol (lanes 6, 7) at optimal alcohol concentrations (see Fig. 7). Control incubations in the absence of any alcohol (lane 1) or with boiled protein (lane 8) are presented. The developed TLC plate was illuminated with UV light and photographed with a Polaroid camera as described in the text. Lane designated St contained C$_6$-NBD-PA standard.

of incubation of C$_6$-NBD-PC with a cholate extract of brain membranes. In the absence of an alcohol (Fig. 2, lane 1), a major product formed during the incubation is C$_6$-NBD-PA. In the presence of ethanol, 1-propanol, or 1-butanol, formation of C$_6$-NBD-phosphatidylethanol (C$_6$-NBD-PEt), C$_6$-NBD-PPr, or C$_6$-NBD-phosphatidylbutanol (C$_6$-NBD-PBu) is shown to occur (Fig. 2). Thus, C$_6$-NBD-PC is a substrate for both the hydrolytic and the transphosphatidylation reactions catalyzed by PLD (see Fig. 1).

Because the solubilization is carried out in cholate (0.8%), the protein fraction to be assayed is always added in the presence of the detergent. At concentrations above 0.1%, cholate strongly inhibits the enzyme activity (Fig. 3). This inhibition is not due to the surface diluting effect of cholate on PLD activation by sodium oleate (see below), since the surface concentration of the latter was maintained at a molar ratio of 15% of total surfactants

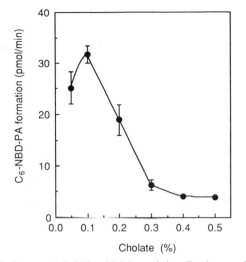

FIG. 3 Effect of cholate on solubilized PLD activity. Brain membranes were solubilized in 1% cholate. Approximately 15 μg protein/tube was incubated for 10 min at 37°C in the presence of 0.1 mM C_6-NBD-PC, 1 mM $MgCl_2$, sodium oleate, and increasing amounts of cholate. The latter was added directly to the assay mixture to give the final concentrations indicated. The sodium oleate concentration was adjusted to maintain a sodium oleate/surfactant molar ratio of 15%.

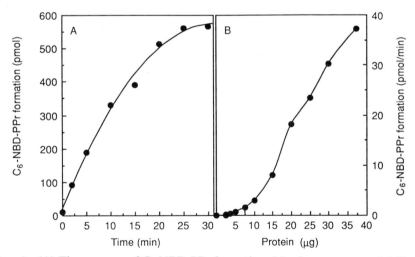

FIG. 4 (A) Time course of C_6-NBD-PPr formation. Membranes were solubilized in 0.8% cholate. Extract (37.5 μg protein/tube) was incubated at 37°C for various time periods under standard assay conditions in the presence of 150 mM 1-propanol and 1.0 mM $MgCl_2$. (B) Dependence of C_6-NBD-PPr formation on protein concentration. Membrane proteins solubilized in 0.8% cholate were diluted to give the exact concentrations indicated, keeping the final cholate concentration at 0.1%.

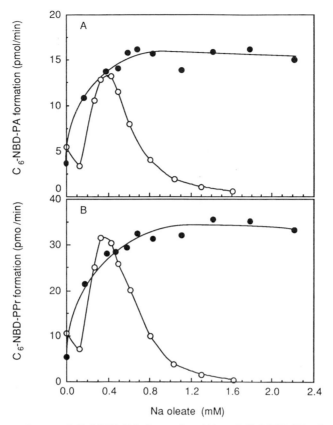

FIG. 5   Dependence of C_6-NBD-PA formation (A) and C_6-NBD-PPr formation (B) on sodium oleate concentration. Membranes were solubilized in 0.8% cholate. Extract (22 μg protein/tube) was incubated for 5 min in the presence of 150 mM 1-propanol, 0.1 mM C_6-NBD-PC (open circles) or 1.0 mM C_6-NBD-PC (filled circles), and with increasing concentrations of sodium oleate.

present (cholate, sodium oleate, and C_6-NBD-PC). Activity of solubilized PLD depends on the time of incubation and protein concentration (Fig. 4). The PLD activity is a linear function of protein amount above 10 μg/tube.

We have previously shown that the neutral brain PLD is stimulated by sodium oleate (5). The hydrolysis and transphosphatidylation reactions catalyzed by the cholate-solubilized PLD are similarly stimulated by sodium oleate (Fig. 5). In the presence of 0.1 mM C_6-NBD-PC, PLD activity is inhibited at sodium oleate concentrations above 0.4 mM. This inhibition does not take place at 1.0 mM C_6-NBD-PC (Fig. 5).

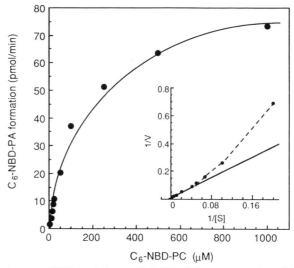

FIG. 6   Dependence of PLD activity on C_6-NBD-PC concentration. Membranes were solubilized in 0.8% cholate. Extract (22 μg protein/assay) was incubated for 5 min with increasing C_6-NBD-PC concentrations while sodium oleate was maintained at a sodium oleate/surfactant molar ratio of 15% (see text). C_6-NBD-PA was measured in the absence of alcohol. The Lineweaver–Burk plot (inset) shows the reciprocal values of all of the points, but the regression line represents the results for C_6-NBD-PC concentrations above 50 μM only.

Figure 6 shows the formation of C_6-NBD-PA in response to increasing substrate concentrations. To minimize the surface-diluting effect of varying C_6-NBD-PC concentrations on the stimulation by sodium oleate, the latter was maintained at a molar ratio of 15% of the total surfactants present. The Lineweaver–Burk plot (Fig. 6, inset) shows that the dependence on substrate concentration is not linear at C_6-NBD-PC concentrations below 50 μM. The apparent K_m and V_{max} values derived from the plot are 160 μM and 87 pmol C_6-NBD-PA/min (3.95 nmol/min/mg), respectively. The average apparent K_m and apparent V_{max} in five independent experiments are 175 $\pm$ 68 μM and 128 $\pm$ 39 pmol/min (mean $\pm$ S.D.), respectively. The nonlinear dependence below 50 μM C_6-NBD-PC may be explained by substrate cooperatively at these low concentrations; however, other explanations cannot be excluded at present. A detailed kinetic analysis of PLD activity will be carried out as soon as purified enzyme preparations become available.

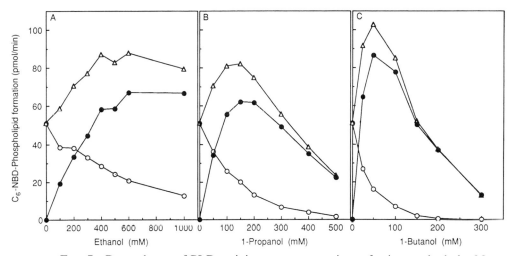

FIG. 7   Dependence of PLD activity on concentrations of primary alcohols. Membranes were solubilized with 1% cholate. Approximately 30 μg protein/tube was incubated for 5 min with 0.1 mM C_6-NBD-PC, 0.4 mM sodium oleate, 1.0 mM MgCl$_2$ and in the absence or presence of increasing concentrations of ethanol (A), 1-propanol (B), or 1-butanol (C). The formation of C_6-NBD-PA (open circles), the relevant C_6-NBD-phosphatidyl alcohol (filled circles), and their sum (open triangles) was determined.

The dependence of phosphatidyl alcohol production on alcohol concentration is shown in Fig. 7. The transphosphatidylation reaction occurs at the expense of C_6-NBD-PA formation but is not accompanied by its complete suppression. In addition, 1-propanol and 1-butanol inhibit PLD activity (sum of C_6-NBD-PA and C_6-NBD phosphatidyl alcohol) at high concentrations. In this series of alcohols, the longer the alcohol the lower is its optimal concentration as a PLD substrate. Because butanol inhibits PLD activity at relatively low concentrations, and C_6-NBD-PEt is not as well resolved from C_6-NBD-PA as the other products (cf. Fig. 2), the formation of C_6-NBD-PPr is most convenient and is routinely utilized.

Comments and Conclusions

The use of C_6-NBD-PC for assaying solubilized PLD activity offers significant advantages over our previous assay employing ^{3}H-labeled PC (5). In addition to the convenience of a water-soluble short-chain substrate, the new assay is more sensitive (the signal-to-noise ratio under standard conditions is around 50 instead of 5 in the previous assay) and safer (nonradioactive). Using the present assay we have measured high PLD activity in solubilized membranes isolated from Swiss/3T3 fibroblasts (11). C_6-NBD-PC may also be utilized as a PLD substrate in assays of membrane-bound (nonsolubilized) PLD, where PLD activity is likewise dependent on sodium oleate (H. Möhn, unpublished results). Introduction of the short chain C_6-NBD-PC molecule into intact cells [as described by Pagano and Sleight (12)] may additionally open the possibility of measuring PLD activity *in vivo*.

Acknowledgments

This work was supported in part by grants from the United States–Israel Binational Science Foundation, the Minerva Foundation, and the Irwin Green Research Fund in the Neurosciences. H. M. is a recipient of a Minerva Fellowship. M. L. is a recipient of an Yigal Allon Fellowship and the incumbent of the Shloimo and Michla Tomarin Career Development Chair in Membrane Physiology in the Department of Hormone Research, The Weizmann Institute of Science (Rehovot, Israel).

References

1. M. Saito and J. Kanfer, *Arch. Biochem. Biophys.* **169,** 318 (1975).
2. J. Kanfer, *Can. J. Biochem.* **58,** 1370 (1980).
3. M. Liscovitch, *Biochem. Soc. Trans.* **19,** 402 (1992).
4. J. Balsinde, E. Diez, B. Fenandez, and F. Mollinedo, *Eur. J. Biochem.* **186,** 717 (1989).
5. V. Chalifa, H. Möhn, and M. Liscovitch, *J. Biol. Chem.* **265,** 17512 (1990).
6. P. Wang, J. C. Anthes, M. I. Siegel, R. W. Egan, and M. M. Billah, *J. Biol. Chem.* **266,** 14877 (1991).
7. M. Liscovitch, V. Chalifa, M. Danin, and Y. Eli, *Biochem. J.* **279,** 319 (1991).
8. H. Möhn, V. Chalifa, and M. Liscovitch, *J. Biol. Chem.* **267,** 11131 (1992).
9. Y. Kagawa and E. Racker, *J. Biol. Chem.* **246,** 547 (1971).
10. G. L. Peterson, *Anal. Biochem.* **83,** 346 (1977).
11. H. Eldar, P. Ben-Av, U. S. Schmidt, E. Livneh, and M. Liscovitch, *J. Biol. Chem.* in press (1993).
12. R. E. Pagano and R. G. Sleight, *Science* **229,** 1051 (1985).

[3]   Soluble Phospholipase D

M. Motasim Billah, John C. Anthes, and Peng Wang

Introduction

Phospholipase D has emerged as an important component in cellular signal transduction mechanisms (1). The enzyme is activated in many cells in response to a wide variety of receptor agonists. Phospholipase D catalyzes the hydrolysis of phospholipid substrates to generate phosphatidic acid and water-soluble bases. Phosphatidic acid and its dephosphorylated product diacylglycerol are important intracellular messengers.

Mammalian phospholipase D acts on several phospholipids including phosphatidylcholine (PC), phosphatidylethanolamine (PE), and phosphatidylinositol (PI) (2). A unique property of phospholipase D is its ability to catalyze a transphosphatidylation reaction by which the phosphatidyl moiety of the phospholipid substrate is transferred to a nucleophilic acceptor such as ethanol (or other primary alcohols) to form phosphatidylethanol (3). This property of phospholipase D provides the basis for a simple and definitive assay of phospholipase D in both intact cells and in cell-free preparations (3, 4). Until recently, it was widely believed that phospholipase D is a membrane-bound enzyme (5). During our recent efforts at purifying phospholipase D from bovine lung, we found that phospholipase D activities are present in both membrane-bound and soluble forms (2). Here, we discuss the detection and characterization of the soluble phospholipase D.

Assay of Soluble Phospholipase D

Materials

1-Stearyl-2-[^{14}C]arachidonylphosphatidylcholine (55 mCi/mmol), 1,2-di[^{14}C]-palmitoylphosphatidylcholine (113 mCi/mmol), 1-palmitoyl-2-[^{14}C]oleoyl-phosphatidylcholine (52 mCi/mmol), and 1,2-[^{14}C]dioleoylphosphatidylcholine (105 mCi/mmol) were from Amersham (Arlington Heights, IL). 1-Palmitoyl-2-[^{14}C]arachidonylphosphatidylcholine (53 mCi/mmol), 1-palmitoyl-2-[^{14}C]linoleoylphosphatidylcholine (50 mCi/mmol), and 1-palmitoyl-2-[^{14}C]arachidonylphosphatidylethanolamine (53 mCi/mmol) were from New England Nuclear (Boston, MA). All of the unlabeled lipids of appropriate fatty acyl composition were obtained from Avanti Polar Lipids (Birmingham,

AL). Mono HR 5/5 prepacked columns were from Pharmacia LKB Biotechnology Inc. (Piscataway, NJ). Silica gel K-6 thin-layer plates were purchased from Whatman (Clifton, NJ). Octylglucoside is from Calbiochem (La Jolla, CA).

Assay Buffer

The assay buffer is 0.1 *M* 2-[*N*-morpholino]ethanesulfonic acid (MES)–NaOH, pH 6.0.

Substrate Solution

To perform 100 assays, phosphatidylcholine (4 μmol) and [^{14}C]phosphatidylcholine (20 μCi) are mixed and dried under a flow of nitrogen gas. Two milliliters of the assay buffer containing 0.5% octylglucoside (w/v) and 6.25% ethanol (v/v) is added. The mixture is vigorously vortexed for 60 sec followed by sonication for 30 sec to obtain a uniform suspension.

Procedure

The assay tubes contain 180 μl of assay buffer, 20 μl of substrate solution, and 50 μl of enzyme sample. Control tubes contain buffer instead of enzyme sample. Tubes are incubated at 37°C for 60 min, and the reaction is terminated by adding 2 ml of chloroform/methanol/HCl (100 : 200 : 0.5, by volume). A mixture of standard phosphatidic acid (10 μg) and phosphatidylethanol (10 μg) is added to each tube, and the phases are separated by adding 0.6 ml of chloroform and 0.85 ml of water, then centrifuging at 4°C for 5 min at 150 *g*. The lower chloroform phase containing the lipids is dried under a flow of nitrogen gas. The dried sample is redissolved in a chloroform/methanol mixture (3 : 1, by volume) and spotted onto a thin-layer plate.

The thin-layer plate is developed using a solvent system consisting of the upper phase of an ethyl acetate/isooctane/acetic acid/water mixture (110 : 50 : 20 : 100, by volume). Phosphatidic acid and phosphatidylethanol are localized by iodine staining, and the area containing phosphatidic acid and phosphatidylethanol are scraped into scintillation vials. Scintillation fluid is added to scintillation vials, and silica gel particles are suspended. The radioactivity in the vials is quantified by liquid scintillation spectrometry.

Preparation of Cytosolic Enzyme

All procedures are performed at 0–4°C. Bovine tissue samples are freshly obtained from a local slaughterhouse, and the tissue is excised, weighed, and cut into small pieces. Homogenization of the tissue (100 g) is done in a Waring blender with 400 ml of buffer containing 20 m*M* Tris-HCl (pH 7.2), 1 m*M* ethylenebis(oxyethylenenitrilo)tetraacetic acid (EGTA), 0.1 m*M* phenylmethylsulfonyl fluoride (PMSF), and 0.02% (w/v) sodium azide. The homogenate is centrifuged at 500 g for 10 min to remove unbroken debris and nuclei. The supernatant is centrifuged again at 105,000 g for 60 min. The supernatant is dialyzed overnight at 4°C against a 20 mM Tris-HCl buffer (pH 8.0) containing 1 mM EGTA, 0.1 mM PMSF, and 0.02% sodium azide, then fractionated on a Mono Q anion-exchange column using a Pharmacia FPLC (fast protein liquid chromatography) system. Proteins were eluted in 1-ml fractions by a linear gradient of NaCl (0–0.3 M) with the same buffer at a flow rate of 1 ml/min.

Properties of Cytosolic Enzyme

Anion-Exchange Chromatography of Soluble Phospholipase D

The activity hydrolyzing phosphatidylcholine to both phosphatidylethanol and phosphatidic acid was eluted from the Mono Q column at 50 mM NaCl. The ratio of phosphatidylethanol to phosphatidic acid was 1.3. This fractionation step enhanced the activity up to 20-fold, suggesting the presence in the soluble fractions of a phospholipase D inhibitory factor(s). Addition of some of fractions lacking phospholipase D activity to the activity peak suppressed the phospholipase D activity. The inhibitory activity could not be destroyed by boiling or by trypsin treatment, suggesting that the inhibitory factor(s) might not be a protein(s). It is likely that the inhibition of radioactive product formation resulted from the dilution of the radiolabeled substrate by endogenous phospholipids.

Molecular Mass

By gel filtration using Bio-Sil SEC-400 columns (Bio-Rad, Richmond, CA), the activity was resolved into two molecular mass species: 30 and 80 kDa. The ratio of the two species varied depending on the presence or absence of octylglucoside. In the presence of octylglucoside, low molecular mass species predominated, suggesting that the native enzyme may exist in a multimeric form.

Stability

Freezing and thawing caused a loss of the enzyme activity. However, the enzyme could be stored without significant loss of activity for up to 2 months at 4°C in 10 mM MES–NaOH, pH 6.0, buffer containing 10% (v/v) glycerol, 1 mM EGTA, 0.1 mM PMSF, and 0.02% sodium azide.

TABLE I   Substrate Specificity of Cytosolic
Phospholipase D[a]

Lipid	Relative activity (%)
1-Stearoyl-2-arachidonyl-PC	100
1-Palmitoyl-2-arachidonyl-PC	210
1-Palmitoyl-2-linoleoyl-PC	107
1-Palmitoyl-2-oleoyl-PC	0
1,2-Dipalmitoyl-PC	0
1,2-Dioleoyl-PC	0
1-Palmitoyl-2-arachidonyl-PE	134

[a] Assays were performed under standard conditions.

pH and Divalent Cation Requirements

The enzyme showed maximal activity at pH 6.0–6.5. The activity rapidly declined with either an increase or decrease in pH. Ca^{2+} was not needed for activity, but the addition of Ca^{2+} enhanced the activity. For example, the presence of 10 mM Ca^{2+} enhanced the activity by about 80%. Mg^{2+} had no effect even at 10 mM. The effects of other divalent cations were not evaluated.

Substrate Specificity

Using phosphatidylcholine as a substrate, the effect of fatty acid composition on the activity was evaluated. The results of a typical experiment are shown in Table I. The nature of the fatty acyl moieties in positions 1 and 2 exerted a profound effect on phospholipase D activity. Phosphatidylcholine with arachidonic acid at position 2 and palmitic acid at position 1 was the most preferred substrate. The enzyme activity was reduced or undetectable when arachidonic acid at position 2 was replaced by a less unsaturated fatty acid (e.g., oleic acid, linoleic acid) or by saturated fatty acids (e.g., palmitic acid, stearic acid). The polar head group also affected phospholipase D activity. The following order of activity was established using pure substrates with defined fatty acid composition: phosphatidylcholine > phosphatidylethanolamine > phosphatidylinositol. Sphingomyelin was not a substrate, and phosphatidylglycerol has not been tested.

Detergents

Octylglucoside (0.075–0.25%) enhanced the activity, whereas various other detergents including Triton X-100, sodium dodecyl sulfate (SDS), and CHAPS were inhibitory.

Tissue Distribution

Of bovine tissues, the richest sources of cytosolic phospholipase D activity was the lung. The rank order of the tissues was as follows: lung > brain = spleen > heart = kidney > thymus > liver.

References

1. M. M. Billah, and J. C. Anthes, *Biochem. J.* **269**, 281 (1990).
2. P. Wang, J. C. Anthes, M. I. Siegel, R. W. Egan, and M. M. Billah, *J. Biol. Chem.* **266**, 14877 (1991).
3. J.-K. Pai, M. I. Siegel, R. W. Egan, and M. M. Billah, *J. Biol. Chem.* **263**, 12472 (1988).
4. J. C. Anthes, S. P. Eckel, M. I. Siegel, R. W. Egan, and M. M. Billah, *Biochem. Biophys. Res. Commun.* **163**, 657 (1989).
5. R. J. Chalifour and J. N. Kanfer, *Biochem. Biophys. Res. Commun.* **96**, 742 (1980).

[4] Phosphatidylethanol Formation as Index of Phospholipase D Activity in Rat Brain Cortex Slices

Silvia Llahi and John N. Fain

Introduction

Many hormone and neurotransmitter receptors transduce signals into cells through the activation of specific phospholipases, resulting in the production of phospholipid-derived second messengers (1). Although phospholipases A_2 and C have received much attention, evidence gathered over the last few years indicates that the receptor-mediated activation of phospholipase D (PLD) may constitute an important novel signal transduction mechanism (2–4). The hydrolytic activity of PLD (EC 3.1.4.4) acts on the terminal phosphodiester bond of glycerophospholipids, generating the free polar head group of the phospholipid and phosphatidic acid (PA), which may itself act as a lipid second messenger (5). PA can be further degraded by a specific phosphohydrolase to diacylglycerol, a well-established second messenger. In fact, the slow and sustained generation of diacylglycerol detected in many cells after stimulation, which may imply the prolonged activation of protein kinase C (PKC), has been associated with the activation of PLD (2, 3, 6).

Most of the available information about PLD comes from studies on phosphatidylcholine (PC) breakdown, since it seems to be hydrolyzed in preference to phosphatidylinositol and phosphatidylethanolamine (4). PLD activity has been identified in a wide variety of mammalian cells, where its stimulation by receptor agonists, phorbol esters, and Ca^{2+} ionophores has been extensively documented.

Most of the receptor agonists associated with the activation of PLD also stimulate phosphoinositide-specific phospholipase C (PLC). Because PLD activity is also stimulated by tumor-promoting phorbol esters, which activate PKC, and by an increase in intracellular Ca^{2+}, it has been suggested that PLD activity may be secondary to the activation of PLC (3, 4). Some evidence coming from experiments using GTPγS (a nonhydrolyzable GTP analog) and pertussis toxin has indicated the possible involvement of guanine nucleotide-binding proteins (G proteins) in the

Methods in Neurosciences, Volume 18

receptor-mediated activation of PLD (2, 3). The activation of PLD by GTPγS, under experimental conditions in which PLC activation was virtually abolished, has been reported in permeabilized HL-60 granulocytes, where the activation of PKC, an increase in Ca^{2+}, and a G protein seem to be required to produce the full activation of PLD (7). Moreover, although different mechanisms of activation of PLD by receptor agonists and phorbol esters have been reported in many cells (8–10), the stimulation of PLD activity as a event secondary to the activation of PKC has also been proposed for all agents (11). However, both PKC-dependent (2, 3) and PKC-independent (8, 12) mechanisms have been reported for the effect of phorbol esters on PLD. Furthermore, the receptor-mediated activation of PLD as the result of an increase in intracellular Ca^{2+} and its regulation by tyrosine kinases have also been suggested (3, 13, 14). Thus, PLD may be coupled to receptors by several different mechanisms and/or multiple isoforms of PLD may exist. However, some discrepancies about its activation may possibly be attributed to the different methodologies employed to assess PLD activity in some preparations.

As mentioned above, the hydrolytic activity of PLD leads to the generation of the free polar head group (base) of the phospholipid (e.g., choline) and PA, which can be metabolized to diacylglycerol. PA is also generated by either *de novo* synthesis from glycerol precursors (15) or the combined actions of a phospholipase C and diacylglycerol kinase (4). Moreover, increased release of phospholipid bases may be due to the base exchange enzymatic activities. Thus, measuring PLD activity by monitoring the generation of either free bases or PA may lead to some uncertainty. However, in addition to its hydrolytic activity, PLD has the unique ability to catalyze a transphosphatidylation reaction in which a primary alcohol such as ethanol is transferred to the phosphatidyl group of the phospholipid substrate, generating the corresponding phosphatidyl alcohol (e.g., phosphatidylethanol) (16, 17). The generation of phosphatidylethanol (PEt), a product with a high degree of metabolic stability, has been taken as an unequivocal indicator of PLD activity, since PEt results exclusively from PLD-catalyzed transphosphatidylation and is formed neither by base exchange enzymatic activities nor by *de novo* synthesis (18–22).

Although PLD activity has been reported in a wide variety of cells, little is known about its receptor-mediated activation in intact cells of the nervous system. To gain further insight into the mechanism of PLD activation in brain, we have adapted an assay to assess PLD activity in rat brain cortical slices, based on the production of PEt (23). In this chapter, we describe this assay method and summarize our major findings about the mechanisms involved in the activation of PLD in rat brain cortex.

Experimental Procedures

Materials

Ortho[^{32}P]phosphoric acid (carrier-free, 8800 Ci/mmol) was obtained from Du Pont New–England Nuclear (Boston, MA). Silica gel HL plates were supplied by Analtech (Newark, DE). All other drugs and chemicals were from Sigma (St. Louis, MO).

Prelabeling of Brain Cortical Slices

Adult male Sprague-Dawley rats are sacrificed by decapitation. Cerebral cortices are dissected free of meninges and white matter on an ice-cold plate and cross-chopped into 350×350 μm slices. Cortical slices are dispersed in Krebs–Henseleit buffer without added phosphate (116 mM NaCl, 4.7 mM KCl, 1.2 mM MgSO$_4$, 25 mM NaHCO$_3$, 11 mM glucose, 1 mM CaCl$_2$), at pH 7.4, equilibrated with O$_2$/CO$_2$ (95 : 5, v/v). After dispersion, slices are washed and incubated in an orbital shaking water bath in the same buffer for 3 hr at 37°C in the presence of radiolabeled inorganic phosphate (^{32}P$_i$, 75 μCi/ml). To preserve cells, slices should be maintained under a well-oxygenated atmosphere. The ^{32}P$_i$ not incorporated into slices is then removed by extensive washing with the same buffer.

Assay of Phospholipase D Activity

Cortical slices prelabeled with ^{32}P$_i$ are packed under gravity and 50-μl aliquots incubated at 37°C in an orbital shaking water bath for 30 min (or the indicated times) with the appropriate additions in a final volume of 250 μl of phosphate-free Krebs–Henseleit buffer and in the presence or absence of 170 mM ethanol (or the indicated concentration). Reactions are stopped by adding 1.2 ml of chloroform/methanol (1 : 2, v/v).

In experiments designed to determine PLD activity in response to the adrenergic receptor agonist norepinephrine (NE), slices should be preincubated for about 15 min at 37°C in the presence of 50 μM pargyline to inhibit irreversibly monoamine oxidase activity. After that, slices should be extensively washed prior to the assay for PLD activity. NE needs to be dissolved in the presence of ascorbic acid (0.1 mg/ml, final concentration) in order to avoid any oxidation.

Lipid Extraction and Thin-Layer Chromatography

Fifteen minutes after reactions are stopped, lipids are extracted by adding chloroform (0.5 ml) and 0.25 M HCl (0.5 ml). Two phases are then separated by centrifugation at 2300 g for 15 min. To quantify the production of [^{32}P]PEt in each assay, 550-μl aliquots of the lower organic phases are dried by centrifugation under vacuum and resuspended in 40 μl of chloroform/methanol (9 : 1, v/v). Aliquots are then carefully spotted on heat-activated silica gel HL plates. PEt is separated from the other lipids by thin-layer chromatography with the solvent system chloroform/methanol/acetic acid (65 : 15 : 2, by volume) (20). In this solvent system PEt (R_f 0.4) migrates above PA (R_f 0.1–0.2) and other phospholipids (R_f 0–0.1). Plates are analyzed by autoradiography, and the areas corresponding to the [^{32}P]PEt are identified by comparison to the PEt standard and by their appearance only in the presence of ethanol. Regions containing [^{32}P]PEt are then carefully scraped and counted by liquid scintillation spectrometry.

To correct for variations in sample size and for differential uptake of ^{32}P into phospholipids, it is recommended to quantify total lipid labeling by directly counting for radioactivity a 50-μl aliquot of the organic phases. In our experiments total lipid labeling was around $2.2 \pm 0.3 \times 10^6$ counts/min (cpm) for 50 μl of cortical slices. All data are expressed as the fractional conversion to PEt of ^{32}P label in total phospholipids multiplied by 10^4 because of the low rate of conversion.

Phosphatidylethanol Standard

PEt standard is prepared by transphosphatidylation of phosphatidylcholine with cabbage PLD, basically as described by Reinhold et al. (10). In brief, 1 mM phosphatidylcholine is incubated for 30 min at 37°C in 0.1 M sodium acetate buffer (pH 5.6) containing 170 mM ethanol, 140 mM CaCl$_2$, and 10 units/ml of PLD (type I from cabbage). As a control for PEt formation, some incubations are carried out in the absence of ethanol. After stopping with chloroform/methanol (1 : 2, v/v), lipids are extracted and separated by thin-layer chromatography as described above. Thin-layer chromatography plates are then stained with iodine vapor, and PEt is identified by its R_f value (0.4) and by its unique appearance in assays run in the presence of ethanol. A PEt standard is also available from Avanti Polar Lipids (Birmingham, AL).

Results and Comments

The mechanism(s) involved in the regulation of PLD activity is a subject of increasing interest. Several different approaches have been developed to assess PLD activity in mammalian cells. Some available information about PLD comes from studies in which the products of its hydrolytic activity have been quantified by mass determination or by methodologies that involve labeling of cellular phospholipids. However, as mentioned earlier, the metabolites generated by the hydrolytic activity of PLD in intact cells may be common among intracellular phospholipases or generated *de novo* through other enzymatic pathways. For this reason, it is now accepted that transphosphatidylation provides a more specific assay for the study of PLD in intact cells.

A conclusive demonstration that PEt is exclusively formed from PLD activity comes from a series of studies on HL-60 granulocytes. First, granulocytes incubated with [3H]alkyllyso-PC, which incorporate label in endogenous alkyl-PC (1-*O*-alkyl-2-acyl-*sn*-glycero-3-phosphatidylcholine), and with [32P]P$_i$ (to label ATP) were stimulated in the presence of ethanol. In contrast to the case for [3H]PA, 32P was not incorporated into [3H]PEt, indicating that PEt was not generated from diacylglycerol (21). Moreover, this finding was further strengthened by developing a methodology to label granulocytes in endogenous alkyl-PC with [32P]P$_i$ without labeling cellular ATP, and by double-labeling cells with [3H]alkyllyso-PC and alkyllyso[32P]PC (20). These studies have definitively demonstrated that PEt is generated exclusively from PLD activity. In fact, for the last few years most reports have been based on the study of the PLD-catalyzed transphosphatidylation reaction. Ethanol has been widely employed for transphosphatidylation reactions, but other alcohols like butanol or propanol can be also used.

Another approach has been developed to quantify the transphosphatidylation activity of PLD in intact cells (24). This assay method is based on the incubation of cells in the presence of high specific activity 1-[3H]butanol, which is incorporated into [3H]phosphatidylbutanol after stimulation of PLD activity. This procedure allows the use of a small concentration of alcohol and does not require prelabeling of phospholipid substrates. However, 1-[3H]butanol is incorporated into at least three different products which have not yet been identified.

We have used a simple assay for PLD activity in rat brain cortical slices, taking advantage of its unique transphosphatidylation activity (23). Slices provide a functionally intact system where PLD activity can be investigated under more physiological conditions. Thus, the production of [32P]PEt in cortical slices labeled with 32P$_i$ was monitored as a measure of PLD activity. As shown in Fig. 1, basal [32P]PEt accumulation increases as a function of the ethanol concentration. When the modulation of PLD activity by receptor agonists was investigated, we found that NE enhances the production of PEt with near-maximal levels around 200 mM ethanol (Fig. 1A). PLD-mediated [32P]PEt accumulation in response to NE increases with time and is already apparent after 5 min of incubation (Fig. 1B). The effect of NE is dose dependent, and it is mediated by α_1-adrenoceptors, as inferred by the use of specific antagonists.

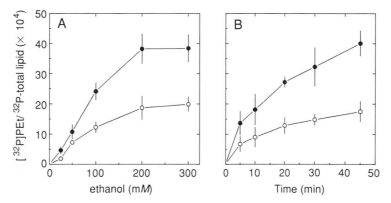

FIG. 1   Effect of ethanol concentration and time course for norepinephrine stimulation of PLD-mediated phosphatidylethanol (PEt) formation. Cortical slices were labeled with $^{32}P_i$ and incubated in the absence (open circles) or presence (filled circles) of 100 μM norepinephrine for 30 min at 37°C with the indicated concentrations of ethanol (A) or with 170 mM ethanol for the indicated times (B). Data are means ± S.E. of three experiments run in duplicate. (Reproduced by permission from Ref. 23.)

As it has been proposed that the receptor-mediated activation of PLD may be secondary to the previous activation of phosphoinositide-specific PLC, we investigated the effect of the muscarinic receptor agonist carbachol on PLD activity in rat cortical slices (23). In contrast to NE, carbachol does not stimulate PLD-mediated PEt production in our preparation (Fig. 2). Similar results for both agonists are observed after addition of phosphate (1.2 mM KH$_2$PO$_4$) to the assay buffer. Under the same experimental conditions used to assay PLD activity, and in the presence or absence of either added phosphate or ethanol (170 mM), NE and carbachol stimulate the accumulation of [^{3}H]inositol phosphates with no major variations between each experimental condition (23). Thus, carbachol does not appear to stimulate PLD activity in rat cortical slices.

The Ca^{2+} ionophore ionomycin and the phorbol ester PMA (phorbol 12-myristate 13-acetate) also stimulate PLD-mediated PEt formation in rat brain cortical slices (23). The effects of both PMA and ionomycin are strongly reduced or completely inhibited by treatment of cortical slices with some PKC inhibitors, such as staurosporine and H-7. Under the same conditions, PKC inhibitors have no effect on the response to NE. Furthermore, the effect of PMA is slower in onset (near-maximal effect is reached after 20 min of incubation) and is not modified by the concentration of extracellular Ca^{2+}, in contrast to the reduction observed in the effect due to NE when assays are run in the presence of no added calcium and EGTA (40 μM). Interestingly, the effects of NE and PMA are additive, even after treatment

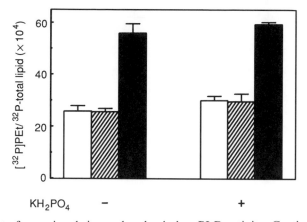

FIG. 2   Effect of norepinephrine and carbachol on PLD activity. Cortical slices were labeled with $^{32}P_i$, washed, and incubated for 30 min at 37°C in buffer with or without added phosphate (1.2 mM KH_2PO_4). Assays were carried out in the absence (open bars) or in the presence of 1 mM carbachol (striped bars) or 100 μM norepinephrine (solid bars). (Reproduced by permission from Ref. 23.)

with PKC inhibitors. From these results it could be concluded that NE and PMA stimulate PLD activity in rat cerebral cortex through two different mechanisms, one independent of and one dependent on PKC. An α_1-adrenoceptor-mediated activation of PLD independent of the prior activation of PKC is also corroborated by the finding that carbachol, which stimulates phosphoinositide breakdown under our experimental conditions, has no effect on PLD activity in rat cortical slices.

Accumulation of [^{32}P]PEt as a measure of PLD activity has also been investigated in slices from rat cerebellum and hippocampus labeled with $^{32}P_i$, with the same assay conditions as described for cerebral cortical slices (23). Interestingly, whereas NE also stimulates PLD activity in hippocampal slices, no effect is detected in slices from cerebellum, where a low density of α_1-adrenoceptors has been reported (25).

In summary, by monitoring PEt formation as an index of PLD activity in rat brain cortical slices, we have reported the first demonstration for the involvement of α_1-adrenoceptors in receptor-mediated activation of PLD. Our observations strongly suggest that PLD activity can be regulated by both PKC-dependent and PKC-independent mechanisms. Furthermore, this assay provides a useful and highly reproducible method for the study of PLD activity.

References

1. E. A. Dennis, S. G. Rhee, M. M. Billah, and Y. A. Hannun, *FASEB J.* **5,** 2068 (1991).
2. M. M. Billah and J. C. Anthes, *Biochem. J.* **269,** 281 (1990).
3. J. H. Exton, *J. Biol. Chem.* **265,** 1 (1990).
4. S. D. Shukla and S. P. Halenda, *Life Sci.* **48,** 851 (1991).
5. S. B. Bocckino, P. B. Wilson, and J. H. Exton, *Proc. Natl. Acad. Sci. U.S.A.* **88,** 6210 (1991).
6. M. Fallman, M. Gullberg, C. Hellberg, and T. Anderson, *J. Biol. Chem.* **267,** 2656 (1992).
7. B. Geny and S. Cockcroft, *Biochem. J.* **284,** 531 (1992).
8. M. M. Billah, J.-K. Pai, T. J. Mullmann, R. W. Egan, and M. I. Siegel, *J. Biol. Chem.* **264,** 9069 (1989).
9. M. Liscovitch and A. Amsterdam, *J. Biol. Chem.* **264,** 11762 (1989).
10. S. L. Reinhold, S. M. Prescott, G. A. Zimmerman, and T. M. McIntyre, *FASEB J.* **4,** 208 (1990).
11. W. J. van Blitterswijk, H. Hilkmann, J. de Widt, and R. L. van der Bend, *J. Biol. Chem.* **266,** 10344 (1991).
12. Y.-Z. Cao, C. C. Reddy, and A. M. Mastro, *Biochem. Biophys. Res. Commun.* **171,** 955 (1990).
13. N. T. Thompson, R. W. Bonser, and L. G. Garland, *Trends Pharmacol. Sci.* **121,** 404 (1991).
14. I. J. Uings, N. T. Thompson, R. W. Randall, G. D. Spacey, R. W. Bonser, A. T. Hudson, and L. G. Garland, *Biochem. J.* **281,** 597 (1992).
15. R. V. Farese, T. S. Konda, J. S. Davis, M. L. Standaert, R. J. Pollet, and D. R. Cooper, *Science* **236,** 586 (1987).
16. R. M. C. Dawson, *Biochem. J.* **102,** 205 (1967).
17. M. Kobayashi and J. N. Kanfer, *J. Neurochem.* **48,** 1597 (1987).
18. J. N. Kanfer, *Can. J. Biochem.* **58,** 1370 (1980).
19. L. Gustavsson and C. Alling, *Biochem. Biophys. Res. Commun.* **142,** 958 (1987).
20. J.-K. Pai, M. I. Siegel, R. W. Egan, and M. M. Billah, *J. Biol. Chem.* **263,** 12472 (1988).
21. J.-K. Pai, M. I. Siegel, R. W. Egan, and M. M. Billah, *Biochem. Biophys. Res. Commun.* **150,** 355 (1988).
22. M. Liscovitch, *J. Biol. Chem.* **264,** 1450 (1989).
23. S. Llahi and J. N. Fain, *J. Biol. Chem.* **267,** 3679 (1992).
24. R. W. Randall, R. W. Bonser, N. T. Thompson, and L. G. Garland, *FEBS Lett.* **264,** 87 (1990).
25. R. D. Johnson and K. P. Minneman, *Brain Res.* **341,** 7 (1985).

[5] Agonist Stimulation of Phosphoinositide Breakdown in Brain Membranes

Enrique Claro, Fernando Picatoste, and John N. Fain

Introduction

A variety of neurotransmitter receptors are coupled to activation of phosphoinositidase C (PLC) (1, 2), which results in the generation of the intracellular second messengers inositol 1,4,5-trisphosphate [$Ins(1,4,5)P_3$] and 1,2-diacylglycerol (3, 4). Coupling between the receptor and the effector enzyme takes place through a guanine nucleotide regulatory protein or G_q protein (5, 6). To study such functional coupling, it is necessary to use either permeabilized cells or membrane preparations, in order to facilitate access of guanine nucleotides to their binding site in the G protein. In this chapter we focus on various methodological procedures we have adapted, using washed brain membrane preparations, that allowed us to show the direct coupling of muscarinic cholinergic, and 5-HT$_2$-serotonergic receptors to PLC.

Assay with Membranes Made from [^{3}H]inositol-Prelabeled Brain Slices

Gonzales and Crews (7) first reported that addition of guanine nucleotides to brain cortical membranes from slices prelabeled with [^{3}H]inositol ([^{3}H]Ins) resulted in the generation of [^{3}H]Ins phosphates. Subsequently, Chiu *et al.* (8) and Claro *et al.* (9) demonstrated agonist effects in the presence of hydrolysis-resistant GTP analogs.

Preparation of Membranes

Rat brain cortical slices (350 × 350 μm) are incubated for 2 hr at 37°C in 5 volumes of Krebs–Henseleit buffer (composition, in mM: NaCl, 116; NaHCO$_3$, 25; glucose, 11; KCl, 4.7; MgSO$_4$, 1.2; KH$_2$PO$_4$, 1.2), pH 7.4, equilibrated with O$_2$/CO$_2$ (95 : 5, v/v), and [^{3}H]Ins (2–50 μCi/ml). Calcium is omitted from the buffer since this results in substantially higher lipid labeling. After the labeling incubation, slices are washed 5 times with 20 volumes of ice-cold 20 mM Tris-HCl buffer, pH 7.0, containing 1 mM EGTA (Tris/EGTA buffer), then homogenized in 20 volumes of the same buffer

Methods in Neurosciences, Volume 18

using a glass homogenizer with a Teflon pestle. We originally used 10 hand strokes but have found that 20 strokes with a motor-driven pestle at maximum setting results in greater agonist effects. The homogenate is centrifuged for 15 min at 40,000 g. The pellet is then resuspended in Tris/EGTA buffer, rehomogenized, and centrifuged again. This procedure is repeated twice more. The final membranes (about 60 mg protein/g of tissue) contain less than 1% of the original lactate dehydrogenase (LDH) activity, and 90–95% of the total radioactivity is in the lipid fraction. Membranes can be either assayed fresh or kept frozen until use. We normally aliquot the membranes in microcentrifuge tubes and keep the pellets at $-80°C$. There is no variation in PLC responsiveness to GTPγS and agonists for at least 6 months of storage.

Phosphoinositidase C Assay

Membrane pellets are resuspended at a concentration of 2.5 mg protein/ml in a cold buffer consisting of 25 mM Tris–maleate, 5 mM ATP, 15 mM MgCl$_2$, and 25 mM LiCl, pH 6.8 (adjusted with KOH). Reactions (100 µl total volume) are initiated by adding 40 µl of membranes [100 µg protein, 20,000–500,000 disintegrations/per min (dpm)] to tubes containing 5 µl of 20 mM sodium deoxycholate in water, 15 µl of GTPγS and agonists in 25 mM Tris–maleate (pH 6.8), and 40 µl of 7.5 mM EGTA in Tris–maleate buffer containing CaCl$_2$. The EGTA/calcium solution is prepared separately from 7.5 mM EGTA in Tris–maleate (which we keep at 4°C for 3–4 weeks) and concentrated CaCl$_2$ in water. For instance, addition to the assay tubes of 40 µl of a solution made with 34 µl of 0.1 M CaCl$_2$ and 5 ml of 7.5 mM EGTA/ 25 mM Tris-maleate (pH 6.8) will yield a free calcium concentration in the assay of 100 nM, assuming a calcium–EGTA dissociation constant of 10^{-6} M at pH 6.8 (10).

Tubes are incubated at 37°C for 10–20 min (accumulation of [³H]Ins phosphates is linear for up to 30 min). The reactions are stopped with 1.2 ml chloroform/methanol (1 : 2, v/v), then 0.5 ml each of chloroform and 0.25 M HCl are added to create two phases. After neutralizing the aqueous phase with 1.5 M NH$_4$OH, [³H]Ins phosphates are separated from one another and/or from free [³H]Ins by anion-exchange chromatography with Dowex 1 × 8 (100–200 mesh, formate form) as described by Berridge *et al.* (11), or by high-performance liquid chromatography (HPLC). If sufficient label was incorporated into the membranes and less than 5% is free [³H]Ins, aliquots of the aqueous phases can be counted directly. Column chromatography is needed if individual [³H]Ins phosphates are to be quantified. [³H]Ins(1,4)P$_2$ is the main product (about 85% of the total) that accumulates, even at short incubation times (0.5 min). There is some [³H]Ins(1,4,5)P$_3$, [³H]Ins(4)P, and a little [³H]Ins(1)P, but [³H]Ins(1,3,4,5)P$_4$ or [³H]Ins(1,3,4)P$_3$ are not formed.

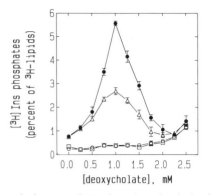

FIG. 1 Effect of deoxycholate on GTPγS and carbachol stimulation of formation of [³H]Ins phosphates by membranes from [³H]Ins-prelabeled rat brain cortical slices. Prelabeled membranes were incubated for 10 min with the indicated concentrations of sodium deoxycholate in the absence (open circles) or presence of 1 mM carbachol (squares), 1 μM GTPγS (triangles), or both (filled circles). Production of [³H]Ins phosphates is expressed as the percentage of total radioactivity in lipids. [Adapted with permission from E. Claro, A. García, and F. Picatoste, *Biochem. J.* **261,** 29 (1989).]

Comments

It is crucial to control the free calcium concentration in the assay. At 100 nM calcium, basal production of [³H]Ins phosphates is negligible and ligand effects are greatest. As the free calcium concentration is increased, basal PLC activity increases and agonist effects become less apparent. The assay is very sensitive to pH changes, as acidification of the medium will release calcium from the EGTA buffer and indirectly stimulate PLC. Thus, all additions should be checked for pH. This is particularly important for agonists, since omission of this control may give false agonist effects. Inclusion of ATP and magnesium is necessary for the synthesis of polyphosphoinositides. We find 2 mM ATP and 6–9 mM MgCl₂ to be optimum. Although there is practically no inositol monophosphatase activity in the membrane preparation, 10 mM LiCl is included in the assay to prevent any inositol polyphosphate 1-phosphatase activity present.

The presence of deoxycholate is required for agonist effects (Fig. 1). In the absence of deoxycholate, GTPγS stimulates PLC, but there is no further effect of neurotransmitter receptor agonists when added together with the nucleotide. With 1 mM (0.04%, w/v) deoxycholate, GTPγS stimulation is potentiated, and agonists, which by themselves have no effect (this should always be checked), become stimulatory in the presence of GTPγS. The range of deoxycholate concentrations that allow agonist effects is very narrow

(0.75–1.5 mM), and we have consistently found 1 mM to be optimal (Fig. 1). Apparently deoxycholate effects, which can be partially reproduced only with cholate, are rather complex. Deoxycholate at 1 mM, well below the critical micellar concentration, is insufficient to stimulate PLC directly but does stimulate phosphatidylinositol (PI) and phosphatidylinositol 4-phosphate (PIP) kinases. It may also permeabilize the artificial membrane vesicles created by the homogenization procedure, allowing GTPγS and receptor agonists to gain access to their respective binding sites which occur in opposite sides of the membrane.

It is also possible to measure the breakdown of endogenous phosphatidylinositol 4,5-bisphosphate (PIP$_2$) using a radioligand binding assay to determine the mass of Ins(1,4,5)P$_3$. In the studies of Lee and Fain (12) the same conditions were used as described above for measuring formation of labeled Ins phosphates except for the use of 300 μg of membrane protein instead of 100 μg per assay tube. Increase of Ins(1,4,5)P$_3$ mass as stimulated by GTPγS and carbachol is maximal at 2 min (about 500% of control). Owing to the larger amount of membranes used and the cost and time required for radioligand binding assays, this procedure will probably be most useful in demonstrating that breakdown of endogenous PIP$_2$ is occurring in membranes.

Assays with Exogenous [^{3}H]Phosphoinositide Substrates

Guanine nucleotide activation of the breakdown of exogenously supplied [^{3}H]phosphatidylinositol 4,5-bisphosphate ([^{3}H]PIP$_2$) by brain membranes was first described by Litosch (13), but the effects of neurotransmitters were not reported. Using a protocol similar to that described for studies with [^{3}H]Ins-prelabeled membranes, we showed that brain membranes hydrolyze all three phosphoinositides added exogenously, in a carbachol-sensitive, GTPγS-dependent fashion (14). Subsequently, we extended our observations to a variety of muscarinic agonists (15) and serotonin analogs (15). In addition to rat brain regions, we have successfully applied the same protocol to rabbit (16), cat (17) and human (18) brain membrane preparations.

Preparation of Membranes

Membranes are prepared exactly as described above. Brain slices can be incubated in Krebs–Henseleit buffer for up to 4–5 hr, allowing a variety of pretreatments. Alternatively, brain regions can be homogenized immediately after dissection. Frozen brain samples, which can be used as well, are thawed in cold Tris/EGTA buffer prior to homogenization.

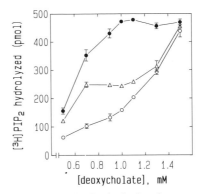

FIG. 2   Effect of deoxycholate on the hydrolysis of exogenous [^{3}H]PIP$_2$ substrate. Rat cortical membranes were incubated for 10 min with 30 μM [^{3}H]PIP$_2$, and with different deoxycholate concentrations as indicated, in the absence (open circles) or presence of 1 μM GTPγS alone (triangles) or in combination with 1 mM carbachol (filled circles). [Reprinted with permission from E. Claro, M. A. Wallace, H. M. Lee, and J. N. Fain, *J. Biol. Chem.* **264,** 18288 (1989).]

Phosphoinositidase C Assay

Optimal conditions for our standard procedure using exogenous [^{3}H]PIP$_2$ substrate are very similar to those described for prelabeled membranes. [^{3}H]PIP$_2$ is mixed with cold PIP$_2$ and evaporated under a stream of N$_2$, then resuspended in 20 mM sodium deoxycholate using a Fisher probe dismembrator (two 15-sec bursts, setting 35) and added in 5 μl to the reaction tubes so that the detergent concentration in the assay is 1 mM (Fig. 2). The final [^{3}H]PIP$_2$ concentration is 30 μM, at a specific activity of 3–6 Ci/mol (20,000–40,000 dpm/tube). Reactions are stopped as before, and 1-ml aliquots of the aqueous phases containing [^{3}H]Ins phosphates are directly counted for radioactivity. Basal PLC activity using exogenous [^{3}H]PIP$_2$ substrate is more sensitive to stimulation by calcium than with endogenous substrate. Therefore, we use 30–50 nM free calcium because agonist effects are greater on a percentage basis. Unlike the assay with prelabeled membranes, the reaction is linear for only 3–5 min. However, we routinely carry out 10-min incubations to maximize the difference between stimulated and basal activities. The membrane preparation contains both phosphoinositide kinases and the corresponding phosphatases. Over the 10-min incubation period, about 20% of the initial [^{3}H]PIP$_2$ appears as [^{3}H]PIP, and 35% as [^{3}H]PI (14). Exogenous PI is poorly hydrolyzed at 30–50 nM free calcium (see below), but PIP is as good a substrate as PIP$_2$ (14). The reaction products include [^{3}H]Ins(1,4)P$_2$, [^{3}H]Ins(4)P, and [^{3}H]Ins(1,4,5)P$_3$, with the latter appearing marginally unless Ins(1,4,5)P$_3$ 5-phosphatase inhibitors (e.g., 2,3-bisphosphoglycerate) are included in the assay.

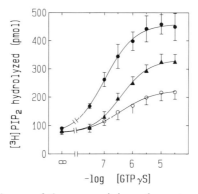

FIG. 3 GTPγS dependency of the muscarinic and serotonergic stimulation of the breakdown of exogenous [³H]PIP₂ by phospholipase C. Rat cortical membranes were incubated with 30 μM [³H]PIP₂ and with the indicated concentrations of GTPγS alone (open circles) or together with 0.3 mM 5-methyltryptamine (triangles) or 1 mM carbachol (filled circles). [Adapted with permission from M. A. Wallace and E. Claro, *J. Pharmacol. Exp. Ther.* **255**, 1296 (1990), © by the American Society for Pharmacology and Experimental Therapeutics.]

In addition to polyphosphoinositides, exogenously added PI can also be hydrolyzed at higher calcium concentrations directly by PLC in a GTPγS and agonist-dependent manner, yielding Ins(1)P as the only reaction product. For optimal agonist effects, free calcium and substrate concentrations are increased to 300 nM and 100 μM, respectively. This assay does not require ATP, and thus the magnesium concentration can be dropped to 1 mM, enough to support G protein activation.

Endogenous PI does not appear to be a good substrate for brain PLC, even at high (above 300 nM) calcium concentrations. Thus, the situation in the intact membrane is best reproduced by using [³H]PI, MgATP to allow [³H]polyphosphoinositide synthesis, and a calcium concentration restrictive for the direct breakdown of [³H]PI (30 nM). Under these conditions, the production of [³H]Ins phosphates, mainly [³H]Ins(1,4)P₂, as stimulated by GTPγS and carbachol is linear for at least 30 min, with a lag of about 5 min consistent with the phosphorylation of [³H]PI prior to the action of PLC.

Comments

The use of exogenous substrates is an obvious advantage over that of [³H]Ins-prelabeled membranes when it is difficult to obtain metabolically active brain tissue. This is particularly true when studies on human brain samples are undertaken, as discussed in Chapter 6 of this volume. Agonist effects are observed just as well in assays with exogenous substrates (Fig. 3). Moreover, although the substrate is presented unnaturally, the specificity of the receptor–agonist interaction is maintained: muscarinic antagonists like atropine and pirenzepine inhibit the stimulation of PLC elicited by muscarinic agonists (carbachol, oxotremorine M) with K_i values similar to those found in the intact tissue, and the same is true for serotonin (and its analogs) and 5-HT$_2$ receptor-selective antagonists (ketanserin).

As already mentioned, in terms of substrate specificity, assays with exogenous [3H]PI do not reflect the situation in the cell. However, the possibility of controlling the flux of the tritium label from [3H]PI either directly to [3H]Ins(1)P or through [3H]PIP–[3H]PIP$_2$ to [3H]Ins(1,4)P$_2$–[3H]Ins(1,4,5)P$_3$ (no ATP and 300 nM free calcium, or ATP and 30 nM free calcium, respectively) allows a clear differentiation between effects on PLC activation and effects on polyphosphoinositide synthesis (19). These assays also offer some cost advantage over those involving [3H]PIP$_2$ and [3H]PIP substrates.

Assays with Membranes Directly Labeled with [3H]Inositol

PI is synthesized from CDP-diacylglycerol and Ins by the action of phosphatidylinositol synthase, in the following reaction:

$$\text{Ins} + \text{CDP-diacylglycerol} \rightleftharpoons \text{PI} + \text{CMP}$$

Taking advantage of the reversibility of the reaction, McPhee *et al.* (20) showed in turkey erythrocyte membranes that, in the presence of CMP, [3H]Ins could be exchanged by the polar head moiety of PI, allowing the direct labeling of endogenous PI. Subsequently we used this approach for a simple assay of brain PLC in membranes using [3H]Ins as labeled presursor (21).

Labeling of Membranes

Rat brain membranes, prepared as described above, are thawed and/or resuspended in 20 mM Tris-HCl, pH 7.0, containing 1 mM EGTA, 6 mM MgCl$_2$, and 1 mM CMP, at a protein concentration of 2.5 mg/ml. [3H]Ins (0.5–5 μCi/ml) is added, and then membranes are incubated for 45 min at 37°C with orbital shaking. Under these conditions, rat cortical membranes incorporate 130,000 to 1,300,000 dpm/mg protein, and in this regard they are very similar to turkey erythrocyte ghosts (22). In the absence of CMP, [3H]Ins incorporation into lipids is about one-third, showing the concurrent participation of both PI synthase and the PI head group exchanging enzyme (which is independent of CMP) in the labeling process. [3H]Ins is incorporated exclusively into PI; however, by adding 2 mM ATP during the last 10 min of incubation,

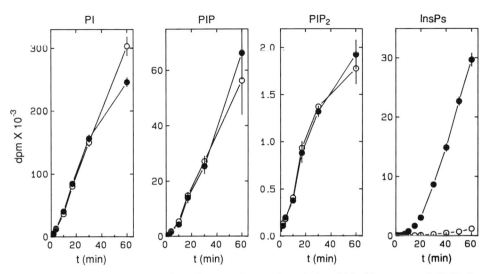

FIG. 4   Concerted activities of PI synthase, phosphoinositide kinases, and GTPγS- and carbachol-stimulated phospholipase C. Rat cortical membranes (100 μg protein) were incubated for the times indicated with [³H]Ins (1.5 μCi/ml) and in the absence (open circles) or presence (filled circles) of 1 μM GTPγS plus 1 mM carbachol. Note that agonists affect only the production of [³H]Ins phosphates. [Adapted with permission from E. Claro, M. A. Wallace, and J. N. Fain, *J. Neurochem.* **58,** 2155 (1992).]

the label equilibrates between PI, PIP, and PIP₂. After labeling, membranes are diluted with the same cold buffer and centrifuged for 15 min at 150,000 *g*, then resuspended at 2.5 mg protein/ml in cold Tris–maleate buffer, pH 6.8, containing 5 mM ATP, 15 mM MgCl₂, and 25 mM LiCl, and assayed exactly as for membranes from [³H]Ins-prelabeled tissue slices. In all aspects (assay conditions, [³H]Ins phosphate products, signal-to-noise ratio) the assay is identical to that with membranes from prelabeled slices.

Concerted Assay of Phosphatidylinositol Synthase, Phosphoinositide Kinases, and Phospholipase C

It is now clear that the washed rat brain membrane preparation described in this chapter contains the machinery required to label PI with [³H]Ins, convert it to [³H]polyphosphoinositides, and hydrolyze them in a GTPγS- and receptor agonist-sensitive manner. Thus, it is possible to monitor the flux of tritium label from free [³H]Ins to [³H]Ins phosphates arising from the concerted activities of PI synthase, PI and PIP kinases, and receptor/G protein-regulated PLC.

Membranes (100 μg protein) are incubated at 37°C in 100 μl of 25 mM Tris–maleate buffer, pH 6.8, containing 0.5–5 μCi of [³H]Ins, 6 mM MgCl$_2$, 10 mM LiCl, 1 mM sodium deoxycholate, 2 mM ATP, 3 mM EGTA and CaCl$_2$ necessary for a free calcium concentration of 100 nM (~0.27 mM), 1 mM CMP, and agonists. After stopping the reaction, it is necessary to remove free [³H]Ins by Dowex chromatography because, after 30 min, about 7% of the total radioactivity is incorporated into lipids and only 0.5% of the total label appears as [³H]Ins phosphates. Although there is no lag in the appearance of [³H]PI, [³H]PIP and [³H]PIP$_2$ appear after 2 min (Fig. 4). [³H]Ins phosphates are formed after a lag of 10 min, then accumulate at a constant rate for up to 60 min (Fig. 4).

TABLE I Comparison of Different Assays for Agonist- and GTPγS-Stimulated Phosphoinositidase C in Brain Membranes

Assay	Cost	Assay conditions	Response to 1 μM GTPγS + 1 mM carbachol[a] (% of basal)	Comments	Ref.
Endogenous breakdown using membranes from [³H]Ins-prelabeled tissue slices	$	100 nM Ca²⁺, 10 min	1500	Linear for 30 min; requires metabolically active tissue; Dowex separation of free [³H]inositol is recommended	9
Endogenous breakdown measuring Ins (1, 4, 5) P$_3$ mass	$$	100 nM Ca²⁺, 2 min	500	Requires more membranes; allows measurement of total Ins (1, 4, 5) P$_3$	12
Exogenous [³H]PIP$_2$–[³H]PIP	$$$	30–50 nM Ca²⁺, 10 min	500	Linear for 3–5 min	14
Exogenous [³H]PI (direct breakdown)	$$	300 nM Ca²⁺, no ATP, 20 min	200	Linear for 30 min; not a physiological substrate; bypass of PI–PIP kinases	14, 16
Exogenous [³H]PI (preconversion to [³H]PIP–[³H]PIP$_2$)	$$	30 nM Ca²⁺, 10 min	500	Linear for 30 min (5-min lag); requires active PI–PIP kinases	19
Membranes labeled directly with [³H]inositol + CMP (concerted assay)	$	100 nM Ca²⁺, 30 min	3000	Linear for 60 min (10-min lag); requires Dowex separation to remove free [³H]Ins; requires active PI–PIP kinases	21

[a] Assays conducted with membranes from rat brain cortex.

In the concerted assay, inclusion of 1 mM deoxycholate is necessary for agonist effects on PLC and results in the inhibition of [^{3}H]Ins labeling of PI through the head group exchanging enzyme by 80%, whereas the CMP-dependent process (due to PI synthase) is stimulated by 20%, so that conversion of [^{3}H]Ins to [^{3}H]Ins phosphates becomes strictly dependent on the presence of CMP. The optimal calcium concentration for agonist effects is again 100 nM. Calcium facilitates agonist stimulation of PLC acting on endogenous substrates, but it also completely inhibits PI synthase at concentrations of 3 μM and higher, with a IC$_{50}$ value of around 200 nM. Therefore, the production of [^{3}H]Ins phosphates due to GTPγS and carbachol is enhanced as calcium concentrations increase up to 100 nM but becomes inhibited at higher concentrations of the ion owing to the inability of the label to flux through the PI synthase step.

Conclusion

The procedures described here are summarized in Table I. With the exception of the Ins(1,4,5)P$_3$ mass determination by radioligand binding assays, the different approaches are characterized basically by the way the labeled phosphoinositide substrate is presented (endogenous or exogenous) and, if using endogenous substrate, in the way [^{3}H]Ins is incorporated. As a reference, we provide data regarding relative cost and the responsiveness of each assay to GTPγS and carbachol when conducted with membranes from rat brain cortex. Procedures involving labeling of endogenous phosphoinositides are more advantageous in terms of cost and signal-to-noise ratio; however, they require either the use of metabolically active tissue or functioning PI synthase and phosphoinositide kinase activities, whereas with exogenous substrates only the receptor–G protein–PLC coupling needs to be preserved.

References

1. S. K. Fisher and B. W. Agranoff, *J. Neurochem.* **48,** 999 (1987).
2. S. K. Fisher, A. M. Heacock, and B. W. Agranoff, *J. Neurochem.* **58,** 18 (1992).
3. M. J. Berridge, *Nature (London)* **361,** 315–325 (1993).
4. Y. Nishizuka, *Nature (London)* **334,** 661 (1988).
5. J. N. Fain, *Biochim. Biophys. Acta* **1053,** 82 (1990).
6. G. Berstein, J. L. Blank, A. V. Smrcka, T. Higashijima, P. C. Sternweis, J. H. Exton, and E. M. Ross, *J. Biol. Chem.* **267,** 8081 (1992).
7. R. Gonzales and F. T. Crews, *Biochem. J.* **232,** 799 (1985).
8. A. S. Chiu, P. P. Li, and J. J. Warsh, *Biochem. J.* **256,** 995 (1988).

9. E. Claro, A. García, and F. Picatoste, *Biochem. J.* **261,** 29 (1989).
10. T. Sasaguri, M. Hirata, and H. Kuriyama, *Biochem. J.* **231,** 497 (1985).
11. M. J. Berridge, C. P. Downes, and M. R. Hanley, *Biochem. J.* **206,** 587 (1982).
12. H. M. Lee and J. N. Fain, *J. Neurochem.* **59,** 953 (1992).
13. I. Litosch, *Biochem. J.* **244,** 35 (1987).
14. E. Claro, M. A. Wallace, H. M. Lee, and J. N. Fain, *J. Biol. Chem.* **264,** 18288 (1989).
15. M. A. Wallace and E. Claro, *J. Pharmacol. Exp. Ther.* **255,** 1296 (1990).
16. H. R. Carter and J. N. Fain, *J. Neurochem.* **56,** 1616 (1991).
17. E. Claro, M. A. Wallace, J. N. Fain, B. G. Nair, T. B. Patel, G. Shanker, and H. J. Baker, *Mol. Brain Res.* **11,** 265 (1991).
18. M. A. Wallace and E. Claro, *Neurochem. Res* **18,** 139 (1993).
19. E. Claro, M. A. Wallace, and J. N. Fain, *Biochem. J.* **268,** 733 (1990).
20. F. McPhee, G. Lowe, C. Vaziri, and C. P. Downes, *Biochem. J.* **275,** 187 (1991).
21. E. Claro, M. A. Wallace, and J. N. Fain, *J. Neurochem.* **58,** 2155 (1992).
22. C. Vaziri and C. P. Downes, *Biochem. J.* **284,** 917 (1992).

[6] Regulation of Phosphoinositide Metabolism in Membranes Prepared from Human Brain Cortex

Michael A. Wallace

Introduction

The phosphoinositide signaling pathway is a major mechanism through which neurotransmitters affect intracellular calcium and diacylglycerol levels, thus playing an important role in neuronal function. Activation of phosphoinositide-specific phospholipase C (PI–PLC) through guanine nucleotide-binding (G) proteins is the proven or suspected pathway of transmembrane signaling for muscarinic cholinergic (M_1, M_3), α_1-adrenergic, serotonergic (5-HT$_2$, 5-HT$_{1c}$), histaminic, peptidergic (e.g., substance P), and possibly D_1-dopaminergic agonists (1, 2). There are at least three distinct types of PI–PLC, each type having multiple isoforms, which catalyze the breakdown of phosphatidylinositol 4,5-bisphosphate (PIP$_2$) (3). The γ isoforms contain *src* sequence similarity and are subject to phosphorylation by tyrosine kinases. This phosphorylation probably stimulates PI–PLC activity when cells respond to hormones such as platelet-derived growth factor (PDGF) or epidermal growth factor (EGF). The β isoforms are regulated by hormones and neurotransmitters which act through G proteins. The mode of regulation for PI–PLC δ is at present unknown but may also be through G proteins. In addition, changes in intracellular calcium levels can affect PI–PLC activity; thus, phosphoinositide degradation is stimulated when neurons are subjected to depolarizing conditions. The ability to assess the functional integrity of the activation by a neurotransmitter of the PI–PLC pathway in human brain could be an important tool in analyzing various disease states.

Kendall and Firth (4) and Nicoletti *et al.* (5) have analyzed the PI–PLC system in biopsied brain samples from humans. They used conditions for studying phosphoinositide turnover in human tissue similar to those routinely used in work with brain tissue slices from rodents. These important studies are limited, though, because biopsy material is not usually available for studying diseases such as Alzheimer's disease or schizophrenia. Using synaptosomal preparations from autopsied material to study phosphoinositide signaling after labeling the endogenous phospholipid with [^{3}H]inositol has not proved generally satisfactory (6). A procedure for assay of PI–PLC with

Methods in Neurosciences, Volume 18

exogenous substrate added to synaptosomal-like preparations has been reported by O'Neill *et al.* (7). Stimulation of PI–PLC by GppNHp and other nucleotides was found, but the effects of neurotransmitters were not analyzed.

Our laboratory has developed an experimental system wherein exogenous tritiated phospholipid substrates for PI–PLC [including phosphatidylinositol (PI), phosphatidylinositol 4-phosphate (PIP), and PIP$_2$] are added to nonvesiculated brain membrane preparations (8). Hydrolysis of the phosphoinositides by PI–PLC is promoted by a variety of neurotransmitters in a guanine nucleotide-dependent manner. This system has been adapted for the routine study of human brain membranes prepared from unfixed samples frozen in liquid N$_2$ at autopsy (9).

When using human brain samples, it is important to be aware of variations that are due to (1) age of patients at death, (2) use of neuroleptics prior to death, (3) postmortem interval prior to tissue freezing, and (4) length of tissue storage prior to assay. The agonal state of the deceased is also relevant. Dodd *et al.* (10) have discussed these issues at length. Whereas the levels of many metabolites change quickly and radically at death, proteins, especially membrane-bound proteins, appear to be much more stable. Thus, although PIP$_2$ levels fall postmortem (11), the functional coupling of at least some neurotransmitter receptors with G protein(s) and PI–PLC is preserved, and the interaction can be monitored by adding back exogenous substrate to the membranes.

Preparation of Membranes

The preparation of membranes from human cortex is similar to the method used for rat or rabbit studies (8, 12, 13). Tissue samples (1–2 g) stored at −70°C are chopped into pieces, and the white matter is removed as the pieces thaw into homogenization buffer held at 4°C. Homogenization buffer contains 20 mM Tris–maleate, pH 7, with 1 mM EGTA. The tissue is homogenized in approximately 10 volumes of buffer using a motor-driven homogenizer with a Teflon pestle. The homogenate is centrifuged at 100 g for 15 min. The supernatant is collected and centrifuged at 39,000 g for 15 min. The resulting pellet is then twice more rehomogenized and recentrifuged at 39,000 g. The final pellet is resuspended into 20 mM Tris–maleate, pH 6.8, at a concentration of 2.5 mg protein/ml. This suspension is distributed into microcentrifuge tubes in 1-ml aliquots, which are spun at 10,000 g for 10 min. The liquid is aspirated and the pellets frozen at −70°C until used for enzyme assays. The frozen pellets retain their PI–PLC activity for at least 6 months.

Assay of Neurotransmitter Stimulation of Phosphoinositide-Specific Phospholipase C

Membrane pellets are thawed into buffer held at 4°C containing 25 mM Tris–maleate, pH 6.8, 15 mM MgCl$_2$, and 5 mM ATP. Resuspension of the pellet is accomplished by trituration, first with a 1-ml plastic pipette tip and then a 1-ml syringe fitted with a 25-gauge needle. Usually the membranes are brought to a concentration of about 1.9 mg protein/ml so that a 40-μl aliquot of the mixture diluted to a final volume of 100 μl yields a final protein concentration of about 0.75 mg/ml (as well as a final concentration of 6 mM MgCl$_2$ and 2 mM ATP). The rest of the reaction mixture components are 3 mM EGTA plus CaCl$_2$ sufficient to obtain 30 nM free Ca^{2+}, 1 mM deoxycholate, and 30 μM [^{3}H]PIP or [^{3}H]PIP$_2$. The PIP or PIP$_2$ substrate is prepared by drying down together the radioactive and unlabeled phospholipids under a stream of N$_2$. The substrate is then sonicated into solution at 20 times the final assay concentration in 20 mM deoxycholate using a Fisher probe dismembrator at setting 35 with three 15-sec bursts. Approximately 30,000 disintegrations/min (dpm) is present in each final 100 μl of reaction mixture (added as a 5-μl aliquot of the deoxycholate/phospholipid solution). EGTA and CaCl$_2$ are added as 40-μl aliquots of 25 mM Tris–maleate, pH 6.8, with 7.5 mM EGTA and CaCl$_2$. The last 15 μl of the reaction mixture is reserved for adding neurotransmitters, guanine nucleotides and other test substances, and vehicle controls as needed. Some neurotransmitters are incubated with membranes on ice prior to initiation of the PI–PLC reactions so that binding may equilibrate prior to addition of the deoxycholate.

The reactions are started by addition of the membranes, and they are generally run for 15 min at 37°C. Addition of 1.25 ml of CHCl$_3$/methanol (1 : 2, v/v) stops the reactions and is followed by 0.5 ml CHCl$_3$ and 0.5 ml 0.25 M HCl. The solutions are thoroughly mixed, and the organic and aqueous phases are then separated by centrifugation at 1400 g for 10 min. The upper aqueous phase thus contains the tritiated inositol phosphates derived from PI–PLC activity. These are conveniently quantified by scintillation counting of 1 ml of the aqueous phase mixed with 4 ml of Ecolume (ICN Biomedicals, Inc., Costa Mesa, CA).

Assays of Phosphatidylinositol Synthase and Phosphatidate Cytidylyltransferase

Phosphatidylinositol synthase (CDPdiacylglycerol–inositol 3-phosphatidyl-transferase) can be measured by the back-reaction of CDPdiacylglycerol + inositol $\rightleftharpoons$ CMP + PI (14, 15). Thus, the final reaction mixture contains 17.5

mM Tris, pH 6.9, with 1 mM MgCl$_2$, 0.7 mM EGTA, and 1 mM CMP. [^{3}H]Inositol is added at a concentration of 2.5 μCi/ml. Membrane pellets prepared as for PI–PLC assays are thawed and resuspended at 5 mg protein/ml into buffer containing 25 mM Tris, pH 6.8, with 1 mM EGTA. Reactions are run in 100 μl final volume for 30 min at 37°C. The incorporation of [^{3}H]inositol into PI is used as an index of PI synthase activity. The reactions are stopped and the extractions performed as described above for PI–PLC assays. However, the initial aqueous phase is discarded and the organic phase washed once with 1.25 ml of methanol/0.1 N HCl (1 : 1, v/v). After centrifugation at 1400 g for 10 min, the aqueous phase is aspirated, and an aliquot of the organic phase is dried down for scintillation counting.

A similar procedure can be used to follow phosphatidate cytidylyltransferase activity, CTP + phosphatidic acid $\rightarrow$ CDPdiacylglycerol + PP$_i$. Here, the incorporation of [^{3}H]CTP into the organic-soluble CDPdiacylglycerol is monitored (16, 17). The reaction buffer contains 10 mM HEPES, pH 8.0, 3 mM MgCl$_2$, 1 mM EGTA, 1 mM [^{3}H]CTP (20 μCi/ml), and 1 mM phosphatidic acid in a final volume of 100 μl. The phosphatidic acid substrate is initially dried out of its organic solvent under a stream of N$_2$ and then sonicated into suspension as a 10 mM solution in water. The cortical membranes are resuspended into 10 mM HEPES, pH 8.0, at 5 mg protein/ml and diluted to the final assay concentration of 1 mg/ml. Reactions are started by the addition of the membranes, and incubations are usually carried out for 30 min at 37°C. Termination of the reactions, extraction of products, and scintillation counting are as described for PI synthase above.

Assay of Phosphatidylinositol 4-Kinase

The phosphatidylinositol 4-kinase activity producing PI(4)P in cortical membranes [PI(4) kinase] is assayed in buffer containing (final concentrations) 20 mM Tris-HCl, pH 7.4, 50 mM NaCl, 10 mM MgCl$_2$, 1 mM EGTA, 0.1 mg/ml PI, and 50 μM [γ^{32}P] ATP (1–10 $\times$ 10^6 dpm/assay) in a total volume of 50 μl. The membrane protein concentration is 20 μg/50 μl (0.4 mg/ml). Reactions are carried out for 2 min at room temperature. The reactions are stopped, and extraction of PI(4)P is as described above for extraction of PI or CDPdiacylglycerol. Three micrograms of PI(4)P are added per assay as carrier before the phases are separated by addition of HCl. Under basal conditions, PI(4)P is nearly the only product labeled with ^{32}P, although traces of labeled phosphatidic acid also appear owing to the activity of diacylglycerol kinase. This can be determined by thin-layer chromatography of the organic phase on silica gel GHL plates (Analtech, Inc., Newark, DE) in a solvent containing CHCl$_3$/methanol/28% ammonium hydroxide/water

(90 : 90 : 10 : 19, by volume). Addition of 0.5% Nonidet P-40 to the assay greatly stimulates ^{32}P incorporation into PI(4)P while completely suppressing phosphatidic acid production. Further, the addition of this detergent should inhibit any PI(3) kinase, which is the enzyme often activated by growth factor receptors that have tyrosine kinase activity (18–20). The product of PI(3) kinase, PI(3)P, is not a substrate for PI–PLC.

Results

To date our experiments with human brain membranes have dealt with samples from prefrontal cortex (e.g., Brodmann's area 9). Thus, it is important to point out that the human cortical samples may be obtained from more homogeneous regions than is often the case with the much smaller rat brain, where the whole cortex is usually employed. Although the methods for analysis of neurotransmitter stimulation of PI–PLC have been successfully used with other brain areas (striatum and hippocampus from rats or mice, for example), we have no experience to date with such areas from human brain.

There are both advantages and disadvantages when using the PI–PLC assays with exogenous substrate to monitor neurotransmitter action. The most obvious advantage is that an assessment of functional coupling between neurotransmitter receptors, G proteins, and PI–PLC can be made under conditions where other factors affecting substrate levels are minimized. Unfixed tissue available from various brain banks is suitable for analysis since the assay does not require the neurons be intact and metabolizing normally, as is the case of biopsies assayed in tissue slices. Thus, the exogenous substrate assay does not require initial labeling of the phospholipid with [^{3}H]inositol in tissue slices as in the method of Claro et al. (21). Further, the assay does not require functional PI synthase and/or PI and PIP kinases.

On the other hand, we have developed a method for looking at concerted coupling of PI synthesis with neurotransmitter activation of PI–PLC in rat cortical membranes (15), which might have been potentially useful for human membranes. In these assays the PI in membranes is labeled with [^{3}H]inositol through the reverse reaction of PI synthase, and this PI is subsequently converted to PI(4)P and PIP$_2$ by the appropriate kinase activities in the presence of ATP. Finally, the newly made [^{3}H]PIP and [^{3}H]PIP$_2$ can be degraded by PI–PLC when stimulated by GTPγS and carbachol. We have, therefore, measured the activities of PI synthase, phosphatidate cytidylyltransferase, and PI(4) kinase in order to determine the feasibility of using the concerted PI synthesis/PI–PLC coupling regimen for analysis of autopsied

TABLE I   Enzymes Important to Phosphatidylinositol and Phosphatidylinositol 4-Phosphate Production in Human Cortical Membranes[a]

Group	PI synthase	Phosphatidate cytidylyltransferase	PI(4) kinase	
			Basal	NP-40
Age-matched controls (n = 3)	4900 ± 130	38 ± 5	49 ± 8	184 ± 14
Alzheimer's patients (n = 6)	3500 ± 300[b]	37 ± 6	23 ± 2[b]	122 ± 11[b]
Parkinson's patients (n = 5)	3600 ± 300[b]	27 ± 8	35 ± 11	145 ± 17
Rats (whole cortex)	21,000	65	285	1700

[a] Data for PI synthase (means ± SEM) are expressed as dpm of [^{3}H] inositol incorporated into PI/min/mg protein in the presence of CMP. Data for phosphatidate cytidylyltransferase (means ± SEM) are in pmol CTP incorporated into CDPdiacylglycerol/min/mg protein. Data for rat cortex are means from single representative experiments. PI(4) kinase data are expressed as pmol ^{32}P incorporated into PI(4)P/min/mg protein in the absence (basal) or presence of 0.5% Nonidet P-40 (NP-40), which stimulates PI(4) kinase and suppresses both PI(3) kinase and diacylglycerol kinase. For humans n values are the number of subjects, each assayed in duplicate for synthase or triplicate for cytidylyltransferase and PI(4) kinase.

[b] Significantly different from age-matched controls, $p \leq 0.05$ in unpaired t-test.

human brain samples. The data presented in Table I indicate that these enzyme activities are low relative to membranes prepared from whole rat cortex. Further, PI synthase is lower in patients with Parkinson's and Alzheimer's disease than in age-matched controls. Thus, overall, the use of the concerted PI synthesis/PI–PLC coupled assay is contraindicated for assessment of G protein/PI–PLC coupling in human autopsy samples.

Jolles et al. (22) have suggested that there may be a significant reduction of PI kinase activity in the cytosol prepared from Alzheimer's patients compared to controls. Most interestingly, the results in Table I confirm and extend that observation. A specific defect in PI(4) kinase was found in membranes prepared from Alzheimer's patients. Whether PI(3) kinase is also altered is not known at this time. Impairment of the PI signaling pathway in Alzheimer's disease might occur owing to low levels of PI(4) kinase activity which provides the PI(4)P for PIP$_2$ synthesis.

Another method for measuring neurotransmitter plus guanine nucleotide stimulated breakdown of PIP$_2$ by PI–PLC in brain membranes was reported by Lee and Fain (23). In this method the PIP$_2$ was not radiolabeled. Rather, the endogenous lipid was used as substrate, and inositol 1,4,5-triphosphate was quantified in a competitive binding assay (24). This PI–PLC assay is conducted under the same experimental conditions as in Claro et al. (8, 21) in the presence of deoxycholate and ATP, but with 3 times more protein per

TABLE II Activation of Phosphoinositide-Specific Phospholipase C in Human Cortical Membranes[a]

Source	Basal	+3.3 μM GTPγS	+3.3 μM GTPγS and 1 mM carbachol
Human	31 ± 13	74 ± 4	145 ± 7
Rat	214 ± 1	305 ± 22	516 ± 4

[a] Data are expressed as pmol PIP$_2$ hydrolyzed/min/mg protein. Human data (means ± SEM) are from three subjects, each assayed 3–5 times in triplicate as in Ref. 9. Rat data (means ± SEM) are from triplicate samples in a representative experiment where assay conditions were identical to those used in human studies but incubations were for 10 min rather than 15 min. There is no effect of carbachol alone on the basal activity.

assay sample. Again, this assay probably relies on the activity of PIP and PI kinases to provide PIP$_2$ for the PI–PLC. Thus, specific changes in PI or PIP kinases could affect the interpretation of results concerning receptor/G protein function.

Assay of PI–PLC using exogenous substrate can yield clear data concerning the integrity of receptor/G protein/PI–PLC coupling in human brain membranes. The data in Table II show that PI–PLC in human cortical membranes is stimulated by GTPγS and by carbachol in a guanine nucleotide-dependent manner. Whereas the absolute activity of PI–PLC is lower in human membranes than in rat membranes, the human preparations are as responsive to agonists in terms of percentage stimulations over basal.

In our studies to date we have found few differences in PI–PLC activation by neurotransmitters in prefrontal cortex among patients with Alzheimer's or Parkinson's disease, schizophrenics, and age-matched controls (9). There is a report that PLC δ identified histologically with anti-PLC δ antibodies, is associated with plaques in the brains of patients with Alzheimer's disease (25). However, we find no major differences between Alzheimer's and control brain membranes for total PI–PLC activity measured at any concentration of Ca^{2+} (from 30 nM up to 10 μM) nor for maximal stimulation of PI–PLC by carbachol in the presence of GTPγS (9). Interestingly, though, PI–PLC in Alzheimer's brain showed a significant increase in sensitivity to GTPγS. Parkinson's membranes differed slightly from others in that they failed to respond to dopamine in the presence of carbachol although their response to dopamine alone remained intact. Schizophrenic brain membranes had highly variable responses to serotonin, but were otherwise similar to the control, Alzheimer's, and Parkinson's tissue (9).

One drawback to the PI–PLC assays is their requirements for a low level of deoxycholate (1 mM, 0.04%, w/v), which is still not fully understood. It is possible that deoxycholate could affect the coupling of receptors and G proteins and result in artifactual data relevant to disease. When added exogenously, PI is a suitable substrate for the agonist-activated PI–PLC (8), although endogenous PI is rarely if ever used as substrate (12, 15, 26). On the other hand, exogenous PI can be used to advantage when attempting to isolate the actions of PI–PLC in the absence of PIP_2 or PIP phosphomonoesterase activities (e.g., when the actions of dopamine were analyzed on the phosphoinositide pathway as in Ref. 27). Our initial studies indicated that exogenously added PI is an acceptable but rather poor substrate for PI–PLC in human cortical membranes.

In conclusion, with the exogenous substrate assay for PI–PLC activation it is possible to get functional data from autopsied human tissue concerning the coupling of neurotransmitter receptors to G proteins and then to PI–PLC. Questions regarding the feasibility of neurotransmitter replacement therapies for activation of PI–PLC in conditions such as Alzheimer's disease can be at least partially answered. Clearly, a defect in an enzyme such as PI(4) kinase, which seems to occur in Alzheimer's disease, may profoundly affect signal transduction through the phosphoinositide system. Careful comparisons of results from autopsy studies with those from animal model studies have the potential of yielding important data about how disease processes and various therapeutic treatments may affect signaling throughout the PI–PLC pathway.

Acknowledgments

Tissue specimens were obtained from the National Neurological Research Bank, VAMC Wadsworth Division (Los Angeles, CA 90073), which is sponsored by NINDS/NIMH, National Multiple Sclerosis Society, Huntington's Disease Foundation, Comprehensive Epilepsy Program, Tourette Syndrome Association, Dystonia Medical Research Foundation, and Veterans Health Services and Research Administration, Department of Veterans Affairs; and from the Alzheimer's Disease Research Center, Sanders-Brown Center on Aging, University of Kentucky (Lexington, KY 40536). The authors thank W. W. Tourtellotte, Iris Rosario, and Bob Kao at the National Neurological Research Bank and Dr. W. R. Markesbury, Dr. W. K. Wekstein, and Paula Thomason at the Alzheimer's Disease Research Center for help in collection of samples used in this work.

References

1. S. K. Fisher, A. M. Heacock, and B. W. Agranoff, *J. Neurochem.* **58,** 18 (1992).
2. C. J. Fowler and G. Tiger, *Neurochem. Int.* **19,** 171 (1991).
3. S. G. Rhee and K. D. Choi, *J. Biol. Chem.* **267,** 12393 (1992).

4. D. A. Kendall and J. L. Firth, *Br. J. Clin. Pharmacol.* **100,** 37 (1990).
5. F. Nicoletti, P. L. Canonico, A. Favit, G. Nicoletti, and V. Albanese, *Eur. J. Pharmacol.* **160,** 299 (1989).
6. C. J. Fowler, C. O'Neill, A. Garland, and R. F. Cowburn, *Trends Pharmacol. Sci.* **11,** 183 (1990).
7. C. O'Neill, C. J. Fowler, B. Wiehager, I. Alafuzoff, and B. Winblad, *Brain Res.* **543,** 307 (1991).
8. E. Claro, M. A. Wallace, H.-M. Lee, and J. N. Fain, *J. Biol. Chem.* **264,** 18288 (1989).
9. M. A. Wallace and E. Claro, *Neurochem. Res.* **18,** 139 (1993).
10. P. R. Dodd, J. W. Hambley, R. F. Cowburn, and J. A. Hardy, *J. Neurochem.* **50,** 1333 (1988).
11. C. E. Stokes and J. N. Hawthorne, *J. Neurochem.* **48,** 1018 (1987).
12. M. A. Wallace, E. Claro, H. R. Carter, and J. N. Fain, *in* "Methods in Enzymology" (E. A. Dennis, ed.) Vol. 197, p. 183. Academic Press, San Diego, 1991.
13. H. R. Carter, M. A. Wallace, and J. N. Fain, *Biochim. Biophys. Acta* **1054,** 119 (1990).
14. F. McPhee, G. Lowe, C. Vaziri, and C. P. Downes, *Biochem. J.* **275,** 187 (1991).
15. E. Claro, M. A. Wallace, and J. N. Fain, *J. Neurochem.* **58,** 2155 (1992).
16. M. A. Wallace and J. N. Fain, *in* "Methods in Enzymology" (L. Birnbaumer and B. W. O'Malley, eds.), Vol. 109, p. 469. Academic Press, Orlando, Florida, 1985.
17. J. R. Carter and E. P. Kennedy, *J. Lipid Res.* **7,** 678 (1966).
18. G. Endemann, S. N. Dunn, and L. Cantley, *Biochemistry* **26,** 6845 (1987).
19. M. Whitman, D. Kaplan, T. Roberts, and L. Cantley, *Biochem. J.* **247,** 165 (1987).
20. C. Carpenter, B. C. Duckworth, K. R. Auger, B. Cohen, B. Schaffhausen, and L. Cantley, *J. Biol. Chem.* **265,** 19704 (1990).
21. E. Claro, A. Garcia, and F. Picatoste, *Biochem. J.* **261,** 29 (1989).
22. J. Jolles, J. Bothmer, M. Markerink, and R. Ravid, *J. Neurochem.* **58,** 2326 (1992).
23. H.-M. Lee and J. N. Fain, *J. Neurochem.* **59,** 953 (1992).
24. P. H. Nibbering, T. P. L. Zomerdijk, P. J. M. van Haaster, and R. van Furth, *Biochem. Biophys. Res. Commun.* **170,** 755 (1990).
25. S. Shimohama, Y. Homma, T. Suenaga, S. Fugimoto, T. Taniguchi, W. Araki, Y. Yamaoka, T. Takenawa, and J. Kimura, *Am. J. Pathol.* **139,** 737 (1991).
26. S. Fisher, A. M. Heacock, E. B. Sequin, and B. W. Agranoff, *Mol. Pharmacol.* **38,** 54 (1990).
27. M. A. Wallace and E. Claro, *Neurosci. Lett.* **110,** 155 (1990).

[7] Purification of Phospholipase C-β3 from Rat Brain

Deok-Young Jhon, Dongeun Park, and Sue Goo Rhee

Introduction

Phosphoinositide-specific phospholipase C (PLC) plays a central role in transmembrane signaling. The enzyme catalyzes the hydrolysis of phosphatidylinositol 4,5-bisphosphate [PtdIns(4,5)P$_2$] and thereby generates two second messenger molecules, namely, inositol 1,4,5-trisphosphate (IP$_3$) and diacylglycerol, in response to the binding of various ligands to their cell surface receptors.

A number of distinct PLC enzymes have been purified from a variety of mammalian tissues, and several forms have been molecularly cloned and sequenced (1). Comparison of deduced amino acid sequences and immunological cross-reactivities indicated that mammalian PLCs could be divided into three types: PLC-β, PLC-γ, and PLC-δ, each of which is a discrete gene product (1). Although the overall amino acid sequence similarity between the three types of PLC is low, a significant similarity is apparent in two regions, one of approximately 170 amino acids and the other of around 260 amino acids, which are designated the X and Y regions, respectively. Each of the three types of PLCs contains an amino-terminal sequence of about 300 amino acids that precedes the X region. Sequence similarity in this region is insignificant. Whereas PLC-β and PLC-δ contain short sequences of 50 to 70 amino acids separating the X and Y regions, PLC-γ instead has a long sequence of around 400 amino acids, which contains the so-called *src* homology (SH2 and SH3) domains, domains first identified as noncatalytic regions common to a variety of tyrosine kinases in the *src* family. Furthermore, whereas the carboxyl-terminal sequence following the Y region is approximately 450 amino acids long in PLC-β, this region is almost nonexistent in PLC-δ. Thus, PLC-δ is much smaller than PLC-β and PLC-γ.

To date, three unique members of PLC-β (PLC-β1, PLC-β2, and PLC-β3), two members of PLC-γ (PLC-γ1 and PLC-γ2), and three members of PLC-δ (PLC-δ1, PLC-δ2, and PLC-δ3) have been identified. The distinct structural features of the different PLC types appear to be related to specific mechanisms underlying the receptor-mediated enzyme activation. PLC-γ1 and PLC-γ2 are specifically activated by receptor or nonreceptor protein tyrosine kinases (1). Activation of the β-type isozymes is achieved by a

Methods in Neurosciences, Volume 18

completely different mechanism. The α subunit of the G_q class of guanine nucleotide-binding proteins (G proteins) has been shown to activate PLC-β isozymes in the order of PLC-β1 $\geq$ PLC-β3 $\gg$ PLC-β2 (2), whereas the $\beta\gamma$ subunits of G proteins activate them in the order of PLC-β3 $>$ PLC-β2 $>$ PLC-β1 (3).

A rich source of PLC isozymes is mammalian brains. PLC-β1 (4–8), PLC-γ1 (4–8), PLC-δ1 (4–7),*,† and PLC-δ2 (8) were purified from either rat or bovine brains. PLC-γ2 was purified from bovine spleen (9, 10). PLC-β2 was purified from extracts of HeLa cells that had been transfected with vaccinia virus containing PLC-β2 cDNA (11). The distribution of PLC-β2 is not known except that cDNA corresponding to PLC-β2 was derived from HL-60 cells (12). PLC-δ3 is known only at cDNA levels (12). We have purified two new β-type enzymes, PLC-β3 (2) and PLC-β4 from rat brain and bovine retina, respectively. We describe the procedures for the purification of PLC-β3 in this chapter and PLC-β4 in [8] of this volume.

Phospholipase C Assay

Enzyme activity during purification is measured at 37°C in a 200-μl reaction mixture containing 20,000 counts/min (cpm) of [^{3}H]phosphatidylinositol (PtdIns, Du Pont–NEN Research Products, Boston, MA), 150 μM soybean PtdIns, 0.1% (w/v) sodium deoxycholate, 3 mM CaCl$_2$, 2 mM EGTA, 50 mM HEPES (pH 7.0), and a source of enzyme.

The amount of PLC-β3 is extremely low compared to other PLC isoenzymes, especially compared to PLC-β1 in brains, which are one of the most abundant sources of PLC-β3. Thus, it is necessary to monitor the progress of purification by immunoblotting with antibodies to PLC-β3. For this purpose, antiserum to a peptide corresponding to PLC-β3 amino acid residues 1206–1217 (ADSESQEENTQL) is used.

Phospholipase C-β3 Purification Procedure

Frozen brains harvested in liquid nitrogen are obtained from Bioproducts for Science (Indianapolis, IN). All operations are carried out at 4°C unless otherwise specified.

---

* The molecules referred as PLC-I, PLC-II, and PLC-III in Refs. 4–6 are now known as PLC-β1, PLC-γ1, and PLC-δ1, respectively.

† The molecules referred as PLC-β, PLC-γ, and PLC-δ in Ref. 7 are, more specifically, now known as PLC-β1, PLC-γ1, and PLC-δ1, respectively.

*Step 1: Extraction of Phospholipase C-β3 from Rat Brain
Particulate Fraction*

One thousand rat brains are washed twice with cold homogenization buffer [50 mM Tris-HCl, pH 7.0, 1 mM EDTA, 1 mM phenylmethylsulfonyl fluoride (PMSF), 5 μg/ml leupeptin, and 1 mM dithiothreitol (DTT)] and then homogenized with a Polytron (Brinkmann Instruments, Westbury, NY) (three times, each time for 10 sec) in 8 liters of homogenization buffer. The homogenate is centrifuged for 10 min at 1000 g to remove debris. The supernatant is further centrifuged for 90 min at 23,000 g, and the resulting pellet was suspended in 4 liters of homogenization buffer with a Teflon pestle and then centrifuged for 60 min at 23,000 g. The new pellet is washed and stored frozen at $-70°$C.

The final washed pellets from two identical preparations (corresponding to 2000 rat brains) are thawed and suspended in 6 liters of homogenization buffer containing 2 M KCl. The suspension is stirred for 2 hr at 4°C and then centrifuged for 60 min at 23,000 g. The supernatant is brought to 60% saturation with ammonium sulfate by adding solid salt. The suspension is stirred for 1 hr at 4°C and then centrifuged for 20 min at 16,000 g. The resulting pellet is suspended in 1 liter of homogenization buffer and dialyzed overnight against homogenization buffer. The dialyzed solution is centrifuged for 30 min at 13,000 g to remove insoluble particles, and the supernatant is diluted by adding homogenization buffer (final volume ~3 liters) to reduce the conductivity of the protein solution below 4 mho.

Step 2: Heparin-Sepharose CL-6B Column Chromatography

Three liters of dialyzed membrane extract (3.6 g of protein) are applied to a heparin-Sepharose CL-6B column (5.9 × 11 cm, Pharmacia, Piscataway, NJ) that had been equilibrated with 20 mM HEPES (pH 7.0), 1 mM EGTA, and 0.1 mM DTT (Fig. 1). Unbound proteins are washed wtih 680 ml of equilibration buffer. Bound proteins are eluted from the column with a linear gradient from 0 to 1 M NaCl in 2 liters of equilibration buffer. Fractions (26 ml) are collected every 3 min and assayed for PtdIns-hydrolyzing activity and PLC-β3 protein [by sodium dodecyl sulfate–polyacrylamide gel electrophoresis (SDS-PAGE) followed by immunoblotting with antibodies to PLC-β3]. Peak fractions (75 to 93) of PLC-β3 are pooled and concentrated to 32 ml on an Amicon (Danvers, MA) concentrator.

*Step 3: First Reversed-Phase Chromatography on TSK
Phenyl-5PW Column*

Solid NaCl is added to the concentrated fractions from Step 2 to give a concentration of 2.5 M, and the mixture is then centrifuged to remove insoluble particles. The supernatant is applied to high-performance liquid chroma-

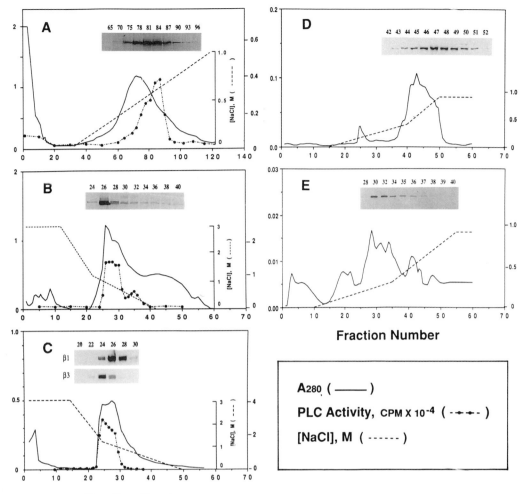

Fraction Number

FIG. 1   Purification of PLC-β3 on a heparin-Sepharose CL-6B column (A), a preparative HPLC TSK phenyl-5PW column (B), an analytical HPLC TSK phenyl-5PW column (C), an HPLC heparin-5PW column (D), and an HPLC Mono Q column (E). Detailed procedures are described in the text.

tography (HPLC) preparative phenyl-5PW column (21.5 × 150 mm, Toso-Haas, Montgomeryville, PA) equilibrated with 20 mM HEPES (pH 7.0), 1 mM EGTA, and 3 M NaCl. Proteins are eluted, at a flow rate of 5 ml/min, by successive application of (1) the equilibrium buffer for 10 min, (2) a decreasing NaCl gradient from 3 to 1.2 M for 10 min, and (3) a decreasing

NaCl gradient from 1.2 to 0 *M* for 25 min. Finally, the column is washed with NaCl-free buffer. Fractions (5 ml) are collected and assayed for PtdIns-hydrolyzing activity and PLC-β3 protein. Peak fractions (25 to 27) of PLC-β3 are pooled and adjusted to 2 *M* NaCl by adding solid salt.

Step 4: Second Reversed-Phase Chromatography on TSK Phenyl-5PW Column

The pooled fractions (28 mg of protein in 15 ml) from Step 3 are applied to an HPLC analytical TSK phenyl-5PW column (7.5 × 75 mm) equilibrated with the same buffer as used for the preparative column. Proteins are eluted at a flow rate of 1 ml/min by application of the same decreasing NaCl gradients as used for the preparative column. Peak fractions (23 to 25) are pooled, concentrated to 1 ml, and then diluted to 3 ml by addition of 20 m*M* HEPES (pH 7.0) containing 1 m*M* EGTA.

Step 5: Absorption of Phospholipase C-β1 on Monoclonal Anti-PLC-β1 Antibody Affinity Gel

An immunoaffinity gel is prepared by covalently attaching 3 mg of anti-PLC-β1 monoclonal antibody (Upstate Biotechnology Inc., Lake Placid, NY) per milliliter of Affi-Gel 10 (Bio-Rad, Richmond, CA) according to the manufacturer's instructions. The pooled fractions (3 ml) from the second TSK phenyl-5PW column are incubated with 0.5 ml of immunoaffinity gel for 1 hr at 4°C in a rotary mixer. Unbound proteins are removed by filtration through a sintered glass funnel and washing of the gel with 4 ml of 20 m*M* HEPES (pH 7.0) containing 1 m*M* EGTA. The filtrate is combined with the washing solution. The immunoabsorption procedure is repeated to ensure complete removal of PLC-β1.

Step 6: Chromatography on Heparin-5PW

The unbound proteins (2.2 mg) from the immunoaffinity gel are applied to an HPLC heparin-5PW column (7.5 × 75 mm, TosoHaas) equilibrated with 20 m*M* HEPES (pH 7.0) containing 1 m*M* EGTA and 0.1 m*M* DTT. Proteins are eluted at a flow rate of 1.0 ml/min by sequential application of equilibration buffer for 15 min and increasing linear NaCl gradients from 0 to 0.4 *M* for 25 min and from 0.4 to 0.9 *M* for 10 min. Peak fractions (46 to 48) are identified by immunoblotting with antibodies to PLC-β3, pooled, concentrated to 0.5 ml in a Centricon-100 microconcentrator (Amicon, Danvers, MA), and diluted to 8 ml to reduce the salt concentration.

Step 7: Ion-Exchange Chromatography on Mono Q Column

The diluted PLC-β3 sample (8 ml) from Step 6 is applied to Mono Q column (7 × 60 mm, Pharmacia) equilibrated with 20 m*M* Tris-HCl (pH 7.4) containing 1 m*M* EGTA and 0.1 m*M* DTT. Proteins are eluted at a flow rate of

TABLE I Purification of Phospholipase C-β3

Step	Protein (mg)		PLC-β3[a] (mg)	Yield (%)	Purification (-fold)
KCl extract of pellet	3600	[b]	0.62	100	1
Heparin-Sepharose	230	[b]	0.45	73	12
Phenyl, preparative	30	[b]	0.32	51	62
Phenyl, analytical	2.2	[b]	0.12	19	310
Heparin	0.32[b]		0.05	8	850
Mono Q	0.04[c]		0.04	6	5900

[a] Determined by immunoblot with the use of ^{125}I-labeled protein A.
[b] Determined by the method of Bradford.
[c] Estimated using an average absorptivity of $A_{280}^{0.1\%} = 1.14$.

1 ml/min by a linear NaCl gradient from 0 to 0.3 M for 25 min. Peak fractions (30 to 32) are identified by immunoblotting, pooled, and concentrated to 0.4 ml. The final sample is divided into aliquots and stored at $-70°$C. A summary of the purification steps (see Fig. 1) is presented in Table I.

References

1. S. G. Rhee and K. D. Choi, *J. Biol. Chem.* **267,** 12393 (1992).
2. D.-Y. Jhon, H.-H. Lee, D. Park, C.-W. Lee, K.-H. Lee, O. J. Yoo, and S. G. Rhee, *J. Biol. Chem.* in press (1993).
3. D. Park, D.-Y. Jhon, C.-W. Lee, K.-H. Lee, and S. G. Rhee, *J. Biol. Chem.* in press (1993).
4. S. H. Ryu, K. S. Cho., K. Y. Lee, P. G. Suh, and S. G. Rhee, *Biochem. Biophys. Res. Commun.* **141,** 137 (1986).
5. S. H. Ryu, K. S. Cho, K. Y. Lee, P. G. Suh, and S. G. Rhee, *J. Biol. Chem.* **262,** 12511 (1987).
6. S. H. Ryu, P. G. Suh, K. S. Cho, K. Y. Lee, and S. G. Rhee, *Proc. Natl. Acad. Sci. U.S.A.* **84,** 6649 (1987).
7. S. G. Rhee, S. H. Ryu, K. Y. Lee, and K. S. Cho, *in* "Methods in Enzymology" (E. A. Dennis, ed.), Vol. 197, p. 502. Academic Press, San Diego, 1991.
8. E. Meldrum, M. Katan, and S. J. Parker, *Eur. J. Biochem.* **182,** 673 (1989).
9. Y. Homma, Y. Emori, F. Shibasaki, K. Suzuki, and T. Takenawa, *Biochem. J.* **269,** 13 (1990).
10. T. Takenawa, Y. Homma, and Y. Emori, *in* "Methods in Enzymology" (E. A. Dennis, ed.), Vol. 197, p. 511. Academic Press, San Diego, 1991.
11. D. Park, D.-Y. Jhon, R. Kriz, J. Knopf, and S. G. Rhee, *J. Biol. Chem.* **267,** 16048 (1992).
12. R. Kriz, L.-L. Lin, L. Sultzman, C. Ellis, C.-H. Heldin, T. Pawson, and J. Knopf, *in* "Proto-Oncogenes in Cell Development," Ciba Foundation Symp. 150, p. 112. Wiley, Chichester, 1990.

[8] Purification of Phospholipase C-β4 and Phospholipase C-δ2 from Bovine Retinas

Chang-Won Lee, Kweon-Haeng Lee, and Sue Goo Rhee

Introduction

Although the specific role of phospholipase C (PLC) in photoreceptor cell function remains unclear, light is known to activate PLC in frog rod outer segments (ROS) (1, 2), rat ROS (3), and chick ROS (3). Anderson and co-workers (4) showed that bovine ROS contain at least two PLC isozymes on the basis of immunoblots with antipeptide antibodies to the conserved PLC sequences in the X and Y regions. In addition, the same group (5) provided evidence that PLC activity in bovine ROS can be activated by arrestin, suggesting a possible novel mechanism by which rhodopsin is coupled to PLC.

In an effort to understand the role of PLC in the phototransduction system, we have identified PLC isozymes in bovine retina. Retina proteins were separated on a high-performance liquid chromatography (HPLC) heparin column and immunoblotted with various isozyme-specific antibodies to PLC. We detected PLC-β1, PLC-β3, PLC-γ1, PLC-δ1, and PLC-δ2, but not PLC-β2, PLC-γ2, and PLC-δ3. In addition, a novel β-like PLC, PLC-β4, was identified in the retina extracts. Here we describe the procedures for the purification of PLC-β4 and PLC-δ2.

Materials

Frozen bovine retinas are purchased from Pel-Freez Biologicals (Rogers, AR) and stored at −70°C until use.

Phospholipase C Assay

The assay procedure is as described in [7] of this volume.

Purification Procedure

All manipulations are done in a 4–6°C cold room or on ice, unless indicated otherwise.

Methods in Neurosciences, Volume 18

Step 1: Preparation of Particulate and Soluble Fractions of Retinas

Four thousand retinas are thawed in 10 liters of homogenization buffer [10 mM Tris-HCl, pH 7.4, 1 mM EGTA, 1 mM EDTA, 1 mM phenylmethylsulfonyl fluoride (PMSF), 2 μg/ml leupeptin, 4 μg/ml each of calpain inhibitors I and II] and homogenized with a Polytron (Brinkmann Instruments, Westbury, NY) and then in a glass homogenizer fitted with a motor-driven Teflon pestle. The homogenate is centrifuged at 1000 g for 10 min. The supernatant is further centrifuged at 23,000 g for 1 hr. Both the particulate and supernatant fractions are saved for the purification of PLC-β4 and PLC-δ2, respectively.

Purification of Phospholipase C-β4

All chromatographic buffers used in the purification of PLC-β4 contain 2 μg/ml each of calpain inhibitors I and II.

Step 2: Extraction of Phospholipase C-β4 from Retinal Particulate Fraction

The precipitate from Step 1 is resuspended with a glass homogenizer in 4 liters of homogenization buffer and centrifuged at 23,000 g for 1 hr. The washed pellet is suspended in 4 liters of homogenization buffer containing 2 M KCl, stirred for 2 hr, and centrifuged at 23,000 g for 1 hr. The supernatant (~3.4 liters) containing 6.8 g proteins is dialyzed overnight against 40 liters of 20 mM HEPES, pH 7.0, 1 mM EGTA, 0.1 mM dithiothreitol (DTT), and calpain inhibitors. Insoluble materials are removed by centrifugation at 16,000 g for 20 min.

Step 3: Heparin-Sepharose CL-6B Column Chromatography

The slightly turbid supernatant from Step 2, which contains 3.4 g protein and about 0.2 M KCl as estimated by conductivity, is applied at a flow rate of 10 ml/min to a heparin-Sepharose CL-6B column (5 × 13 cm, Pharmacia LKB Biotechnology Inc., Piscataway, NJ) equilibrated with 20 mM HEPES, pH 7.0, 0.2 M NaCl, 1 mM EGTA, 0.1 mM DTT, and calpain inhibitors. The column is washed with 400 ml of equilibration buffer, at the end of which the absorbance of effluent drops to near zero. Bound proteins are eluted at a flow rate of 6 ml/min with a linear gradient from 0 to 1.6 M NaCl in a total volume of 2 liters of equilibration buffer. Fractions of 18 ml are collected and assayed for [³H]phosphatidylinositol ([³H]PI)-hydrolyzing activity. Two PLC activity peaks are eluted as shown in Fig. 1A. The first peak (fractions 32–39), which contains PLC-β4, is pooled and concentrated

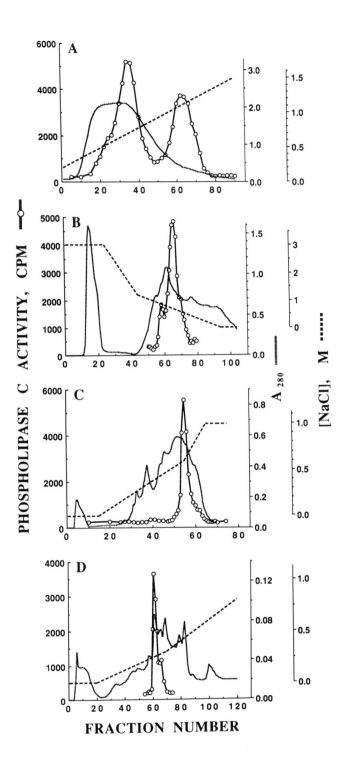

to approximately 20 ml on an Amicon concentrator (Danvers, MA). The second peak is due to PLC-δ2.

Step 4: Reversed-Phase Chromatography on TSK Gel Phenyl-5PW Column

Solid KCl is added to the concentrated solution of PLC-β4 from Step 3 to give a final salt concentration of approximately 3 *M*, and any insoluble materials are removed by centrifugation. The clear supernatant (~270 mg protein) is injected into a preparative TSK gel phenyl-5PW HPLC column (21.5 × 150 mm, TosoHaas, Montgomeryville, PA) equilibrated with 20 m*M* HEPES, pH 7.0, 3 *M* NaCl, and 1 m*M* EGTA. Proteins are eluted, at a flow rate of 5 ml/min, by successive application of the equilibration buffer for 12 min, a decreasing linear gradient from 3.0 to 1.2 *M* NaCl for 10 min, and a decreasing linear NaCl gradient from 1.2 to 0 *M* for 25 min. The column is then washed with NaCl-free buffer. Fractions of 2.5 ml are collected and assayed for [3H]PI-hydrolyzing activity. Peak fractions (63–68) are pooled and washed with 20 m*M* HEPES, pH 7.0, 1 m*M* EGTA in a Centriprep-100 (Amicon) to lower the salt concentration below 0.2 *M*.

Step 5: Chromatography on TSK Gel Heparin-5PW Column

The desalted fractions (~8 mg protein) from Step 4 are applied to TSK gel Heparin-5PW HPLC column (7.5 × 75 mm, TosoHaas) equilibrated with 20 m*M* HEPES, pH 7.0, 1 m*M* EGTA, and calpain inhibitors. Proteins are eluted at a flow rate of 1.0 ml/min by the application of the equilibration buffer for 15 min, then a linear gradient from 0 to 0.64 *M* NaCl for 40 min, followed by a second NaCl gradient from 0.64 to 1.0 *M* for 10 min. Finally, the column is washed with the equilibration buffer containing 1.0 *M* NaCl. One-milliliter fractions are collected and assayed for [3H]PI-hydrolyzing activity. Peak fractions (54–56) are concentrated and washed with 50 m*M* Tris-HCl, pH 7.4, 1 m*M* EGTA in a Centricon-100 to reduce its salt concentration below 50 m*M*.

Step 6: Ion-Exchange Chromatography on Mono Q FPLC Column

The desalted PLC-β4 sample (~1 mg protein) from Step 5 is applied to a Mono Q FPLC (fast protein liquid chromatography) column (7 × 60 mm, Pharmacia LKB Biotechnology Inc.) equilibrated with 50 m*M* Tris, pH 7.4,

FIG. 1   Purification of PLC-β4 on a heparin-Sepharose CL-6B column (A), an HPLC TSK gel phenyl-5PW column (B), an HPLC TSK gel heparin-5PW column (C), and a Mono Q FPLC column (D). Details of the purification procedures are described in the text.

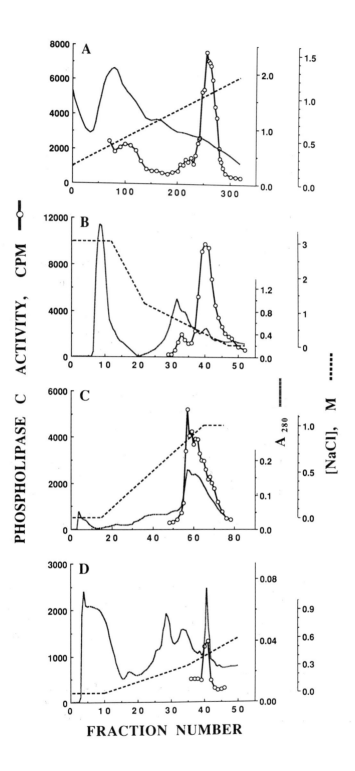

1 mM EGTA, and calpain inhibitors. Proteins are eluted as a flow rate of 1.0 ml/min by successive application of the equilibration buffer for 10 min, a linear NaCl gradient from 0 to 0.3 M for 25 min, and a linear NaCl gradient from 0.3 to 0.9 M in 30 min. Fractions of 0.5 ml are collected. Peak fractions (60–63) are concentrated, and aliquots are stored at −70°C.

This procedure yields about 150 μg of PLC-β4 from 4000 retinas. Sodium dodecyl sulfate–polyacrylamide gel electrophoresis (SDS-PAGE) of the purified preparation shows one major of 130 kDa and two minor bands slightly separate from the major band. None of the three protein bands is recognized by isoform-specific antibodies to known PLCs (PLC-β1, −β2, −β3, −γ1, −γ2, and −δ1). All three bands, however, react with antipeptide antibodies raised against conserved PLC sequences in the X (GCRCVELDCW) and Y (LSRIYPKG) regions. Thus, the two minor proteins are likely to be PLC enzymes that are closely related to PLC-β4. Previously, purified PLC-β1 has been shown to contain several proteins which are proteolytic fragments of PLC-β1 (6) and a product of alternatively spliced PLC-β1 mRNA (7).

Purification of Phospholipase C-δ2

Step 7: Dialysis of Retinal Soluble Fraction

The supernatant from Step 1 is brought to 60% ammonium sulfate saturation by adding solid salt. The suspension is centrifuged at 16,000 g for 20 min, and the pellet is kept frozen at −70°C. The frozen pellet is suspended in 1 liter of 20 mM HEPES, pH 7.0, 1 mM EGTA and dialyzed overnight against 20 liters of the same buffer. The turbid dialyzate (~1.7 liters), with a conductivity approximately equivalent to that of 0.2 M NaCl solution, is centrifuged at 16,000 g for 30 min to remove insoluble materials.

Step 8: Heparin-Sepharose CL-6B Column Chromatography

The clear supernatant from Step 7 (~16 g protein) is applied at a flow rate of 6 ml/min to a heparin-Sepharose CL-6B column (9 × 14 cm) equilibrated with 20 mM HEPES, pH 7.0, 0.2 M NaCl, 1 mM EGTA. The column is washed with 2 liters of equilibration buffer. Bound proteins are eluted at a flow rate of 6.7 ml/min by a linear NaCl gradient from 0 to 1.3 M in a total

FIG. 2   Purification of PLC-δ2 on a heparin-Sepharose CL-6B column (A), an HPLC TSK gel phenyl-5PW column (B), an HPLC TSK gel heparin-5PW column (C), and a Mono Q FPLC column (D). Details of the purification procedures are described in the text.

volume of 8 liters of the equilibration buffer. Fractions of 20 ml are collected and assayed for [^{3}H]PI-hydrolyzing activity. PLC-δ2 is eluted as the major activity peak (Fig. 2A). Peak fractions (241–277) are pooled, concentrated to about 20 ml on an Amicon concentrator, and centrifuged to remove insoluble materials.

Step 9: Reversed-Phase Chromatography on TSK Gel Phenyl-5PW Column

Solid KCl is added to the cleared concentrate of PLC-δ2 from Step 8 to give a final salt concentration of approximately 3 M, and any insoluble materials are removed by centrifugation. The supernatant containing about 50 mg protein is applied to a preparative TSK gel phenyl-5PW HPLC column (21.5 × 150 mm) equilibrated with 20 mM HEPES, pH 7.0, 3 M NaCl, and 1 mM EGTA. Proteins are eluted, at a flow rate of 5 ml/min, by the application of the same salt gradients used in Step 4. Fractions of 5 ml are collected and assayed for [^{3}H]PI-hydrolyzing activity. Peak fractions (39–41) are pooled and washed in a Centriprep-30 (Amicon) with 20 mM HEPES, pH 7.0, 1 mM EGTA to lower the salt concentration below 0.2 M.

Step 10: Chromatography on TSK Gel Heparin-5PW Column

The washed fractions (~4 mg protein) from Step 9 are applied to a TSK gel heparin-5PW HPLC column (7.5 × 75 mm) equilibrated with 20 mM HEPES, pH 7.0, 1 mM EGTA. Proteins are eluted at a flow rate of 1.0 ml/min by application of the equilibration buffer for 15 min, then a linear gradient from 0 to 1.0 M NaCl for 50 min. The column is washed with the equilibration buffer containing 1.0 M NaCl. One-milliliter fractions are collected and assayed for [^{3}H]PI-hydrolyzing activity. The PLC activity is eluted as a peak with a maximum at fraction 58. The activity profile nearly coincides with the protein profile (Fig. 2C). Analysis by SDS-PAGE indicates that, although the earlier fractions (53–58) contain an apparently homogeneous (>95%) preparation of 85-kDa protein, the later fractions contained contaminating proteins. The impure fractions (59–70) are pooled, washed with 50 mM Tris-HCl, pH 7.4, 1 mM EGTA in a Centricon-30 concentrator to reduce the salt concentration below 50 mM, and subjected to further purification.

Step 11: Ion-Exchange Chromatography on Mono Q Column

The washed, impure fractions (~1.5 mg protein) from Step 10 are applied to a Mono Q FPLC column (7 × 60 mm) equilibrated with 50 mM Tris, pH 7.4, 1 mM EGTA. Proteins are eluted at a flow rate of 1.0 ml/min by washing with the equilibration buffer for 10 min, then applying a linear NaCl gradient of 0 to 0.3 M for 25 min and a second linear NaCl gradient of 0.3 to 0.9 M

in 30 min. Fractions of 1 ml are collected and assayed for [^{3}H]PI-hydrolyzing activity. PLC-δ2 is eluted as a sharp peak at fractions 40 and 41. The peak fractions are combined with fractions 57–59 from Step 10, concentrated, and stored in aliquots at −70°C. A total of 320 μg of homogeneous PLC-δ2 is obtained.

References

1. A. J. Ghalayini and R. E. Anderson, *Biochem. Biophys. Res. Commun.* **124,** 503 (1984).
2. F. Hayashi and R. Amakawa, *Biochem. Biophys. Res. Commun.* **128,** 954 (1985).
3. F. A. Millar, S. C. Fisher, C. A. Muir, E. Edwards, and J. N. Hawthorne, *Biochim. Biophys. Acta* **970,** 205 (1988).
4. A. Ghalayini, A. P. Tarver, W. M. Mackin, C. A. Koutz, and R. E. Anderson, *J. Neurochem.* **57,** 1405 (1991).
5. A. Ghalayini and R. E. Anderson, *J. Biol. Chem.* **267,** 17977 (1991).
6. D. Park, D.-Y. Jhon, C.-W. Lee, S. H. Ryu, and S. G. Rhee, *J. Biol. Chem.* **268,** 3710 (1993).
7. S. H. Ryu and P. G. Suh, personal communication.

[9] Purification of $\alpha_{q/11}$ from Brain

Alan V. Smrcka and Paul C. Sternweis

Introduction

Guanine nucleotide-binding proteins (G proteins) are intermediaries in the transduction of many types of extracellular signals across the plasma membrane to the interior of the cell. Transmembrane receptors at the cell surface detect extracellular ligands and subsequently activate G proteins at the inside surface of the cell membrane. The G proteins, in turn, regulate enzymes or ion channels to effect intracellular processes. G proteins are composed of three subunits: an α subunit of about 40–45 kDa, a 35- to 36-kDa β subunit, and a 9-kDa γ subunit. Activated receptors catalyze the dissociation of GDP from the α subunit, thereby allowing the activating nucleotide, GTP, to bind. The activated α subunits more readily dissociate from the $\beta\gamma$ subunit dimer, thereby generating two potential signaling molecules. The α subunits have been the best characterized as activators of enzymes (for reviews, see Refs. 1–3), but increasing evidence indicates that the $\beta\gamma$ subunits can also activate second messenger systems (4–6).

G protein α subunits from the G_q subfamily have been shown by our group and others to regulate the phosphatidylinositol-specific phospholipase C (PI–PLC) β enzymes (for reviews, see Refs. 1 and 2). Here we describe the purification of the α subunits of G_q and G_{11} from bovine brain. The protein purified in this way has been shown to activate PI–PLC β (7). The procedure combines conventional chromatography techniques with an affinity chromatography technique based on the interaction of the α subunit with immobilized $\beta\gamma$ subunit dimers (8, 9).

Materials and Assays

Production of Antibodies

The antisera that are available for detection of α_q and its close homolog, α_{11}, were raised to synthetic peptides based on unique amino acid sequences deduced from the cDNA sequences for α_q and α_{11}. Some of the antisera that

Methods in Neurosciences, Volume 18

TABLE I   Antisera to α_q or α_{11}

Code[a]	Specificity	Sequence[b]	Amino acid number[c]	Ref.
X384[d]	$\alpha_{q/11}$	CILQLNLKEYNLV	348–359	e
Z811	$\alpha_{q/11}$	VKDTIQLNLKEYNLV	345–359	f
Z808	$\alpha_{q/11}$	LQLNLKEYNLV	349–359	f
WO82	α_q	EVDVEKVSAFENPYVDAIK	115–133	g
E973	α_q	EVDVEKVSAFENPYVDAIK	115–133	h
C63	$\alpha_{q/11}$	TILQLNLKEYNLV	347–359	h
E976	α_{11}	YLNDLDRVADPSY	160–172	i
—	α_q	KVTTFEHQYVNAIKT	120–134	j
—	α_{11}	KVSAFENPYVDAIKS	120–134	j
QL	$\alpha_{q/11}$	QLNLKEYNLV	350–359	k

[a] Code number assigned to antiserum by investigator that produced that antiserum.

[b] The one-letter amino acid abbreviations are defined as follows: C, Cys; V, Val; K, Lys; D, Asp; T, Thr; I, Ile; L, Leu; Q, Gln; N, Asn; E, Glu; Y, Tyr; S, Ser; A, Ala; F, Phe; P, Pro; R, Arg; H, His.

[c] Numbers correspond to position in the deduced linear sequence of either α_q, α_{11}, or both.

[d] Cys was added to the N terminus of the peptide.

[e] S. Gutowski, A. Smrcka, L. Nowak, D. Wu, M. Simon, and P. C. Sternweis, *J. Biol. Chem.* **266**, 20519 (1991).

[f] A. V. Smrcka and P. C. Sternweis, unpublished, 1992.

[g] I.-H. Pang and P. C. Sternweis, *J. Biol. Chem.* **265**, 18707 (1990).

[h] G. Berstein, J. L. Blank, A. V. Smrcka, T. Higashijima, P. C. Sternweis, J. H. Exton, and E. M. Ross, *J. Biol. Chem.* **267**, 8081 (1992).

[i] S. J. Taylor and J. H. Exton, *FEBS Lett.* **286**, 214 (1991).

[j] D. Wu, C. H. Lee, S. G. Rhee, and M. I. Simon, *J. Biol. Chem.* **267**, 1811 (1992).

[k] A. Shenker, P. Goldsmith, C. G. Unson, and A. M. Spiegel, *J. Biol. Chem.* **266**, 9309 (1991).

are available are listed in Table I. The antiserum that we have used for purification (WO82) was based on an internal sequence (residues 115–133) of α_q. Antisera have also been made to peptide sequences corresponding to the common carboxyl termini of α_q and α_{11}. These antisera are useful for immunoprecipitation of $\alpha_{q/11}$ and for blocking the function of $\alpha_{q/11}$ in membrane assays (10–12).

Peptides were linked to keyhole limpet hemocyanin (Sigma, St. Louis, MO) or the purified protein derivative of tuberculin (PPD) (Statens Seruminstitut, Copenhagen, Denmark) and were used to generate antisera in rabbits by standard procedures (13). To test the sera, cholate extracts from bovine brain membranes are resolved by sodium dodecyl sulfate–polyacrylamide gel electrophoresis (SDS-PAGE) and immunoblotted as described below.

Immunoblotting for $\alpha_{q/11}$

Samples to be assayed for the presence of α_q are treated with *N*-ethylmaleimide (NEM) prior to SDS-PAGE. Samples (30 μl, at pH 7 to 8) are reduced by mixing with 10 μl of a solution containing 5% (w/v)

SDS and 1 mM dithiothreitol (DTT) and heating at 90°C for 3 min. Samples then are alkylated by addition of a fresh solution of 30 mM NEM (10 μl) and incubation at room temperature for 15 min. Finally, 10 μl of 50 mM DTT and 30 μl of sample buffer containing 100 mM Tris-Cl (pH 6.8), 2.5% (w/v) SDS, 50% (w/v) glycerol, and 0.3 mM bromphenol blue are added, and the samples are boiled for 5 min.

Samples (30 μl) are resolved by SDS-PAGE on a 9.5% (w/v) polyacrylamide gel with 3.3% (w/v) cross-linking. After electrophoresis, proteins are transferred to a nitrocellulose membrane (Schleicher and Schuell, Keene, NH) for immunoblot analysis [0.1 A overnight in buffer containing 25 mM Tris, 192 mM glycine, and 20% (v/v) methanol]. The membrane is incubated for 1 h with Blotto [50 mM Tris-Cl, pH 8.0, 80 mM NaCl, 2 mM CaCl$_2$, 5% (w/v) nonfat dry milk, 0.2% (v/v) Nonidet P-40, 0.02% (w/v) sodium azide], followed by incubation with α_q-specific antiserum (WO82, 1 : 2000 dilution in Blotto) for 1 hr. Free antibodies are washed away with Blotto, and the nitrocellulose is incubated for 1 hr with anti-rabbit immunoglobulin G (IgG) coupled with alkaline phosphatase (Pierce, Rockford, IL) at a 1 : 5000 dilution in Blotto. To prepare the solution for color development, 33 μl of 5-bromo-4-chloro-3'-indolylphosphate p-toluidine salt (BCIP) (Pierce) (500 mg/ml in 100% dimethylformamide) and 66 μl of nitro blue tetrazolium chloride (NBT) (Pierce) [500 mg/ml in 70% (v/v) dimethylformamide] are mixed with 10 ml of substrate buffer (100 mM Tris-Cl, pH 9.5, 100 mM NaCl, and 5 mM MgCl$_2$). After washing away the free alkaline phosphatase-coupled antibody, the color development solution is added for 5 min. After the blue color has developed, the reaction is terminated by rinsing with distilled water.

Binding of ^{35}*S-Labeled Guanosine 5'-O-(3-Thio)Triphosphate*

Samples are diluted into 10 mM Na–HEPES, pH 8.0, 1 mM EDTA, 1 mM DTT, and 0.1% (v/v) polyoxyethylene 10 lauryl ether (C$_{12}$E$_{10}$) (Sigma). The diluted samples (30 μl) are added to 30 μl of reaction mix containing 10 mM Na–HEPES, pH 8.0, 1 mM EDTA, 2 mM DTT, 200 mM NaCl, 40 mM MgCl$_2$, 1 μM guanosine 5'-O-(3-thio)triphosphate (GTPγS) (Boehringer-Mannheim, Indianapolis, IN), and [^{35}S]GTPγS (NEN, Boston, MA) [~100,000 counts/min for each sample]. The mixtures are incubated at 30°C for 60 min. The binding reaction is terminated by the addition of 2 ml of ice-cold wash buffer (20 mM Tris-Cl, pH 8.0, 100 mM NaCl, and 25 mM MgCl$_2$). The solution is immediately subjected to vacuum filtration through a 25-mm nitrocellulose filter with a 0.45-μm pore size (BA85, Schleicher and Schluell). The filters are rinsed with three 2-ml aliquots of wash buffer and dried. Filters are then analyzed by mixing with scintillation fluid and liquid scintillation counting. This procedure has been previously published (14).

Purification of $\alpha_{q/11}$

Preparation of Bovine Brain Membranes

Five bovine brains are obtained from the slaughterhouse. Heavily myelinated tissue is removed, and the remaining tissue is homogenized in a Waring blendor with 3 liters of 10 mM Tris-Cl, pH 7.5, 5 mM EDTA, 1 mM EGTA, 10% (w/v) sucrose, and 0.5 mM phenylmethylsufonyl fluoride (PMSF). The homogenate is filtered through two layers of cheesecloth and centrifuged at 30,000 g for 30 min. The pellets are resuspended in wash buffer (10 mM Tris-Cl, pH 7.5, 2 mM EDTA, 10% sucrose, and 0.1 mM PMSF), homogenized with a Potter–Elvehjem tissue homogenizer, and centrifuged at 30,000 g for 30 min. This procedure is repeated, and the final pellet is resuspended in a minimal volume of wash buffer. The suspension is frozen by dripping it into liquid N_2 while stirring. The resulting pellets can be stored indefinitely at $-70°C$.

Extraction of Membranes with Detergent

Frozen membrane pellets are weighed out in a beaker to obtain a total of 12–14 g of membrane protein. The membranes are mixed in a beaker with 1.5 liters of buffer A (20 mM Tris-Cl, pH 8.0, 1 mM EDTA, and 1 mM DTT) at 30°C and stirred while thawing. The beaker can be placed in a 30°C water bath to facilitate the process but must be removed when the membranes are thawed (the temperature of the mixture is not allowed to rise above 4°C). The solution is adjusted to 100 mM in NaCl by addition of 4 M NaCl. Membranes are centrifuged at 30,000 g for 1 hr, and the washed membranes are resuspended with 1 liter buffer A and homogenized in a Potter–Elvehjem tissue homogenizer at 4°C. While stirring the membranes at 4°C, an equal volume of ice-cold buffer A containing 2% sodium cholate is added, and stirring is continued for 45 min at 4°C. The resulting mixture is then centrifuged at 100,000 g for 1.5 hr to remove extracted membranes. The extract (supernatant) is then used for subsequent purification steps.

Chromatography with DEAE-Sephacel

The extract (3 liters) of brain membranes is loaded at 500 ml/hr onto a 1-liter column (6 × 50 cm) of DEAE-Sephacel (Pharmacia LKB, Piscataway, NJ) equilibrated with buffer B (buffer A containing 1%, w/v, sodium cholate and 10 μM GDP). After loading, the column is eluted with a 2-liter gradient from 0 to 300 mM NaCl in buffer B and subsequently washed with 1 liter of 500 mM NaCl in buffer B. Fractions (25 ml) are collected and analyzed by SDS-PAGE and immunoblotting with an α_q-specific antiserum. Fractions (diluted 40-fold) are also assayed for their ability to bind [^{35}S]GTPγS. Bovine

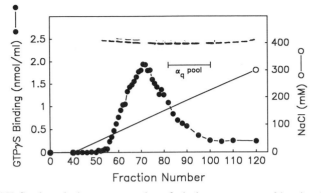

FIG. 1   DEAE-Sephacel chromatography of cholate extracts of bovine brain membranes was conducted as described in the text. The antiserum WO82 was used for immunoblotting as described.

brain contains large amounts of G_o (1% of total membrane protein), less G_i (0.1% of total membrane protein), and relatively small amounts of $G_{q/11}$ (0.01% of total membrane protein). The G_q elutes as a broad peak in the salt gradient, with the majority eluting after the main peak of [^{35}S]GTPγS binding (Fig. 1). The peak of binding sites represents primarily G_i and G_o. For this reason, fractions with G_q immunoreactivity are pooled so that the majority of the [^{35}S]GTPγS binding activity is avoided. The pool of G_q-enriched fractions (400 ml) (Fig. 1) is concentrated to 50 ml by pressure under N_2 on an PM30 filter (Amicon, Beverly, MA). Once the elution profile for $G_{q/11}$ relative to the binding of [^{35}S]GTPγS is established, the binding peak can be used as a marker assay for determining which fractions are enriched in G_q.

Size-Exclusion Chromatography with AcA 44

The concentrated pool from DEAE-Sephacel chromatography is loaded onto a 1-liter (6×50 cm) column of AcA 44 (Pharmacia LKB) equilibrated with buffer B containing 100 mM NaCl. The column is eluted with 1.5 liters of the same solution, and fractions of 15 ml are collected. The column is assayed for immunoreactivity and [^{35}S]GTPγS binding as described. At this stage the immunoreactivity corresponds exactly to the GTPγS binding peak. This peak is pooled (6–7 fractions, 100 ml) and used for hydrophobic chromatography.

Hydrophobic Chromatography on Phenyl-Sepharose

The pool from AcA 44 gel filtration is diluted 5-fold with buffer C (20 mM–HEPES, pH 8.0, 1 mM EDTA, 3 mM DTT, 100 mM NaCl, 10 μM GDP, 30 μM AlCl$_3$, 10 mM MgCl$_2$, and 10 mM NaF) and incubated at 4°C for 2 hr. This dilutes the sodium cholate and allows the α and βγ subunits to dissociate from one another. This diluted pool is loaded onto a 100-ml column on phenyl-Sepharose (Pharmacia LKB) equilibrated with buffer C containing 0.2% sodium cholate and 300 mM NaCl. After loading, the column is washed with 100 ml of buffer C containing 0.2% (w/v) sodium cholate and 300 mM NaCl. The solution that flows through the column and the wash contain most of the free $\alpha_{q/11}$. The majority of the remaining α_i and α_o and all of the remaining $\beta\gamma$ subunits remain bound to the column. A 600-ml gradient from 0.2 to 1% (w/v) sodium cholate in buffer C elutes these remaining G protein subunits in relatively pure form. The flow-through and wash are pooled and concentrated to 3 ml under pressure on an Amicon PM30 filter.

Affinity Chromatography on Immobilized $\beta\gamma$ Subunits

The purification of $\beta\gamma$ subunits (15) and coupling to a solid matrix have been described elsewhere (8) and are not discussed in detail here. In brief, the $\beta\gamma$ subunits are purified by a procedure similar to that described for $\alpha_{q/11}$, except the pool of $\beta\gamma$ subunits from phenyl-Sepharose chromatography is further purified using chromatography on hydroxylapatite prior to synthesis. About 20 mg of purified $\beta\gamma$ is used for coupling to 10 ml of ω-aminobutyl agarose (Sigma). The protein is linked via free sulfhydryl groups using a bifunctional cross-linking reagent, namely sulfosuccinimidyl 4-(p-maleimidophenyl)butyrate (sulfo-SMBP) (Pierce). It is critical that this reagent be very fresh to achieve good coupling of the $\beta\gamma$ to the gel. The resulting affinity matrix generally has a binding capacity of between 4 and 8 nmol of α_o/ml.

The pool of enriched $\alpha_{q/11}$ from phenyl-Sepharose chromatography is gel-filtered into buffer D [20 mM Na–HEPES, pH 8.0, 0.1 mM EDTA, 3 mM DTT, 400 mM NaCl, 0.5% (w/v) $C_{12}E_{10}$, and 10 μM GDP] using a 10-ml prepacked column of BioGel P-6DG (Bio-Rad, Richmond, CA) equilibrated with 10 ml of buffer D. Three milliliters of the pool is loaded on the column and allowed to run into the gel. The flow-through solution is discarded, and the protein is eluted with 4 ml of buffer D.

The $\beta\gamma$ agarose (3 ml) is equilibrated with 10 ml of buffer D and excess buffer removed. The gel is then mixed with the filtered pool of enriched $\alpha_{q/11}$ (4 ml) and incubated for 1 hr with constant mixing at 25°C. The gel is drained and washed 5 times with 3 ml buffer D followed by 20 washes with 3 ml buffer D containing 5 μM GTPγS and 0.2 mM MgCl$_2$. The gel is allowed to sit at 25°C for 5 min between each wash to allow time for the association of GTPγS with α subunits and their subsequent dissociation from the $\beta\gamma$ matrix. Because α_o and α_i bind GTPγS readily under these conditions but $\alpha_{q/11}$ does not, the α_o and α_i subunits elute from the column while the $\alpha_{q/11}$ remains bound. The column is then washed with 3 ml of buffer D containing either 0.5% (w/v) sodium cholate or 1% (w/v) octyl-β-D-glucopyranoside

(OG) (Calbiochem, San Diego, CA). The $\alpha_{q/11}$ is eluted with 3-ml aliquots (5 total) of buffer D containing the desired detergent plus 30 μM AlCl$_3$, 50 mM MgCl$_2$, and 10 mM NaF (AMF). After addition of each aliquot, the matrix is incubated for 5 min at 25°C to allow time for dissociation of the α subunits. All of the washes and elutions are collected as individual fractions and stored on ice until analyzed.

Fractions are analyzed by SDS-PAGE and visualized by both silver staining and immunoblotting. The purified preparation appears as a single polypeptide of about 42,000 Da but may actually contain two highly homologous subunits (α_q and α_{11}) of the α_q subfamily (9). Fractions containing pure $\alpha_{q/11}$ (usually the first three fractions obtained with AMF) are then gel-filtered into a buffer [50 mM Na–HEPES, pH 7.2, 1 mM EDTA, 3 mM EGTA, 1 mM DTT, 5 mM MgCl$_2$, 100 mM NaCl, 10 μM GDP, and either 1% w/v octyl-β-D-glucopyranoside or 0.5% (w/v) sodium cholate] suitable for addition to the phospholipase assay. This is accomplished by using prepacked columns of BioGel P-6DG (Bio-Rad) as described earlier. Purified $\alpha_{q/11}$ can be frozen in liquid N$_2$ and stored at $-70°$C.

The $\beta\gamma$ columns can be reused repeatedly and stored at 4°C for up to 4–6 months before large losses in binding capacity begin to occur. Sometimes the $\alpha_{q/11}$ that elutes from the $\beta\gamma$ column is contaminated to a small extent with other G protein α subunits. By repeating the $\beta\gamma$ affinity chromatography procedure, these contaminants can usually be removed. When frozen at $-70°$C the purified protein is stable for at least 6 months and can be frozen and thawed repeatedly without significant loss of activity.

Reconstitution of Brain $\alpha_{q/11}$ with Phosphatidylinositol-Specific Phospholipase C

Purification of Phosphatidylinositol-Specific Phospholipase C

To assay the functional activity of $\alpha_{q/11}$, a preparation of PI–PLC β is required. There are several published procedures for the purification of PI–PLC β from bovine brain (16, 17), and the following is a modification of one of these (16). Frozen membranes (5 g protein) from bovine brain (prepared as described above) are thawed in buffer E (10 mM Tris-Cl, pH 7.2, 5 mM EGTA, and 0.1 mM DTT) containing 2 mM PMSF, such that the final volume is 250 ml. Buffer A containing 2.5 M KCl (250 ml) is added, and the resulting solution is incubated with stirring. The suspension is then centrifuged at 100,000 g for 3 hr, and the turbid supernatant (400 ml) containing the PI–PLC is collected. The KCl is removed by gel filtration (200 ml at a time) through a 600-ml column of G-25 medium Sephadex (Pharmacia LKB) equilibrated with buffer E. The column is eluted with the same buffer, and fractions are assayed for conductivity and total protein. Fractions containing protein, which are still turbid, are clarified by centrifugation at 100,000 g for 1 hr.

The clarified fractions are loaded on a 1-liter column of DEAE-Sephacel equilibrated with buffer E, and the proteins are eluted with a 2-liter gradient from 0 to 300 mM KCl in buffer E followed by 1 liter of 500 mM KCl in buffer E. Fractions (25 ml) are assayed using the PI–PLC assay described below. The single peak of activity (eluting between 1.5 and 2 liters) is pooled and loaded directly onto a 100-ml column of heparin-Sepharose (Pharmacia LKB) equilibrated with buffer F (20 mM Na–HEPES, pH 7.0, 1 mM EGTA, 0.1 mM DTT, and 100 mM NaCl). The column is eluted with a 1.2-liter gradient from 100 to 600 mM NaCl in buffer F. The fractions (15 ml) are assayed for PI–PLC activity, which elutes around 800 ml. Fractions containing the peak of activity are pooled and concentrated to 5 ml under N_2 pressure on an Amicon PM30 membrane. The concentrated pool is diluted 10-fold with buffer G (20 mM Tris-Cl, pH 7.6, 1 mM EGTA, and 0.1 mM DTT) and reconcentrated to 5 ml.

The concentrated pool is loaded onto a Mono Q column (7 $\times$ 60 mm) (Pharmacia LKB) and eluted at 1 ml/min with a gradient, in buffer G, of 0 to 300 mM NaCl over 20 ml followed by 0.3 to 1 M NaCl over 10 ml. Fractions are assayed for PI–PLC activity and analyzed by SDS-PAGE. The resulting pool is about 90% PI–PLC-β1 which runs as a doublet around 140–150 kDa. Fractions containing the peak of activity are pooled, glycerol is added to 25% (v/v), and aliquots are frozen at $-70°C$. Once aliquots are thawed, they are stable at 4°C for at least 1 week. Repeated freezing and thawing cycles result in significant loss in activity.

Assay of Phosphatidylinositol-Specific Phospholipase C Activity and Activation by $\alpha_{q/11}$

For assay of PI–PLC activity, vesicles formed from sonication of [2-³H-*inositol*]phosphatidylinositol 4,5-bisphosphate (NEN), unlabeled phosphatidylinositol 4,5-biphosphate (PIP$_2$) (Sigma), and bovine brain phosphatidylethanolamine (PE) (Sigma) are used as the substrate. The appropriate amounts of lipid are mixed in the bottom of a 16 $\times$ 100 mm Pyrex tube, and the solvent (chloroform) is evaporated under a stream of N_2. The lipids are suspended in buffer H (50 mM Na–HEPES, pH 7.2, 3 mM EGTA, 80 mM KCl, and 1 mM DTT) such that the final concentrations are 150 μM PIP$_2$, 1500μM PE, and about 500 cpm [2-³H-*inositol*]PIP$_2$/μl. The solution is sonicated in a bath sonicator for 5 min to form vesicles. The resulting solution is a cloudy, uniform suspension without particulate matter.

If fractions from chromatography steps are to be assayed for PI–PLC activity, 10 μl of the substrate vesicles are added to 10 μl of fractions diluted 1 : 100 in buffer H. Five microliters of buffer I (50 mM Na–HEPES, pH 7.2, 1 mM EDTA, 3 mM EGTA, 1 mM DTT, 5 mM MgCl$_2$, 100 mM NaCl, and 10 μM GDP) is then added, followed by 5 μl of buffer H containing 18 mM CaCl$_2$ (free Ca^{2+} concentration is about 10 μM). The samples are transferred from 4° to 30°C for 5 to 10 min. The reactions are terminated by transfer of the samples from 30° to 4°C and addition of 200 μl of 10% cold trichloroacetic acid and 100 μl of 10 mg/ml bovine serum albumin. The samples are vortexed and centrifuged for 5 min at 5000 g at 4°C to remove the precipitated protein and the intact PIP$_2$. The supernatant (300 μl) is then analyzed by liquid scintillation counting.

To assay activation of purified PI–PLC-β by G protein subunits, substrate vesicles (20 μl) are mixed with 20 μl of buffer H containing 0.1–2 ng of purified PI–PLC-β, 1.5 mg/ml bovine serum albumin, 75 μM AlCl$_3$ and 25 mM NaF or 500 μM GTPγS for activation of $\alpha_{q/11}$ (see below), and other additions as desired. Ten microliters of buffer I containing $\alpha_{q/11}$ that has been preactivated with either 200 μM GTPγS or AlF$_4^-$ (10 mM NaF and 30 μM AlCl$_3$) (described below) is then added. The PI–PLC reaction is initiated with 10 μl of buffer H containing 9 to 16 mM Ca^{2+} such that the free concentration of Ca^{2+} in the final assay is between 150 nM and 1 μM. The reactions are initiated by transfer of the samples from 4° to 30°C and terminated for analysis as described above.

Activation of $\alpha_{q/11}$

Relative to other G protein α subunits, activation of $\alpha_{q/11}$ requires high concentrations of GTPγS and long times of incubation. Activation by AlF$_4^-$, on the other hand, is rapid and occurs at concentrations comparable to that required for other G protein α subunits. To preactivate $\alpha_{q/11}$ with GTPγS, an aliquot of the protein in buffer I is incubated for 14 hr at 8°C with 200 μM GTPγS. To activate with AlF$_4^-$, 0.1 volume of a freshly made solution of 300 μM of AlCl$_3$ and 100 mM NaF is added to the solution containing $\alpha_{q/11}$ and incubated at room temperature for 15 min. The level of activation after incubation with GTPγS or AlF$_4^-$ is similar. $\alpha_{q/11}$ activated with GTPγS is resistant to deactivation by $\beta\gamma$ subunits, whereas activation by AlF$_4^-$ is readily reversed by $\beta\gamma$ (18).

Comments

There are several variables that are critical for reproducible activation of PI–PLC-β by $\alpha_{q/11}$. One of these is the concentration and type of detergent. The activation (-fold) of PI–PLC-β1 by $\alpha_{q/11}$ is influenced by the concentration

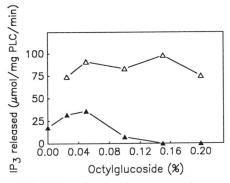

FIG. 2 Dependence of PI–PLC activation by $\alpha_{q/11}$ on the concentration of octyl-β-D-glucopyranoside. Assays were conducted as described in the text, except the concentration of OG was varied as indicated. Assays contained 0.1 ng PI PLC-β1 in the presence ($\triangle$) or absence ($\blacktriangle$) of 20 nM $\alpha_{q/11}$.

of OG (Fig. 2). At all concentrations of OG the activity stimulated by $\alpha_{q/11}$ remains constant, whereas the basal activity is depressed with increasing concentration of detergent. For this reason the degree of activation at a given concentration of $\alpha_{q/11}$ increases greatly as the concentration of OG increases. Cholate can also be used to store $\alpha_{q/11}$ and diluted for addition to this assay; however, larger quantities of PI–PLC-β are required because the residual cholate strongly inhibits the activity of PI–PLC β.

Concentration of the G protein or its gel filtration can lead to loss of $\alpha_{q/11}$ protein. Addition of purified bovine serum albumin (0.5 mg/ml) can reduce this loss, but the recovery from these procedures has to be estimated by silver staining (the presence of bovine serum albumin would interfere with a protein assay). For these reasons, $\alpha_{q/11}$ is eluted in as concentrated a pool as possible from the $\beta\gamma$ affinity matrix.

The order of addition of components to the assay is also important. PI–PLC should always be added to the vesicles first followed by the incubation solution containing the $\alpha_{q/11}$. The Ca^{2+} solution is always added last to start the reaction. We have found the addition of the substrate to start the reaction does not yield potent activation of the PI–PLC by $\alpha_{q/11}$. Finally, the assay should be characterized for linearity with respect to time. We have found that the assay is linear until about 40% of the substrate is hydrolyzed (7).

References

1. J. R. Hepler and A. G. Gilman, *Trends Biochem. Sci.* **17,** 383 (1992).
2. P. C. Sternweis and A.V. Smrcka, *Trends. Biochem. Sci.* **17,** 502 (1992).
3. A. G. Gilman, *Annu. Rev. Biochem.* **56,** 615 (1987).

4. W. J. Tang and A. G. Gilman, *Science* **254,** 1500 (1992).

5. M. Camps, C. Hou, D. Sidiropoulos, J. B. Stock, K. H. Jakobs, and P. Gierschik, *Eur. J. Biochem.* **206,** 821 (1992).

6. A. V. Smrcka and P. C. Sternweis, *J. Biol. Chem.* **268,** 9667 (1993).

7. A. V. Smrcka, J. R. Hepler, K. O. Brown, and P. C. Sternweis, *Science* **251,** 804 (1991).

8. I.-H. Pang and P. C. Sternweis, *Proc. Natl. Acad. Sci. U.S.A.* **86,** 7814 (1989).

9. I.-H. Pang and P. C. Sternweis, *J. Biol. Chem.* **265,** 18707 (1990).

10. S. Gutowski, A. Smrcka, L. Nowak, D. Wu, M. Simon, and P. C. Sternweis, *J. Biol. Chem.* **266,** 20519 (1991).

11. A. Shenker, P. Goldsmith, C. G. Unson, and A. M. Spiegel, *J. Biol. Chem.* **266,** 9309 (1991).

12. R. L. Wange, A. V. Smrcka, P. C. Sternweis, and J. H. Exton, *J. Biol. Chem.* **266,** 11409 (1991).

13. S. M. Mumby, R. A. Kahn, D. R. Manning, and A. G. Gilman, *Proc. Natl. Acad. Sci. U.S.A.* **83,** 265 (1986).

14. J. K. Northup, M. D. Smigel, and A. G. Gilman, *J. Biol. Chem.* **257,** 11416 (1982).

15. P. C. Sternweis and J. D. Robishaw, *J. Biol. Chem.* **259,** 13806 (1984).

16. K.-Y. Lee, S. H. Ryu, P.-G. Suh, W. C. Choi, and S. G. Rhee, *Proc. Natl. Acad. Sci. U.S.A.* **84,** 5540 (1987).

17. S. H. Ryu, K. S. Cho, K.-Y. Lee, P.-G. Suh, and S. G. Rhee, *J. Biol. Chem.* **262,** 12511 (1987).

18. P. C. Sternweis, A. V. Smrcka, and S. Gutowski, *Philos. Trans. R. Soc. London B* **336,** 35 (1992).

Section II

Other Enzymes Involved in Phospholipid Metabolism

[10]   Purification of Phosphatidylinositol Synthase from Brain

Abdallah Ghalayini and Joseph Eichberg

Introduction

The *de novo* biosynthesis of phosphatidylinositol is catalyzed by phosphatidylinositol synthase (cytidinediphosphate-1,2-diacylglycerol-*sn*-glycerol : phosphatidylinositol transferase; EC 2.7.8.11, CDPdiacylglycerol–inositol 3-phosphatidyltransferase) from cytidine diphosphate diacylglycerol (CDPdiacylglycerol) and *myo*-inositol with the concomitant production of CMP. This enzyme activity was first detected in brain (1–3). Subsequent studies by Benjamins and Agranoff (4) showed that phosphatidylinositol synthase activity was present in all guinea pig tissues examined, including liver, lung, brain, kidney, and spleen. Additionally, the highest specific activity in guinea pig (4) and rat brain (5) was associated with microsomes, strongly suggesting that endoplasmic reticulum is the primary site of phosphatidylinositol synthesis. Evidence has also been obtained for the presence of phosphatidylinositol formation in plasma membrane (6).

Rat brain microsomal phosphatidylinositol synthase has been solubilized by several detergents (5), with Triton X-100 (0.5%) being the most effective. In other studies, the solubilized enzyme was successfully purified from rat brain in our laboratory (7) and from *Saccharomyces cerevisiae* (8) using CDPdiacylglycerol affinity resins. This chapter presents the procedure for purification of solubilized phosphatidylinositol synthase from rat brain microsomes.

Preparation of Microsomes and Enzyme Solubilization

To prepare rat brain microsomes, two to three freshly dissected rat brains are homogenized in 9 volumes of ice-cold 0.32 M sucrose in a motor-driven Potter–Elvehjem homogenizer. All subsequent steps are carried out at 4°C unless otherwise indicated. The homogenate is centrifuged at 17,000 g for 20 min and the supernatant obtained is then centrifuged at 105,000 g for 1 hr. The resulting microsomal pellet is resuspended in glycylglycine buffer, pH 8.6, containing 0.6% Triton X-100 and 0.5 mM dithiothreitol (DTT). The suspension is allowed to stand on ice for 1 hr with frequent agitation on a

TABLE I   Solubilization of Phosphatidylinositol Synthase from Rat
Brain Microsomes[a]

Fraction	Protein (mg)	Specific activity (nmol/min/mg protein)	Total activity (nmol/min)	Activity solubilized (%)
Microsomal pellet	8.04	2.25	18.0	—
105,000 g supernatant (no Triton X-100)	1.04	0.38	0.40	2.2
105,000 supernatant (0.6% Triton X-100)	5.36	3.20	17.2	95.6

[a] Rat brain microsomes were prepared and treated in either the absence or presence of Triton X-100 to solubilize phosphatidylinositol synthase as described in the text.

vortex mixer and is then centrifuged at 105,000 g for 1 hr. Using these solubilization conditions, more than 90% of phosphatidylinositol synthase activity is recovered in the resulting supernatant (Table I).

Assay Procedure for Solubilized Phosphatidylinositol Synthase

Solubilized phosphatidylinositol synthase activity is assayed in a mixture containing 1.0 mM CDPdiacylglycerol (prepared by sonication in 10 mM glycylglycine, pH 8.6), 6.0 mM myo-[^{3}H]inositol [50,000 counts/min (cpm)], 0.6% Triton X-100, 48 mM MgCl$_2$, 0.5 mM DTT, and 50 mM glycylglycine buffer (pH 8.6) and 0.2–0.5 mg protein in a final volume of 0.2 ml. Incubations are conducted at 37°C for 30 min and terminated by the addition of 4.8 ml chloroform/methanol (2 : 1, v/v). The lower phase is subsequently washed as described (9), first with 1 ml of 0.01 N HCl, and then twice with 2 ml of 1 mM myo-inositol in 0.01 N HCl/methanol/chloroform (47 : 48 : 3, v/v). An aliquot of the lower phase is dried under nitrogen, and the radioactivity incorporated into phosphatidylinositol is quantified by scintillation counting.

Purification of Solubilized Phosphatidylinositol Synthase on Cytidine Diphosphate Diacylglycerol Affinity Resin

Materials

CMPmorpholidate as the cyclohexylammonium salt, DTT, cyanogen bromide-activated Sepharose 4B, and adipic acid dihydrazide are purchased from Sigma Chemical Company (St. Louis, MO). Sodium phosphatidate is obtained from Avanti Biochemicals (Birmingham, AL) or prepared by hydrolysis of egg phosphatidylcholine with cabbage phospholipase D (10). CDPdiacylglycerol is chemically synthesized from phosphatidic acid and CMPmorpholidate according to Agranoff and Suomi (11). Alternatively, the liponucleotide can be purchased from commercial sources such as Serdary Research Laboratories (London, Ontario, Canada) or Sigma Chemical Company. Asolectin is a product of American Lecithin Co. (Danbury, CT).

Preparation of Cytidine Diphosphate Diacylglycerol Affinity Resin

The covalent attachment of an oxidized derivative of CDPdiacylglycerol to Sepharose 4B is accomplished essentially as previously described (12). The steps involve the oxidation of the liponucleotide with periodate, attachment of an adipic acid spacer arm to Sepharose 4B, and coupling of the oxidized CDPdiacylglycerol to the spacer.

To oxidize CDPdiacylglycerol, 80 μmol each of CDPdiacylglycerol and $NaIO_4$ are added to 25 ml of 0.1 M sodium acetate buffer, pH 4.5, and incubated first at room temperature for 1 hr and then overnight at 4°C. Excess periodate is then destroyed by the addition of 5 ml of 20% (v/v) glycerol. A portion of the reaction mixture is subjected to thin-layer chromatography in a solvent system containing chloroform/methanol/glacial acetic acid/water (25:14:2:4, v/v). After development, the plate is either exposed to iodine or sprayed with a phospholipid-detecting reagent (13). As judged by the appearance of a new spot with an R_f greater than that of CDPdiacylglycerol, more than 90% of the liponucleotide is converted to the corresponding dialdehyde under these conditions.

To attach the spacer arm, cyanogen bromide-activated Sepharose 4B (28 ml) is mixed with 20 ml of 0.1 M Na_2CO_3 (pH 9.5) containing 2.5 g of adipic acid dihydrazide for 20 hr at 4°C. The resin is then washed extensively first with 1 M NaCl and then with water and is tested for the presence of covalently bound unsubstituted hydrazide (14).

To couple CDPdiacylglycerol to the immobile support, the oxidized liponucleotide (80 μmol) is mixed with Sepharose 4B containing the adipic acid spacer arm (28 ml), and the mixture is stirred gently overnight at 4°C in 50 ml of 0.1 M sodium acetate buffer, pH 5.0, containing 0.5% Triton X-100. The resin is then washed with copious amounts of 0.5 M KCl followed by deionized water and finally resuspended in buffer A in preparation for column chromatography (see below). The yield of coupled liponucleotide is 0.4–0.5 μmol of covalently bound CDPdiacylglycerol/ml of packed Sepharose 4B as determined by phosphorus analysis (15). Figure 1 shows the proposed structure of the affinity ligand.

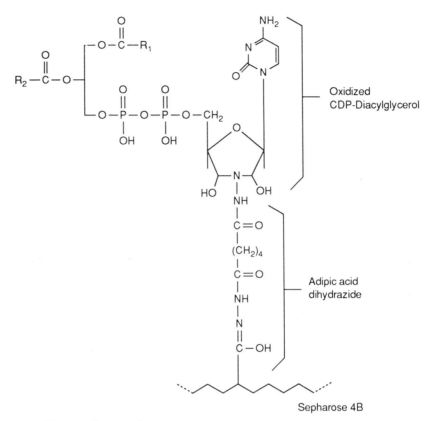

FIG. 1   Proposed structure of CDPdiacylglycerol affinity resin.

Affinity Chromatography of Phosphatidylinositol Synthase

Buffers

Buffer A: 10 mM glycylglycine, pH 8.6, 0.6% Triton X-100, and 0.5 mM DTT

Buffer B: 10 mM glycylglycine, pH 8.6, 0.6% Triton X-100, 0.5 mM DTT, 1.0 mM CDPdiacylglycerol, and 0.3 mM phosphatidylcholine or 10 μg lipid P/ml asolectin

Chromatography Procedure

A CDPdiacylglycerol-Sepharose 4B column (1 × 8 cm) is packed and equilibrated at 4°C with buffer A by extensive washing (4–5 column volumes). Solubilized rat brain microsomes (15–20 mg protein) in buffer A (3–4 ml)

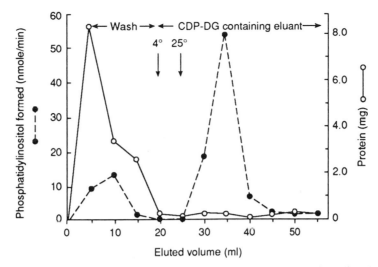

FIG. 2   Elution profile of phosphatidylinositol synthase from a CDPdiacylglycerol (CDP-DG) affinity column [A. Ghalayani, Ph.D. Dissertation, University of Houston, Houston, Texas (1982)]. The elution procedure was carried out as described in the text.

are loaded onto the affinity column which is then washed with 15–20 ml of the same buffer at a flow rate of 0.25 ml/min. Elution is then begun with buffer B in fractions of 0.5–1.0 ml and continued until 5–7 ml of effluent is collected. The column is allowed to stand for 60–90 min and then transferred from 4°C to room temperature and allowed to equilibrate for another 20 min. Elution is resumed at room temperature until 5–6 ml of column fractions is collected. Fractions are assayed for phosphatidylinositol synthase activity and the protein content determined (16). A representative affinity chromatography separation is shown in Fig. 2, and the purification achieved is summarized in Table II.

Assay Procedure for Purified Phosphatidylinositol Synthase

The activity of the purified enzyme is assayed in a mixture containing 50 mM glycylglycine buffer (pH 8.6), 0.3% Triton X-100, 0.5 mM DTT, 5–10 μg phosphorus/ml asolectin or phosphatidylcholine, 1–4 μg enzyme protein, 10 mM MgCl$_2$, 0.5 mM EGTA, 6.0 mM myo-[^{3}H]inositol (30,000–50,000 cpm), and 0.5 mM CDPdiacylglycerol in a final volume of 0.2 ml. Incubations are carried out at 37°C for 8–15 min.

TABLE II   Purification of Rat Brain Phosphatidylinositol Synthase[a]

Fraction	Total enzyme units (nmol/min)	Total protein (mg)	Specific activity (nmol/min/mg protein)	Purification (-fold)	Yield (%)
Homogenate	1546	537	2.9	1.0	100
Microsomal Triton X-100 extract	236	21.5	11.0	3.7	15.2
CDPdiacylglycerol affinity column					
Void volume + wash (4°C)	25	15.1	1.6	—	1.6
CDPdiacylglycerol elution (25°C)[b]	54	0.2	270	93	3.5

[a] Phosphatidylinositol synthase was solubilized from microsomes and purified on a CDPdiacylglycerol affinity column as described in the text. Asolectin was present in the elution buffer.

[b] The activity eluted by CDPdiacylglycerol shown was present in one fraction and constituted 23% of the activity applied to the column (see Fig. 2). Approximately 10% of the enzyme activity applied to the column was eluted in the preceding fraction but was less highly purified.

Properties of Purified Phosphatidylinositol Synthase

Phosphatidylinositol synthase activity is linear with time up to 15 min at 37°C when assayed under conditions described for the purified enzyme. The apparent K_m of the enzyme for *myo*-inositol under these conditions is 4.6 mM, and the highest enzyme activity is obtained at 0.35–0.4 mM CDPdiacylglycerol. The purified enzyme is activated maximally by 10 mM Mg^{2+}, whereas 10 mM Mn^{2+} is about 25% as effective. Enzyme activity is not detectable in the absence of either cation. EGTA (0.5–1.0 mM) stimulates phosphatidylinositol synthase up to 2-fold, presumably by chelation of inhibitory cations, particularly Ca^{2+}. Increasing the assay buffer concentration from 10 to 55 mM glycylglycine (pH 8.6) also stimulates enzyme activity up to 3-fold. The purified enzyme displays optimal activity at pH 8.5–9.0. The highest specific activity of phosphatidylinositol synthase purified and assayed as described is about 600 nmol/min/mg protein. Purified phosphatidylinositol synthase preparations contain less than 1% of measured specific activities for CDPdiacylglycerol hydrolase and phosphatidylglycerophosphate synthase activities, enzymes that also utilize CDP diacylglycerol as substrate (7). Polyacrylamide gel electrophoresis of purified phosphatidylinositol synthase under denaturing conditions revealed three protein bands following Coomassie blue staining.

Comments

Under the conditions described, solubilized phosphatidylinositol synthase binds readily to the CDPdiacylglycerol affinity column. The most critical step in the purification procedure is the elution of the enzyme from the column. Several important manipulations are necessary for successful elution: (1) after loading the solubilized phosphatidylinositol synthase, the column must be allowed to stand at 4°C for at least 1 hr in buffer B in order to allow ample time for the competing ligand (CDPdiacylglycerol) to interact with the bound enzyme on the column; (2) the affinity column should be warmed to room temperature before resumption of elution with buffer B in order to accelerate the elution and enhance the recovery of phosphatidylinositol synthase; and (3) the inclusion of both CDPdiacylglycerol and phosphatidylcholine or asolectin in buffer B is also essential. The CDPdiacylglycerol is absolutely required for the effective elution of the enzyme, whereas the other lipids may help in stabilizing the purified phosphatidylinositol synthase.

In our experience with this procedure, purification of the enzyme has ranged from 87- to 192-fold and with yields of 3–7% based on the brain homogenate. The extent of purification may be underestimated because of the difficulty encountered in assaying recovered protein. We found that the presence of CDPdiacylglycerol interfered with protein analysis by the standard Lowry procedure, and consequently we used a method involving protein precipitation and resolubilization (16).

Alternative Purification Approaches

For Mammalian Enzyme

Phosphatidylinositol synthase activity solubilized from rat brain microsomes has been reported to be enriched up to 60-fold by precipitating the deoxycholate-solubilized enzyme with $MgCl_2$ (48 mM) and resolubilizing the enzyme activity with Triton X-100 (5). In another report (17), the rat liver enzyme was purified using a multistep procedure including ammonium sulfate precipitation, sucrose density centrifugation, and DEAE-cellulose chromatography. This procedure gave a 28-fold purification over microsomes with 3.3% yield of total activity.

For Yeast Enzyme

Phosphatidylinositol synthase from *Saccharomyces cerevisiae* has been purified 1000-fold from microsomes using a combination of CDPdiacylglycerol affinity chromatography and chromatofocusing (8). The highest enrichment of enzyme activity (~400-fold) was obtained in the CDPdiacylglycerol affinity chromatography step. Yeast phosphatidylinositol synthase has been cloned, and its sequence has been deduced (19). The open reading frame indicates the enzyme is composed of 220 amino acids, with a calculated molecular weight of 24,823.

References

1. H. Paulus and E. Kennedy, *J. Am. Chem. Soc.* **80,** 6689 (1958).
2. B. Agranoff, R. Bradley, and R. Brady, *J. Biol. Chem.* **233,** 1077 (1958).
3. H. Paulus and E. Kennedy, *J. Biol. Chem.* **235,** 1303 (1960).
4. J. Benjamins and B. Agranoff, *J. Neurochem.* **16,** 513 (1969).
5. R. Rao and K. Strickland, *Biochim. Biophys. Acta* **348,** 306 (1974).
6. A. Imai and M. Gershengorn, *Nature* (*London*) **325,** 726 (1982).
7. A. Ghalayini and J. Eichberg, *J. Neurochem.* **44,** 175 (1985).
8. A. Fischl and G. Carman, *J. Bacteriol.* **154,** 304 (1983).
9. J. Folch, *J. Biol. Chem.* **177,** 497 (1949).
10. M. Kates and P. Sastry, *in* "Methods in Enzymology" (J. M. Lowenstein, ed.), Vol. 14, p. 197. Academic Press, New York, 1969.
11. B. Agranoff and W. Suomi, *Biochem. Prep.* **10,** 47 (1963).
12. T. Larson, T. Hirabayashi, and W. Dowhan, *Biochemistry* **15,** 197 (1976).
13. V. Vaskovsky and E. Kostetsky, *J. Lipid Res.* **9,** 396 (1968).
14. P. Cuatrecasas, *J. Biol. Chem.* **245,** 3059 (1970).
15. G. Bartlett, *J. Biol. Chem.* **234,** 466 (1959).
16. A. Bensadoun and D. Weinstein, *Anal. Biochem.* **70,** 241 (1976).
17. T. Takenawawa and K. Egawa, *J. Biol. Chem.* **252,** 5419 (1977).
18. A. Ghalayini, Ph.D. Dissertation, University of Houston, Houston, Texas (1982).
19. J. Nikawa, T. Kodaki, and S. Yamashita, *J. Biol. Chem.* **262,** 4876 (1987).

[11] Phosphatidylinositol 4-Kinase from Bovine Brain

Akio Yamakawa and Tadaomi Takenawa

Introduction

Phosphatidylinositol (PI) kinase (1) plays an important role in polyphospho-inositide turnover which produces two second messengers, inositol 1,4,5-trisphosphate (IP_3) and diacylglycerol (DG), since phosphorylation of PI is a rate-limiting step in phosphatidylinositol 4,5-bisphosphate (PIP_2) synthesis. This PI kinase catalyzes the formation of phosphatidylinositol 4-phosphate (PIP) through phosphorylation at the 4-position of the inositol ring in PI. PIP is further phosphorylated to PIP_2 by PIP 5-kinase. The resultant lipid is hydrolyzed by phospholipase C in response to various hormones and mitogens.

In addition to this type of PI kinase, a new type of PI kinase was found to be present as complexes with middle $T/pp60^{c\text{-}src}$, $pp60^{v\text{-}src}$, platelet-derived growth factor receptor, colony stimulation factor-1 receptor, and insulin receptor (2, 3). This enzyme catalyzed the formation of new inositol lipids, namely, PI 3-phosphate, PI 3,4-bisphosphate, and PI 3,4,5-trisphosphate, through phosphorylation at the 3-position of inositol ring in PI, PIP, and PIP_2 (4, 5). However, considering that inositol 1,4,5-trisphosphate is produced only through the hydrolysis of PIP_2 by phospholipase C, the PI kinase which participates in the formation of second messengers should be PI 4-kinase. Therefore, PI 4-kinases play a crucial role in the usual signal transduction pathway of hormones and neurotransmitters. So far, several PI 4-kinases have been purified to homogeneity from bovine uterus, rat brain, and A431 cells (6–8). Here we describe the purification and characterization of PI 4-kinase from bovine brain.

Assay for Phosphatidylinositol 4-Kinase Activity

Principle

Enzyme activity is assayed by measuring the formation of [^{32}P]PIP from PI and [γ-^{32}P]ATP. The formed PIP can be conveniently extracted with chloroform/methanol/concentrated HCl (200 : 100 : 1, v/v). However, for the estimation of the activity of crude enzymes, [^{32}P]PIP must be separated by thin-layer chromatography to avoid contamination with other ^{32}P-labeled lipids. The participation of PI 3-kinase activity is negligible because PI 3-kinase activity is diminished in the presence of detergents.

Reagents

Phosphatidylinositol (soybean), 5 mM dispersed with sonication in 10 mM Tris-HCl buffer (pH 7.4)

Tris-HCl buffer, 250 mM (pH 7.4), containing 100 mM MgCl$_2$, 5 mM EGTA, and 2% Triton X-100 (v/v)

[γ-^{32}P]ATP, 500 μM

Procedure

The standard incubation mixture contains 50 mM Tris-HCl (pH 7.4), 20 mM MgCl^2, 1 mM EGTA, 0.4% Triton X-100, 1 mM PI, 200 μM [γ-^{32}P]ATP (1.0–0.5 μCi), and 1–100 μg of enzyme protein in a total volume of 50 μl. The reaction is started by the addition of [γ-^{32}P]ATP, continued for 10 min at 30°C, and then stopped by the addition of 2 ml of chloroform/methanol/concentrated HCl (200 : 100 : 1, v/v). Then, 0.5 ml of 1 N HCl is added, and the mixture is vortexed and separated into two phases by centrifugation at 2000 g for 5 min at room temperature. The upper phase is discarded, and the lower phase is washed with 0.5 ml of the synthetic upper phase. After centrifugation, the resultant lower phase is removed and dried under a nitrogen gas stream.

Thin-Layer Chromatography

After 10 μg PIP is added as carrier, PIP is separated from other phospholipids with one-dimensional thin-layer chromatography. Prior to the experiments, thin-layer plates (Merck, Darmstadt, Germany) are treated with methanol/water (2 : 3, v/v) containing 1% sodium oxalate and then activated for 1 hr at 110°C. The lipids are spotted on the plates and developed with chloroform/methanol/4.3 M NH$_4$OH (90 : 65 : 20, v/v). The spots are visualized with iodine vapor and then scraped off the plates for measuring the radioactivity.

Enzyme Purification

Homogenization and Preparation of Bovine Brain Membrane Fractions

Bovine brains (~5 kg) are homogenized with a blender in 2 volumes of cold buffer A (10 mM Tris-HCl, pH 7.4, 10 mM 2-mercaptoethanol, 5 mM EDTA, and 0.1 mM phenylmethylsulfonyl fluoride). Homogenates are centrifuged at 8000 g for 20 min at 4°C, and then the supernatant is centrifuged at 100,000 g

for 60 min. Resultant pellets (~300 g) are pooled as microsome fractions and stored in a freezer at −70°C.

Solubilization of Microsome Fraction

Frozen microsome fractions are thawed and homogenized with a Polytron homogenizer (Brinkmann Instruments, Westbury, NY) in 3 volumes of cold buffer A. Then, 1 volume of 10% Triton X-100 solution (v/v) is added to make a final Triton X-100 concentration of 2%. The mixture is stirred at 4°C for 1 hr and centrifuged at 100,000 g for 60 min. The supernatant is used as starting material for subsequent chromatographic purification.

Q Sepharose Fast Flow

All procedures are carried out at 4°C. The supernatant is applied to a Q Sepharose fast flow column (7 × 24 cm), equilibrated with TEG buffer [10 mM Tris-HCl, pH 7.4, 1 mM dithiothreitol, 1 mM EDTA, 0.1 mM phenylmethylsulfonyl fluoride, and 10% glycerol (v/v)] containing 0.5% Triton X-100 (v/v). After washing the column with 3 liters of TEG buffer containing 0.5% Triton X-100, proteins are eluted from the column with a linear gradient of NaCl (0–0.6 M) in 3 liter TEG buffer containing 0.5% Triton X-100 (v/v). PI 4-kinase activity is eluted between 0.15 and 0.2 M NaCl (Fig. 1A).

P11 Cellulose Phosphate

The active fractions from the Q Sepharose Fast Flow column are pooled and diluted 2-fold with HEG buffer (20 mM HEPES–NaOH, pH 7.4, 1 mM dithiothreitol, 1 mM EDTA, 0.1 mM phenylmethylsulfonyl fluoride, and 10% glycerol) containing 0.2% Triton X-100 (v/v) and applied to a P11 cellulose phosphate column (5 × 8 cm) equilibrated with HEG buffer containing 0.2% Triton X-100 (v/v) . After washing the column with 1 liter of HEG buffer containing 0.2% Triton X-100 (v/v), proteins are eluted from the column with a linear gradient of NaCl (0–0.6 M) in 1 liter HEG buffer containing 0.2% Triton X-100 (v/v). The activity is eluted between 0.3 and 0.4 M NaCl (Fig. 1B).

Affi-Gel Blue

The active fractions from the P11 column are pooled, diluted 2-fold with HEG buffer containing 0.2% Triton X-100 (v/v), and applied to an Affi-Gel Blue column (2 × 18 cm). After washing the column with 300 ml of HEG buffer containing 0.2% Triton X-100 (v/v) and 0.4 M NaCl, elution is performed with a linear gradient of NaCl from 0.4 to 1.2 M in 500 ml of HEG buffer containing 0.2% Triton X-100. The activity is eluted between 0.6 and 0.8 M (Fig. 1C).

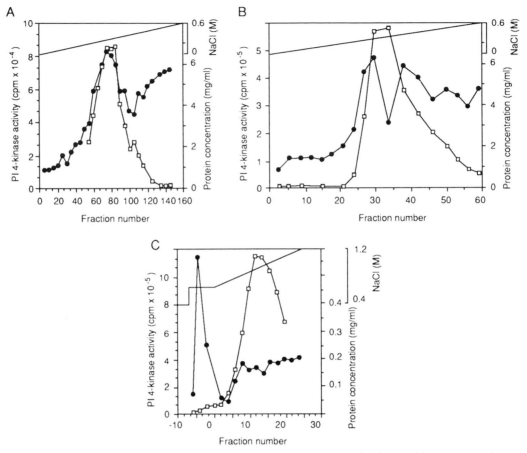

FIG. 1   Chromatography of bovine PI 4-kinase. Bovine brain PI 4-kinase was purified via chromatography on Q Sepharose fast flow (A), P11 cellulose phosphate (B), and Affi-Gel Blue (C) as described in the text. (●), protein; (□), protein 4-kinase.

Toyopearl 55 Superflow

The active fractions obtained from the Affi-Gel Blue column are pooled, and solid ammonium sulfate is added to a final 50% saturation. The mixture is stirred for 60 min and centrifuged at 100,000 *g* for 30 min at 4°C. Resultant pellets are resuspended and homogenized with 4 ml of TEG buffer containing 0.1% Triton X-100 (w/v), then applied to a Toyopearl 55 Superflow (Toso, Tokyo, Japan) column (3 × 95 cm) equilibrated with TEG buffer containing 0.1% Triton X-100 and 0.1 *M* NaCl (Fig. 2A). The column is eluted with the same buffer at a flow rate of 0.3 ml/min.

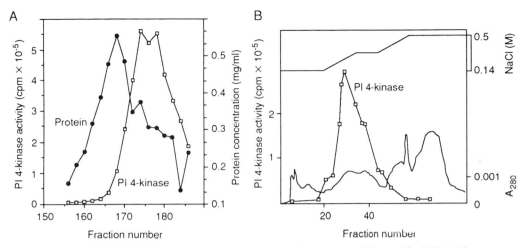

FIG. 2 Chromatography of bovine PI 4-kinase. Partially purified PI 4-kinase was further purified by chromatography on Toyopearl 55 Superflow (A) and Blue Sepharose HiTrap (B). (●), protein; (□), PI 4-kinase.

First Heparin-Sepharose HiTrap

The active fractions are diluted with an equal volume of HEG buffer containing 0.2% Triton X-100 and applied to a heparin-Sepharose HiTrap column (Pharmacia LKB Biotechnology, Tokyo, Japan) equilibrated with the same buffer. After washing the column with 30 ml of HEG buffer containing 0.2% Triton X-100 and 0.14 M NaCl at a flow rate of 1.5 ml/min, the proteins are eluted at a flow rate of 1 ml/min by successive application of increasing NaCl gradients from 0.14 to 0.28 M for 20 min, 0.28 M for 10 min, and then from 0.28 to 0.4 M for 20 min (Fig. 2B).

Blue Sepharose HiTrap

The active fractions from the previous step are directly applied to a Blue Sepharose HiTrap column (2 ml) equilibrated with HEG buffer containing 0.2% Triton X-100. After washing the column with 30 ml of HEG buffer containing 0.2% Triton X-100 and 0.6 M NaCl at a flow rate of 1.5 ml/min, the proteins are eluted at a flow rate of 1 ml/min with 30 ml of a NaCl linear gradient (0.6–1.0 M) in HEG buffer containing 0.2% Triton X-100.

Second Heparin-Sepharose HiTrap

The active fractions from the Blue Sepharose HiTrap column are diluted with 9 volumes of HEG buffer containing 0.2% Triton X-100 and applied to the Heparin-Sepharose HiTrap column (1 ml) equilibrated with the same

TABLE I   Purification of Phosphatidylinositol 4-Kinase from Bovine Brain

Purification step	Total protein (μg)	Total activity (nmol/min)	Specific activity (nmol/min per mg)	Purification (-fold)	Yield (%)
Triton X-100 lysate	18,000,000	120	0.0066	1.0	—
Q Sepharose fast flow	6,000,000	216	0.036	5.4	100
P11 cellulose phosphate	1,200,000	194	0.161	24.3	89.8
Affi-Gel Blue	30,000	69	2.3	345	32
Toyopearl 55	6000	29	4.83	725	13.4
First heparin HiTrap	210	13	62	9300	6
Blue HiTrap	10	4.2	420	70,000	1.9
Second heparin HiTrap	2	2.1	1,050	150,000	0.8

buffer, and rechromatography is performed with the same elution gradients. The active fractions are pooled and stored at 4°C.

Comments on Purification Procedures

Our previous study on the distribution of PI 4-kinase activity in rat or bovine brain has shown that 90% of the total activity of the brain homogenate was associated with the membrane fractions. About one-third of the total membrane-associated PI 4-kinase activity was recovered in microsomal fractions (8000–100,000 g fraction), and this differential centrifugation step gave about 5-fold purification.

In both the Triton X-100 solubilization and Q Sepharose Fast Flow steps, yields were larger than 100%, and inhibitors seemed to be removed in these steps. Therefore, purification yields were calculated on the basis of the activity of Q Sepharose fast flow fractions as 100%. About 30% of the activity passed through the Q Sepharose fast flow column, and this fraction was not retained by rechromatography on the same column at pH 7.4. At the P11 cellulose phosphate step, a large portion of proteins did not bind to the cationic ion-exchange gel at neutral pH. However, PI 4-kinase was retained rather tightly on this column, presumably through the affinity of the protein to the phosphate group of the gel. Two group-specific affinity chromatographies using heparin and Cibachron Blue were found to be very useful for the purification of PI 4-kinase. In the Blue HiTrap chromatography step, PI 4-kinase activity was retained more tightly than with Affi-Gel Blue, and almost homogeneous PI 4-kinase was successfully obtained using the differential affinity between Blue HiTrap and Affi-Gel Blue. The final heparin

HiTrap column removed small amounts of contaminating proteins of higher molecular weights.

The purified PI 4-kinase appeared as a single band using silver staining on sodium dodecyl sulfate–polyacrylamide gel electrophoresis (SDS-PAGE), and its molecular weight was 55,000. The specific activity of the purified enzyme was 1.05 μmol/min/mg, and 15,000-fold purification was achieved starting from the Triton X-100 lysate. Table I summarizes the purification procedure. To confirm the correlation between the 55K protein and enzyme activity, the purified sample was electrophoresed through an SDS–polyacrylamide gel, and gel slices were extracted in a small volume of buffer. Although this preparative SDS-PAGE gave only poor recovery (0.1–0.2%), a consistent amount of activity coeluted with the 55K band in SDS-PAGE. These results show that the purified 55K protein has PI 4-kinase activity.

References

1. G. Endemann, S. Dunn, and L. Cantley, *Biochemistry* **26,** 6845 (1987).
2. M. Whitman and L. Cantley, *Biochim. Biophys. Acta* **948,** 327 (1988).
3. D. R. Kaglan, D. C. Pallas, W. Morgan, B. Schaffhausen, and T. M. Roberts, *Biochim. Biophys. Acta* **948,** 345 (1988).
4. C. L. Carpenter, B. C. Duckworth, K. R. Auger, B. Cohen, B. S. Schaffhausen, and L. C. Cantley, *J. Biol. Chem.* **265,** 19704 (1990).
5. F. Shibaski, Y. Homma, and T. Takenawa, *J. Biol. Chem.* **266,** 8108 (1991).
6. F. D. Porter, Y.-S. Li, and T. F. Deuel, *J. Biol. Chem.* **263,** 8989 (1988).
7. A. Yamakawa and T. Takenawa, *J. Biol. Chem.* **263,** 17555 (1988).
8. D. H. Walker, N. Doughery, and L. J. Pike, *Biochemistry* **27,** 6504 (1988).

[12] Phosphatidylinositol 3-Kinase

Stephen P. Soltoff, David R. Kaplan, and Lewis C. Cantley

Introduction

Phosphatidylinositol 3-kinase (PtdIns 3-kinase) is a lipid kinase that is activated by a number of growth factors and takes part in the cascade of signal transduction events involved in cell growth and transformation. It associates with activated protein tyrosine kinases, including growth factor receptors that are autophosphorylated on tyrosine residues in response to the binding of the specific ligands at the plasma membrane. In addition to being activated by growth factors [including colony stimulatory factor-1, insulin, insulin-like growth factor-1 (IGF-1), epidermal growth factor (EGF), hepatocyte growth factor (HGF), and platelet-derived growth factor (PDGF)], PtdIns 3-kinase is activated in cells transformed by polyomavirus middle T antigen and the product of the *abl* oncogene, and in terminally differentiated cells (platelets, neutrophils) exposed to various agonists (fMet-Leu-Phe, thrombin) (reviewed in Refs. 1 and 2).

We have reported that nerve growth factor (NGF), a differentiation-inducing factor, also promotes the activation of PtdIns 3-kinase activity in PC12 cells (3). NGF stimulates the differentiation of the rat pheochromocytoma PC12 cell line into cells that resemble sympathetic neurons (4). gp140^{trk}, the protein product of the *trk* protooncogene, contains intrinsic tyrosine kinase activity and is activated by the binding of NGF (5, 6). NGF promotes the association of PtdIns 3-kinase with gp140^{trk} and the tyrosine phosphorylation of one of the subunits of PtdIns 3-kinase (3; see below). PtdIns 3-kinase is one of several cytoplasmic proteins that are recruited to the inner face of the plasma membrane and that associate with activated tyrosine kinases. Other proteins include *ras* GAP (GTPase-activating protein), c-*raf*, and PtdIns-specific phospholipase C-γ. The involvement of these proteins in cell proliferation and their recruitment to the plasma membrane have been reviewed (1). The ligand-activated protein tyrosine kinases and the cytosolic targets, including PtdIns 3-kinase, may be coimmunoprecipitated using antibodies specific for the proteins present in the complexes or by antiphosphotyrosine (anti-P-Tyr) antibody. This chapter describes several of the techniques used by our laboratory to identify the PtdIns 3-kinase protein and to measure its activity using lipid kinase assays of anti-P-Tyr-immunoprecipitated enzyme and *in vivo* labeling of the products of PtdIns 3-kinase.

Methods in Neurosciences, Volume 18

PtdIns 3-kinase catalyzes the formation of a family of phosphoinositides that contain phosphate at the D-3 position of the inositol ring, namely, phosphatidylinositol 3-phosphate [PtdIns(3)P], phosphatidylinositol 3,4-bis-phosphate [PtdIns(3,4)P$_2$], and phosphatidylinositol 3,4,5-trisphosphate [PtdIns(3,4,5)P$_3$]. The products of PtdIns 3-kinase are distinct from other lipids that are involved in the canonical signaling cascade, such as phosphati-dylinositol 4,5-bisphosphate [PtdIns(4,5)P$_2$]. In addition, the lipid products of PtdIns 3-kinase are not hydrolyzed by PtdIns-specific phospholipases C (7), suggesting that these lipids themselves may act as signaling molecules.

PtdIns 3-kinase has been purified and found to be a heterodimeric enzyme that consists of subunits of 85 (p85) and 110 kDa (p110) (8). The cDNAs for p85 (9–11) and p110 (12) have been cloned, sequenced, and expressed. The p85 subunit appears to function as a targeting protein involved in the recruit-ment of PtdIns 3-kinase via the binding of the *src* homology 2 (SH2) domain of p85 to activated protein tyrosine kinases (reviewed in Ref. 1). The kinase activity of PtdIns 3-kinase appears to reside in the p110 subunit (12). Although the physiological and biochemical roles of these products have not yet been determined, p110 has sequence similarity with VPS34p (12), a protein in *Saccharomyces cerevisiae* that is involved in the targeting of proteins to the vacuole (13). This raises the possibility that PtdIns 3-kinase may play a role in membrane trafficking.

Evidence that PtdIns 3-kinase was associated with cell transformation came from early findings that demonstrated enhanced levels of PtdIns kinase activity in immunoprecipitates made using middle T- or pp60^{c-src} specific antisera from cells transformed with polyomavirus (14). Subsequent studies reported that two different PtdIns kinases were found in fibroblasts (15) and other cells (reviewed in Ref. 16). One enzyme phosphorylated PtdIns at the D-3 position of the inositol ring, making PtdIns(3)P (17), and this enzyme was designated PtdIns 3-kinase to distinguish it from PtdIns 4-kinase. The two PtdIns kinases were distinguishable by their susceptibility to inhibition by detergent: only PtdIns 3-kinase was blocked by nonionic detergents, such as Nonidet P-40 (NP-40) (15). Cells exposed to growth factors (PDGF) and transformed cells (by polyomavirus middle T antigen) exhibited both in-creased PtdIns kinase activity and tyrosine phosphorylation of the 85 kDa subunit (18). Subsequent studies demonstrated that PDGF stimulated the production of PtdIns(3,4)P$_2$ and PtdIns(3,4,5)P$_3$ *in vivo* in PDGF-treated ra-diolabeled cells and in anti-P-Tyr immunoprecipitates of PDGF-treated cells (19), and similar studies have been performed in a variety of cells exposed to different growth factors.

Thus, the production of these lipids can be measured using *in vitro* lipid kinase assays of immunoprecipitates of growth factor-treated cells or by measuring the *in vivo* production of lipids in radiolabeled cells. We have utilized these techniques on a variety of cultured cell lines, including studies of the effects of NGF on PC12 cells. For the purposes of this chapter, we specify protocols that we used with NGF on PC12 cells, but similar techniques have been applied to other cells and using other growth factors. The methods of labeling cells with ortho[^{32}P]phosphate and myo-[^{3}H]inositol have been described previously (20).

Lipid Kinase Assays of Anti-P-Tyr Immunoprecipitated Proteins

Several techniques are commonly employed to measure the production of the novel lipid products. Because PtdIns 3-kinase associates with the PDGF receptor, middle T/pp60$^{c\text{-}src}$ tyrosine kinase, and other receptors that are phosphorylated on tyrosine in response to growth factors, it became and still remains an established technique to immunoprecipitate this kinase using anti-P-Tyr antibodies.

PC12 cells are grown in 100-mm dishes in 10 ml of Dulbecco's modified Eagle's medium (DMEM; GIBCO BRL, Gaithersburg, MD) supplemented with 5% (v/v) horse serum plus 5% (v/v) calf serum at 37°C in a 95%/5% air/CO$_2$ mixture (by volume). When the cells are nearly confluent, they are serum-starved overnight in DMEM supplemented with 0.1% bovine serum albumin (BSA). On the day of the experiment, the volume of medium is diminished to 4 ml so that the amount of added growth factor can be minimized. Cells are treated with NGF (100 ng/ml) for varying lengths of time, washed twice with ice-cold buffer A (137 mM NaCl, 20 mM Tris, 1 mM MgCl$_2$, 1 mM CaCl$_2$, 0.2 mM vanadate, pH 7.5), and exposed to 1 ml of lysis buffer [buffer A plus 10% glycerol (v/v), 1% NP-40 (v/v), and 1 mM phenylmethylsulfonyl fluoride]. The cells are scraped off the dish using a cell scraper, added to a 1.5-ml microcentrifuge tube, vortexed thoroughly, and centrifuged at 16,000 g in an Eppendorf 5414 centrifuge for 15 min at 4°C. The cleared supernatant is transferred to a fresh 1.5-ml microcentrifuge tube and incubated with anti-P-Tyr antibody (5 μg/ml lysate, Upstate Biotechnology, Inc., Lake Placid, NY, No. 05-321) and protein A-Sepharose (4 mg/ml lysate; see below) for 3–4 hr at 4°C. The immunoprecipitates are washed three times in phosphate-buffered saline (PBS: 137 mM NaCl, 15.7 mM NaH$_2$PO$_4$, 1.47 mM KH$_2$PO$_4$, and 2.68 mM KCl, pH 7.4)/1% NP-40, two times in 0.5 M LiCl/0.1 M Tris (pH 7.5), and two times in TNE (10 mM Tris, 100 mM NaCl, 1 mM EDTA, pH 7.5). Vanadate (200 μM) is present in all wash solutions.

Two variations of a lipid kinase assay are usually performed, and both are done in a final volume of 50 μl. We leave around 30 μl (~20 μl of protein A-Sepharose beads plus ~10 μl TNE) in the microcentrifuge tube after the last wash and add 10 μl of a lipid mixture combined with 10 μl of a [γ-^{32}P]ATP (DuPont–NEN, Boston, MA, specific activity 3000 Ci/mmol) mixture to initiate the assay. One PtdIns kinase assay is performed by adding 10 μl containing 20–40 μCi [γ-^{32}P]ATP (in 250 μM ATP, 25 mM MgCl$_2$, and 5 mM HEPES, pH 7.5) and 10 μl of sonicated PtdIns (1 mg/ml in 10 mM HEPES, 1 mM EGTA, pH 7.5) to the immunoprecipitates for 10 min at room temperature. Lipid stocks are stored in chloroform at $-70°$C. Stock lipid is added to a microcentrifuge tube, dried under a stream of N$_2$, and resuspended in the HEPES/EGTA solution. The lipid mixture is sonicated for 5 min just prior to use. Note that the lipids and nonradiolabeled ATP get diluted to one-fifth their concentration, and thus the final concentration of PtdIns is 0.2 mg/ml and ATP is 50 μM. In a variation of the assay, a mixed lipid composition [PtdIns, PtdIns(4)P, PtdIns(4,5)P$_2$, and phosphatidylserine in 10 mM HEPES/1 mM EGTA, pH 7.5] is added with the [^{32}P]ATP mixture described above. The relative phosphorylation of the different phosphatidyl-inositol lipids will depend on the relative ratio of lipids. A sufficient mixture to demonstrate a readily observable phosphorylation of all three lipids must be empirically determined, but one that works well with PC12 and other cells is 1 : 1 : 1 : 1 (0.4 mg total lipid/ml final concentration in the lipid kinase assay). Frequently, excellent results may be obtained using a crude phospho-inositide mixture (Sigma, St. Louis, MO, No. P 6063) that contains these four lipids (Dr. C. L. Carpenter, personal communication, 1992).

The reaction is stopped by adding 80 μl of HCl (1 M) and vortexing the sample. Subsequently, 160 μl of methanol/chloroform (1 : 1, v/v) is added, and the sample is vortexed thoroughly. The sample is centrifuged briefly ($\sim$10 sec) to separate the organic and aqueous layers. The lipid-containing chloroform phase (below the aqueous phase) is spotted onto oxalate-coated aluminum-backed thin-layer chromatography (TLC) plates (silica gel 60, 0.2 mm thickness, EM Separations, EM Industries, Gibbstown, NJ). The plates are coated in 1% (w/v) potassium oxalate in 50% (v/v) methanol, then baked in a drying oven at 100°C for at least 30 min prior to use.

Two different solvent systems are used, depending on the lipid mixture. If the lipid kinase assay is performed using PtdIns alone, the samples are spotted onto 20 × 20 cm TLC plates that are cut in half and developed (10 cm vertical) in a mixture of chloroform/methanol/water/ 7.7 N NH$_4$OH (60 : 47 : 11.3 : 2, v/v). (Note: Attention should be paid that the solvent constituents form a single phase when mixed. To promote this, chloroform should be added last). The solvent is allowed to migrate nearly to the top, which this takes approximately 30 min. This solvent system resolves PtdIns, PtdInsP, and PtdInsP$_2$, but PtdIns(3,4,5)P$_3$ and ATP remain at the origin. Authentic PtdIns(4)P is spotted as a standard and visualized using iodine vapor. Usually a substantial amount of unreacted PtdIns remains in the assay samples and is visualized by iodine, and [^{32}P]PtdInsP appears just below the

A

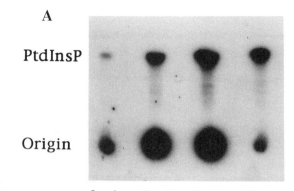

PtdInsP

Origin

0 min   1 min   5 min   15 min

FIG. 1   Separation by TLC of products of PtdIns 3-kinase produced in assays of anti-P-Tyr immunoprecipitates of NGF-treated PC12 cells. (A) Lipid kinase assays were performed using [^{32}P]ATP and PtdIns (0.2 mg/ml) on the anti-P-Tyr immunoprecipitates of untreated PC12 cells (0) or cells treated with NGF (100 ng/ml) for 1, 5, or 15 min. The products of the assay were extracted with chloroform/methanol (1 : 1, v/v), and the chloroform layer was spotted on oxalate-coated TLC plates and developed using a chloroform/methanol/water/NH$_4$OH solvent system as described in the text. The radioactivity was visualized using X-ray film (11-hr exposure without an intensifying screen). In this experiment, the quantification of the PtdInsP products by Cerenkov radiation was as follows: 79 counts/min (cpm) (0), 1034 cpm (1 min), 2716 cpm (5 min), and 1650 cpm (15 min). When the PtdInsP products were deacylated and subjected to HPLC (not shown), PtdIns(3)P accounted for approximately 90% of the radioactivity. (B) Lipid kinase assays were performed on anti-P-Tyr immunoprecipitates of untreated cells (−) and cells exposed to NGF (100 ng/ml, 15 min) using [^{32}P]ATP and PtdIns, PtdIns(4)P, PtdIns(4,5)P$_2$, and phosphatidylserine (1 : 1 : 1 : 1, v/v, 0.4 mg total lipid/ml) as substrates. The products of the assay were extracted with chloroform/methanol (1 : 1, v/v), and the TLC plate was developed using a 2-propanol/acetic acid solvent system. The positions of authentic PtdIns, PtdIns(4)P, and PtdIns(4,5)P$_2$ are shown, as is the position of PtdInsP$_3$. The TLC spots were visualized using a PhosphorImager (Molecular Dynamics, Sunnyvale, CA). The Molecular Dynamics PhosphorImager uses storage phosphor screens to detect and quantify radioactivity. The advantages to using this technology instead of standard autoradiography using X-ray film are that the exposure period can be greatly reduced (to one-tenth the time) and the sensitivity is greater. Radioactivity at the origin represents ATP or related products and is contributed from the aqueous layer of the extracted samples. The larger amounts of radioactivity at this spot in some of the NGF-treated lanes is coincidental. The radioactive spot immediately below PtdInsP$_3$ is phosphate.

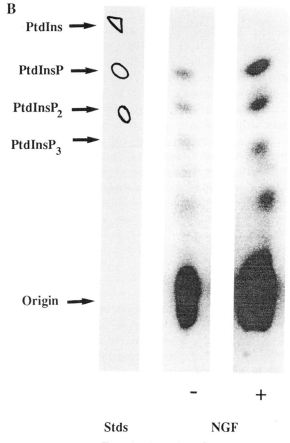

FIG. 1   (*continued*)

nonradiolabeled PtdIns (Fig. 1A). The [^{32}P]PtdInsP spots are excised and quantified by scintillation counting or by measuring Cerenkov radiation.

PtdIns(3)P is not separable from PtdIns(4)P using this technique. However, in experiments with various growth factors and a variety of cell lines, the majority of the radioactivity of the PtdInsP spot is [^{32}P]PtdIns(3)P, the product of PtdIns 3-kinase. This should be confirmed by high-performance liquid chromatography (HPLC) analysis of the deacylated lipid and/or sensitivity of the lipid kinase assay to NP-40 detergent (see Introduction). [In detergent experiments, NP-40 is added to the lipid mixture at 2.5% (v/v) of the mixture (0.5% final concentration in lipid kinase assay) prior to sonication of lipid.] Some batches of PtdIns appears to contain small amounts of PtdIns(4)P;

therefore, minor amounts of [^{32}P]PtdInsP$_2$ [which migrates identically to authentic PtdIns(4,5)P$_2$] may appear as a separate spot below [^{32}P]PtdInsP on the TLC plate. In experiments in which a combination of lipids [including PtdIns(4,5)P$_2$] are added, a 2-propanol/2 M acetic acid (65 : 35, v/v) solvent system is used to separate PtdIns(3,4,5)P$_3$ and the other lipids. The solvent is allowed to migrate nearly to the top of a 20 × 20 cm TLC plate, a process that takes 4–6 hr. Authentic PtdIns, PtdInsP, and PtdInsP$_2$ are used as standards, and they are oriented in descending order from the solvent front (Fig. 1B) as with the other solvent system. The production of [^{32}P]PtdIns(3,4,5)P$_3$, which is found just below PtdInsP$_2$, confirms the presence of PtdIns 3-kinase activity. In addition, sensitivity of the lipid kinase to NP-40 strongly suggests that the PtdIns lipids are the products of PtdIns 3-kinase and are phosphorylated at the D-3 position. More accurate identification must rely on HPLC techniques (20).

Preparation of Protein A-Sepharose

We use commercially prepared protein A-Sepharose (Sigma Chemical Co., No. P-3391) blocked with BSA as follows. The resin (1.5 g) is suspended in 50 ml distilled, deionized water and maintained on ice for 10 min. After centrifugation at 500 g for 2 min, the pelleted beads are mixed with approximately 50 ml of blocking solution (1% BSA, 10 mM Tris, pH 7.5) and maintained on ice for 30 min. The beads are washed three times with 50 ml distilled, deionized water. The swollen beads (~6.5 ml) are suspended in an equal volume of PBS/0.02% (w/v) NaN$_3$ and are distributed into smaller aliquots that are kept at 4°C. Immediately prior to use, the beads are resuspended by vortexing. Usually, we add 40 μl to each 1 ml of lysate.

Identification of D-3 Phosphorylated Lipids *in Vivo* in Ortho[^{32}P]phosphate-Labeled Cells

The most accurate way to demonstrate that growth factors or other agonists promote the production of D-3 phosphorylated lipids under physiological conditions is to measure them *in vivo* in radiolabeled cells. We have done this in PC12 cells and found that NGF stimulates large increases in the production of [^{32}P]PtdIns(3,4)P$_2$ and [^{32}P]PtdIns(3,4,5)P$_3$ (3). PDGF produces similar large changes in NIH fibroblasts (19). In these experiments, the cells are labeled with ortho[^{32}P]phosphate, and the lipids are deacylated and analyzed by HPLC.

PC12 cells are grown in 100-mm dishes to confluence or nearly confluence in DMEM containing 5% horse serum plus 5% (v/v) calf serum, and they are then cultured overnight in serum-free DMEM containing 0.1% (w/v) BSA. The cells are washed once and incubated with 5 ml phosphate-free DMEM (supplemented with 0.1% BSA) for 15 min, then exposed to the same medium plus carrier-free ortho[^{32}P]phosphate (Du Pont–NEN, specific activity 8500–9120 Ci/mmol). We use 100 μCi/ml (500 μCi/dish) for PC12 cells, but larger amounts of radioactivity may be required if the cells do not incorporate sufficiently high levels of radiolabeled lipids. Cells are exposed to the radioisotope at 37°C for 4 hr in a humidified atmosphere containing 5% CO_2, which is the normal conditions under which they are maintained. After the cells are exposed to the agonist, they are washed twice with ice-cold buffer A and 750 μl of 1 M HCl/methanol (1 : 1, v/v) added. The cells are scraped using a cell scraper, and the mixture is placed in a 1.5-ml microcentrifuge tube and vortexed vigorously. After the addition of 380 μl chloroform, the mixture is vortexed and mixed on a rocker for 15 min. The samples are centrifuged briefly at 16,000 g. The aqueous (upper) layer is removed, and the chloroform (lower) phase is extracted two times with an equal volume of methanol/EDTA (0.1 M, pH 7.5) in a 1 : 0.9 (v/v) ratio. The organic (lower) phase is removed and stored at -70°C under N_2 until deacylation (below). The samples are kept behind plexiglass shields throughout these procedures, including the ortho[^{32}P]phosphate incorporation in the tissue culture incubator. A typical acrylic bench-top shield for β emitters is used for bench-top work, and an acrylic box is used during the ortho[^{32}P]phosphate incorporation of the cells in the tissue culture incubator.

In some cells, such as smooth muscle cells (19), fibroblasts (21), and *S. cerevisiae* cells (22), *myo*-[^{3}H]inositol may be used to label the D-3 lipids, as well as the inositol polyphosphates. The protocol for these studies generally employ a 3-day labeling period during which the cells are in inositol-free medium. We have found that it is difficult to incorporate a sufficient amount of label into PC12 cells so that the lipids have high enough levels of radioactivity to be subjected to HPLC analysis (S. P. Soltoff, unpublished results, 1992). For details on the *myo*-[^{3}H]inositol labeling, see Serunian *et al.* (20).

Deacylation of Lipids

The organic phase of the extracted sample is placed in a 20-ml glass, screw-capped scintillation vial and dried under N_2. Methylamine reagent (1.8 ml) is added to hydrolyze the lipids, and the vials are incubated at 53°C for 50 min, taking care to cap the vials tightly. Methylamine reagent is composed of the following (by volume): 26.8% of 40% methylamine (Aldrich Chemical Co., Milwaukee, WI), 45.7% methanol, 11.4% n-butanol, and the remainder (16%) distilled water. For TLC-purified [^{32}P]PtdInsP samples that are to be subjected to HPLC, the PtdInsP area of the TLC plate is excised and placed in a 20-ml scintillation vial, and a small amount (~5 μg) of phospholipid [PtdIns, PtdIns(4)P, or a mixture of crude phospholipids] is added as a carrier to enhance the recovery. Methylamine (1.8 ml) is then added. After cooling to room temperature, the contents of the vials (minus the portion of the TLC plate) are transferred to 2-ml microcentrifuge tubes and dried under a vacuum. A trap of concentrated sulfuric acid in a flask placed on dry ice is placed between the lyophilizer and the vacuum pump to prevent damage to the equipment from methylamine vapor. A flask containing NaOH pellets is placed between the sulfuric acid trap and the vacuum pump to neutralize any acid. After drying the samples (~3–4 hr), 1.8 ml of distilled, deionized water is added to the dried contents and the sample is redried. The sulfuric acid trap is removed prior to drying the distilled, deionized water. In a departure from our earlier description of this process (20), we have found that this step (the addition of distilled, deionized water and redrying) may be skipped if the methylamine is completely evaporated. The dried contents are resuspended in approximately 2 ml distilled, deionized water, transferred to a 13 × 100 mm disposable test tube, and extracted two times with an equal volume of n-butanol/light petroleum ether/ethyl formate (20 : 4 : 1, v/v) to remove fatty acyl groups. The lower (aqueous) phase is removed and dried *in vacuo*, and the samples are stored at −70°C prior to analysis by HPLC.

Chromatographic Separation of Deacylated Phospholipids (Glycerophosphoinositides)

The glycerophosphoinositides produced by the deacylation are separated by HPLC using a 12.5-cm Partisphere 5 μm SAX (strong anion-exchange) column (Whatman, Clifton, NJ) and a salt gradient from 0 to 1.0 M (NH$_4$)$_2$HPO$_4$ (pH 3.8). The details of this system have been reported elsewhere (19, 20). In brief, the HPLC system is connected to an on-line continuous flow liquid scintillation detector (Flow-One/Beta CT; Beckman Instruments, Fullerton, CA), that has the capacity to monitor two isotopes simultaneously. This allows tritiated internal standards of deacylated PtdIns(4)P and PtdIns(4,5)P$_2$ to be coinjected with the ^{32}P-labeled samples. A UV monitor is also connected to the system and allows the detection of ADP and ATP standards, which also function as internal markers.

Identification of Phosphatidylinositol 3-Kinase p85 Protein Using Western Blotting Techniques and Enhanced Chemiluminescence

Proteins that are tyrosine phosphorylated can be identified using Western blotting techniques. We have used this method to demonstrate that the p85 subunit of PtdIns 3-kinase is phosphorylated on tyrosine in PC12 cells exposed to NGF (3). In these experiments, immunoprecipitated proteins are separated by sodium dodecyl sulfate–polyacrylamide gel electrophoresis (SDS–PAGE), transferred to nitrocellulose, and blotted using anti-P-Tyr antibody. The nitrocellulose filters can be stripped and reprobed with other antibodies, including anti-p85 antibody. The specific protocols are described below. Using these protocols and reagents (particularly the antibodies), we found that the tyrosine phosphorylation of p85 is easily and reproducibily observed in PC12 cells in response to NGF and in NIH 3T3 fibroblasts in response to PDGF, although others reported that p85 tyrosine phosphorylation was detected only in cells in which both the PDGF receptor and PtdIns 3-kinase were overexpressed (23).

To determine whether p85 is tyrosine phosphorylated, p85 is immunoprecipitated using a polyclonal anti-p85 antibody (Cat.No. 06-195, Upstate Biotechnology) that was raised in rabbits by Dr. B. Schaffhausen (Tufts University). It is actually a mixture of antibodies against glutathione S-transferase fusion proteins containing the full-length 85-kDa subunit as well as glutathione S-transferase protein containing the N-terminal SH2 domain of the 85-kDa subunit. To maximize visualization of the proteins, cells are grown in 150-mm dishes with 22 ml of medium and are used when they are nearly confluent. In some experiments, cells are exposed to serum-free DMEM (containing 0.1% BSA) overnight. On the day of the experiment, the volume of medium is diminished to 2–8 ml so that the amount of added growth factor can be minimized (the higher end of this range is used for extended time courses). After exposure to NGF (100 ng/ml), the cells are washed twice with ice-cold PBS, and 900 μl of ice-cold lysis buffer is added. In some studies, cells are scraped off the dish using a cell scraper, and the lysis buffer and cells are added to a 1.5-ml microcentrifuge tube and vortexed briefly. A small volume of the PBS wash solution may remain on the 150-mm dishes prior to the addition of lysis buffer, so that the total volume transferred may be slightly greater than 1 ml. Alternatively, after the lysis buffer is added to the dishes, the plates are rocked at 4°C for 20 min, and the supernatant (but not the attached cellular material) is transferred to a microcentrifuge tube. The advantage to the latter procedure is that cell nuclei remain with the cellular material.

The tubes are then centrifuged at 16,000 g for 15 min at 4°C, and the cleared supernatant is transferred to a fresh microcentrifuge tube. Anti-p85 antibody (2 μl) and protein A-Sepharose (4 mg/ml lysate) are added to the supernatant, and the solution is rocked at 4°C for 3–4 hr. At the end of this time, the beads are pelleted by centrifuging at 1000 g for several seconds, and the tubes are put on ice. The supernatant is removed, and the beads are washed three times in PBS/1% NP-40, twice in 0.5 M LiCl/0.1 M Tris, and twice in TNE. During each of the washes, the beads are vortexed thoroughly, centrifuged at 1000 g, and maintained on ice. After the final washing, the beads are pelleted and most of the solution drawn off, leaving about 20 μl beads and 30 μl TNE. An equivalent volume (50 μl) of loading buffer [62.5 mM Tris, pH 6.8, 10% (w/v) glycerol, 2% (w/v) SDS, 0.71 M 2-mercaptoethanol, 0.0025% (w/v) bromophenol blue] is added, and the samples are vortexed, centrifuged (1000 g) for several seconds, and boiled for 5 min. The samples are centrifuged, and the supernatant is run on a 7% polyacrylamide gel in the presence of SDS using a 3% stacking gel.

At the conclusion of the electrophoresis, the gel is washed with Bjerrum and Schafer-Nielsen transfer buffer [48 mM Tris, 39 mM glycine, 20% methanol, pH ~9.2 (do not titrate; use at the constitutive pH)], and proteins are transferred to 0.2 μm nitrocellulose filters using a Bio-Rad (Richmond, CA) Trans-Blot apparatus with plate electrodes for 30 min at 100 mV. Nitrocellulose filters of a 0.45 μm pore size have also been used successfully, but there is a risk that low molecular weight proteins will be lost. The filter is washed in TBS (20 mM Tris, 137 mM NaCl, pH 7.6) for several minutes and then blocked in TBS/2% BSA at room temperature for 1 hr. For identification of tyrosine-phosphorylated proteins, the filter is exposed to anti-P-Tyr antibody (2 μg/ml in TTBS/1% BSA) overnight at 4°C. Good results have also been obtained when the exposure is performed at room temperature for 1 hr. The filter is washed in TTBS for 5 min, and this is repeated two more times. The filter is exposed to the secondary antibody [anti-mouse horseradish peroxidase (HRP), Boehringer-Mannheim, Indianapolis, IN, No. H605250] at a 1:10,000 dilution in TTBS/1% BSA for 1 hr at room temperature. The filter is washed three times in TTBS (TBS + 0.2% Tween 20) at room temperature and washed two times in TBS (5 min each wash). The filter is then ready for identification of tyrosine phosphorylated proteins using enhanced chemiluminescence (ECL).

The filter is placed on a solid support (an acrylic shield works fine), and most of the solution covering it is removed by gently tapping the support on a table. The two ECL solutions are mixed in a 1:1 ratio according to the manufacturer's specifications (Amersham, Arlington Heights, IL) and applied to the filter. The majority of the ECL solution is removed by gently tapping the support on a table, and the filter is covered with plastic wrap or a plasticine sheet. Multiple exposures are collected at different times using standard X-ray film.

To reprobe the blot to analyze it for another protein, the blot is washed two times with TTBS at room temperature and incubated in 62.5 mM Tris (pH 6.8)/0.1 M 2-mercaptoethanol/2% SDS for 30 min at 70°C. The filter is washed two times in TTBS, washed once in TBS, and reblocked in TBS/2% BSA for 1 hr at room temperature. The blot is washed in TTBS, then exposed to the primary antibody at room temperature. To identify the p85 subunit of PtdIns 3-kinase, the filter is exposed to anti-p85 antibody at a 1 : 3000 dilution in TTBS/1% BSA at 4°C overnight or 1 hr at room temperature. The blot is washed three times in TTBS and exposed to the secondary antibody (goat anti-rabbit immunoglobulin G, Bio-Rad, No. 170-6515, or Boehringer-Mannheim, No. 605-220) at a 1 : 10,000 dilution in TTBS/1% BSA for one hour at room temperature. The filter is then washed in TTBS and TBS as described above, and the proteins are identified using enhanced chemiluminescence (we use Amersham No. RPN 2106).

Acknowledgments

This work has been supported in part by National Institutes of Health Grants GM36624 (L.C.C.) and GM41890 (L.C.C.), the Whitaker Health Sciences Fund (S.P.S.), and the National Cancer Institute, Department of Health and Human Services, under Contract N01-CO-74101 with ABL (D.R.K.).

References

1. L. C. Cantley, K. R. Auger, C. Carpenter, B. Duckworth, A. Graziani, R. Kapeller, and S. Soltoff, *Cell* (*Cambridge, Mass.*) **64,** 281 (1991).
2. K. R. Auger and L. C. Cantley, *Cancer Cells* **3,** 263 (1991).
3. S. P. Soltoff, S. L. Rabin, L. C. Cantley, and D. R. Kaplan, *J. Biol. Chem.* **267,** 14472 (1992).
4. L. A. Greene and A. Tischler, *Proc. Natl. Acad.Sci. U.S.A.* **73,** 2424 (1976).
5. D. R. Kaplan, D. Martin-Zanca, and L. Parada, *Nature* (*London*) **350,** 158 (1991).
6. R. Klein, S. Jing, V. Nanduri, E. O'Rourke, and M. Barbacid, *Cell* (*Cambridge, Mass.*) **65,** 189 (1991).
7. L. A. Serunian, M. Haber, T. Fukui, J. W. Kim, S. G. Rhee, J. M. Lowenstein, and L. C. Cantley, *J. Biol. Chem.* **264,** 17809 (1989).
8. C. L. Carpenter, B. C. Duckworth, K. R. Auger, B. Cohen, B. S. Schaffhausen, and L. C. Cantley, *J. Biol. Chem.* **265,** 19704 (1990).
9. M. Otsu, I. Hiles, I. Gout, M. J. Fry, F. Ruiz-Larrea, G. Panayotou, A. Thompson, R. Dhand, J. Hsuan, N. Totty, A. D. Smith, S. J. Morgan, S. A. Courtneidge, P. A. Parker, and M. D. Waterfield, *Cell* (*Cambridge, Mass.*) **65,** 91 (1991).

10. J. A. Escobedo, S. Navankasattusas, W. M. Kavanaugh, D. Milfay, V. A. Fried, and L. T. Williams, *Cell (Cambridge, Mass.)* **65,** 75 (1991).
11. E. Y. Skolnik, B. Margolis, M. Mohammadi, E. Lowenstein, R. Fisher, A. Drepps, A. Ullrich, and J. Schlessinger, *Cell (Cambridge, Mass.)* **65,** 83 (1991).
12. I. D. Hiles, M. Otsu, S. Volinia, M. J. Fry, I. Gout, R. Dhand, G. Panayotou, F. Ruiz-Larrea, A. Thompson, N. F. Totty, J. J. Hsuan, S. A. Courtneidge, P. J. Parker, and M. D. Waterfield, *Cell (Cambridge Mass.)* **70,** 419 (1992).
13. P. K. Herman and S. D. Emr, *Mol. Cell. Biol.* **10,** 6742 (1990).
14. M. Whitman, D. R. Kaplan, B. Schaffhausen, L. Cantley, and T. M. Roberts, *Nature (London)* **315,** 239 (1985).
15. M. Whitman, D. Kaplan, T. Roberts, and L. Cantley, *Biochem. J.* **247,** 165 (1987).
16. C. L. Carpenter and L. C. Cantley, *Biochemistry* **29,** 11147 (1990).
17. M. Whitman, C. P. Downes, M. Keeler, T. Keller, and L. Cantley, *Nature (London)* **332,** 644 (1988).
18. D. R. Kaplan, M. Whitman, B. Schaffhausen, D. C. Pallas, M. White, L. Cantley, and T. M. Roberts, *Cell (Cambridge, Mass.)* **50,** 1021 (1987).
19. K. R. Auger, L. A. Serunian, S. P. Soltoff, P. Libby, and L. C. Cantley, *Cell (Cambridge, Mass.)* **57,** 167 (1989).
20. L. A. Serunian, K. R. Auger, and L. C. Cantley, *in* "Methods in Enzymology" (D. Barnes, J. P. Mather, and G. H. Sato, eds.), Vol. 198, p. 78. Academic Press, San Diego, 1991.
21. L. A. Serunian, K. R. Auger, T. M. Roberts, and L. C. Cantley, *J. Virol.* **64,** 4718 (1990).
22. K. R. Auger, C. L. Carpenter, L. C. Cantley, and L. Varticovsky, *J. Biol. Chem.* **264,** 20181 (1989).
23. P. Hu, B. Margolis, E. Y. Skolnik, R. Lammers, A. Ullrich, and J. Schlessenger, *Mol. Cell. Biol.* **12,** 981 (1992).

[13] Identification of Phosphatidylinositol Trisphosphate in Rat Brain

Ranganathan Parthasarathy, Lathakumari Parthasarathy, and Robert E. Vadnal

Introduction

In recent years, the role of the inositol phospholipids in cell signaling systems has received prominent attention. The major inositol lipid that serves as the precursor of second messenger is phosphatidylinositol bisphosphate (PIP_2), composed of a triphosphorylated *myo*-inositol group at carbon-3 of glycerol, usually with a stearic acid substitution at carbon-1 and arachidonic acid at carbon-2 (1). When the inositol second messenger system is activated, phospholipase C (PLC) acts on PIP_2 generating two second messengers: (i) inositol 1,4,5-trisphosphate (IP_3) and (ii) diacylglycerol, with IP_3 being involved in the release of intracellular calcium. On the other hand, phosphatidylinositol trisphosphate (PIP_3) is the only novel inositol phospholipid capable of potentially releasing inositol tetrakisphosphate (IP_4), which is also thought to be involved in cellular calcium control (2). Although direct hydrolysis of PIP_3 to IP_4 by a PLC has not yet been demonstrated, it has the potential to generate IP_4. Diacylglycerol released from PIP_2 is capable of activating protein kinase C (3), and *myo*-inositol 1,4,5-trisphosphate (IP_3) releases calcium from nonmitochondrial stores (4). IP_4 has also been shown to be involved in calcium binding to endoplasmic reticulum, and it may also play a role in regulating calcium flux across the plasma membrane (2, 5). Thus, the activation of inositol-linked receptor systems releases a number of lipid derivatives and inositol phosphates, each possessing a potential second messenger activity, and the subsequent rise in intracellular calcium concentration by IP_3 modulates several enzymes and proteins (6).

In general, the traditional inositol phospholipids consist of phosphatidylinositol (PI), phosphatidylinositol 4-phosphate (PIP), and phosphatidylinositol 4,5-bisphosphate (PIP_2). PIP_3, containing inositol tetrakisphosphate (IP_4), was identified in neutrophils (7) stimulated with a hexapeptide agonist for the formyl peptide receptor, *N*-formyl-Nle-Leu-Phe-Nle-Tyr-Lys-fluorescein (FLPEP). Recently other groups have identified PIP_3 in a variety of systems (8–10). Neutrophil-derived PIP_3 was noted to be transient in nature and was observed to have a slightly slower R_f value than PIP_2 by thin-layer chromatography (TLC). The neutrophils were labeled using ^{32}P, and the method of Schacht (11) was used for the extraction of inositol lipids. The TLC band containing the PIP_3 ran very close to the PIP_2 band and also contained lyso-PIP and PIP_2 (7).

We describe a technique involving intraventricular injection of myo-[³H]-inositol into the lateral ventricles of rats (12) and sacrifice using high-power head-focused microwave fixation after 24 hr. Microwave fixation of brain is necessary to obtain a good yield of inositol phospholipids, eliminating losses through ischemia (13). The inositol lipids are extracted using two methods, namely those of Hauser and Eichberg (14) and of Schacht (11). We have identified PIP_3 in both extracts, with the method of Hauser and Eichberg proving superior. Alkaline hydrolysis of PIP_3 produces an inositol tetrakis-phosphate, which is identified by high-performance liquid chromatography (HPLC) techniques. Our studies on the fatty acid composition of PIP_3 indicated a similar profile characteristic of inositol lipids (12).

Isolation of Inositol Phospholipids from Rat Brain

Intraventricular Injections and Microwave Fixation

Male Sprague-Dawley rats, 300–350 g (Harlan Sprague-Dawley, Inc., Indianapolis, IN), are sedated with pentobarbital (50 mg/kg i.p.), then placed on a Kopf stereotactic apparatus. The skull is drilled bilaterally: the lateral ventricles (~2 mm lateral from midline and 0.8 mm posterior to bregma) are injected with 20 μCi of myo-[³H]inositol (23 Ci/mmol, American Radiolabeled Chemicals, St. Louis, MO). Figures 1 and 2 demonstrate the sites of injection of radiolabeled myo-inositol on the skull and the stereotactic coordinates, respectively. The animals are sacrificed after 24 hr, by high-power head-focused microwave fixation (8 kW, 1.2 sec, Cober Electronics, Inc., Stamford, CT); the heads are placed immediately in water mixed with crushed ice.

Lipid Extraction and Thin-Layer Chromatography

Cerebra from several rats are dissected and homogenized initially in a small volume of chloroform/methanol (1 : 1, v/v), with several brains pooled into one homogenate, and equal fractions are taken for each sample. This is carried out to reduce the variation in myo-[³H]inositol incorporation between the individual animals. The lipids are extracted essentially according to the method of Hauser and Eichberg (14) or Schacht (11). Prior to use, it is essential to wash each test tube three times with chloroform/methanol (1 : 1, v/v) to remove possible contaminants. The initial neutral extraction removes primarily PI. In addition, during each step of the lipid extraction, the samples are kept under nitrogen using test tubes with Teflon-lined caps. After the

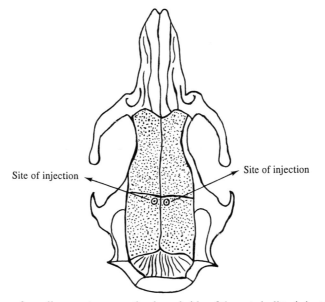

FIG. 1   Sites of needle punctures on the dorsal side of the rat skull to inject [^{3}H]inositol into the lateral ventricles.

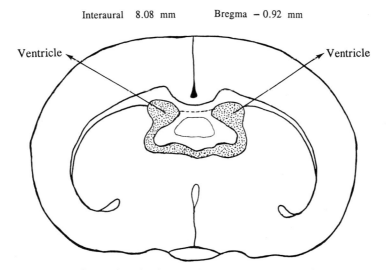

FIG. 2   Coronal sections of rat brain showing stereotactic coordinates and the location of lateral ventricles into which radiolabeled inositol is injected.

acidified chloroform/methanol extraction step, the lipid phases are mixed with 0.2 volume of 1 M HCl, with each phase neutralized immediately with ammonia. The first acidified chloroform/methanol lipid extract is used for all lipid determinations, as this fraction contains most of the polyphosphoinositides.

Silica gel H preoxalated plates (0.25 mm, Analtech, Newark, DE) and silica gel 60 plates (0.5 mm, Merck), oxalated before use, are used to separate the inositol lipids. The plates are prewashed in chloroform/methanol (1 : 1, v/v), then activated at 110°C for 1 hr. The plates are placed in a sealed plexiglass spotting apparatus which allows nitrogen to flow continuously over the plate during spotting. An aliquot is spotted which gives PIP$_2$ radioactive counts of 4000–5000 disintegrations/min (dpm). Two primary solvent systems are used: (i) chloroform/methanol/ammonium hydroxide/water (90 : 90 : 7 : 22, v/v) and (ii) chloroform/methanol/ammonium hydroxide/water (70 : 100 : 15 : 25, v/v) a solvent system developed by us. This latter solvent system is found to provide excellent separation of PIP$_3$ and PIP$_2$ in our experiments and has been tested independently by other groups (15, 16). The R_f values for this system on Merck silica gel 60 (0.5 mm) plates are as follows: PIP$_3$, 0.100; PIP$_2$, 0.366; PIP, 0.500; PI, 0.626. The plates are developed using iodine vapors; the appropriate areas are scraped, and scintillation counting is performed (Packard Instrs., Meriden, CT Model 1900CA). For fatty acid determinations, the plates are not developed in iodine and are kept under a nitrogen atmosphere continuously until ready for gas chromatography (GC) injection. PI, PIP, and PIP$_2$ standards (Sigma, St. Louis, MO) are used in all runs. Flo-Scint IV (Packard) is a useful scintillation fluid with high concentrations of ammonium formate in samples. The radioactive counts are derived using computer programs for both quenching and chemiluminescence (Packard).

Alkaline Hydrolysis of Phosphatidylinositol Trisphosphate

The TLC area with the suspected PIP$_3$ and the known area for PIP$_2$ are scraped, and several lanes are collected in order to have adequate counts [~6000–7000 counts/min (cpm)] prior to alkaline hydrolysis. Silica gel H is extracted with chloroform/methanol/0.2 N HCl (1 : 2 : 0.8, v/v), then exposed to 2 N KOH at 80°C for 60 min. Nonradioactive lipid extract is also added to the mixture as a carrier. Cold 70% perchloric acid is added with samples on ice to neutralize the mixture with the precipitation of potassium perchlorate. The mixture is centrifuged at 4°C for 10 min at 1000 g, and the upper phase is used for anion-exchange column chromatography or HPLC analysis.

Analysis of Inositol Phospholipids

Materials

Bio-Rad (Richmond, CA) AG 1-X8 formate resin, 200–400 mesh, and poly-propylene columns are used to separate the individual inositol phosphates. *myo*-Inositol, insulin, calf intestinal alkaline phosphatase, sodium tetraborate (Borax), phytic acid, Triton X-100 were from Sigma Chemical Company. [^{3}H]Ins(1)P, [^{3}H]Ins(1,4)P$_2$, [^{3}H]Ins(1,4,5)P$_3$, and [^{3}H]Ins(1,3,4,5)P$_4$ were obtained from Amersham Corp. (Arlington Heights, IL. [^{3}H]IP$_6$, *myo*-inositol hexakisphosphate, (10–20 Ci/mmol) in ethanol/water (9 : 1, v/v) was obtained from New England Nuclear (Boston, MA) or Amersham. Toluene, formic acid, and magnesium chloride are the best grade available.

Isolation and Separation of Inositol Phosphates by Anion-Exchange Chromatography

The sample is applied to the anion-exchange resin (Bio-Rad, 2 ml column, AG 1-X8 resin, 200–400 mesh) after diluting twice with water, and the elutions are carried out using different ammonium formate/formic acid solutions as described below.

Bio-Rad anion-exchange resin, AG 1-X8, formate form: Resin (2 ml) is packed in a disposable polypropylene column. After packing, the resin in the columns can be washed in 20% methanol and can be stored at 4°C indefinitely

Inositol, 5 mM: 450 mg of inositol is dissolved in 500 ml of water

Ammonium formate, 3 M stock solution: Ammonium formate (189.09 g) is dissolved in 800 ml of water and the volume is finally made up to 1000 ml with water

Ammonium formate (60 mM) 5 mM sodium tetraborate solution [to isolate glycerophosphoinositol (GPI) from the column]: Three M ammonium formate solutions (10 ml) is added to 400 ml of water; 953 mg of sodium tetraborate (Borax) is dissolved in the above solution, and the volume is finally made up to 500 ml with water

Ammonium formate (0.2 M)/0.1 M formic acid solution (to isolate IP$_1$ from the column): Three M ammonium formate solution (33.3 ml) and 2.2 ml of formic acid (88%) are mixed, and the volume is finally made up to 500 ml with water

Ammonium formate (0.5 M)/0.1 M formic acid solution (to isolate IP$_2$): Three M ammonium formate solution (83.3 ml) and 2.2 ml of 88% formic acid are mixed, and the volume is finally made up to 500 ml with water

Ammonium formate (0.85 M)/0.1 M formic acid solution (to isolate IP$_3$): Three M ammonium formate solution (141.7 ml) and 2.2 ml of 88% formic acid are mixed, and the volume is finally made up to 500 ml with water

Ammonium formate (1.2 M)/0.1 M formic acid solution (to isolate IP$_4$): Three M ammonium formate solution (200 ml) and 2.2 ml of 88% formic acid are mixed, and the volume is finally made up to 500 ml with water

Ammonium formate (2.0 M)/0.1 M formic acid solution (to isolate IP$_6$): Three M ammonium formate solution (333 ml) and 2.2 ml of 88% formic acid are mixed, and the volume is finally made up to 500 ml with water

The column is initially washed with 20–30 ml of distilled water. The pH of the sample is adjusted to 7.0. The radioactive sample is diluted equally with water and loaded on the column, with the sample volume ranging from 1 to 2 ml. If the samples are acidic, it is advisable to buffer the samples with a final concentration of 50 mM tricine, pH 7.8–8.0. After loading the sample, the column is washed with 25 ml of 5 mM myo-inositol solution, and five 5-ml fractions are collected. These samples are counted for unbound labeled inositol. Glycerophosphoinositol, IP$_1$, IP$_2$ are eluted from the column by applying 20 ml of the respective ammonium formate solutions, as described above. IP$_3$ is eluted with 30 ml of 0.85 M ammonium formate solution. The larger volume of ammonium formate solution for IP$_3$ is necessary to separate it as a distinct peak from IP$_2$. IP$_4$ is eluted using 1.2 M ammonium formate solution. In our study, we realized that standard tritiated IP$_6$ (New England Nuclear, Boston, MA) can only be eluted from the column with 2 M ammonium formate/0.1 M formic acid solution. In these experiments, 3.0-ml fractions are collected and standardized with authentic nonradioactive and/or radioactive compounds eluted from the column under the experimental conditions. Samples are mixed with 2 to 3 volumes of Flo-Scint III and counted. The peak fractions are obtained as follows: GPI, 8th fraction; IP$_1$, 16th fraction; IP$_2$, 25th fraction; IP$_3$, 33rd fraction; IP$_4$, 40th fraction; IP$_6$, 2 M ammonium formate eluate.

Comments on Phosphate Analysis

Standardization of the elution patterns of the various individual inositol phosphates was conducted with nonradioactive (cold) inositol phosphates prepared from phytic acid hydrolyzate or chick erythrocytes. The inositol phosphates can be hydrolyzed by acid and alkaline conditions. The phosphate moieties thus liberated from inositol phosphates can be estimated in several ways, the choice depending on the situation confronting the investigator (17). Alternatively, inositol phosphates can be conveniently hydrolyzed by alkaline phosphatase, and the liberated inorganic phosphate can be measured by the colorimetric method using malachite green reagent (18). Selectively, the liberated inositol can also be measured with inositol dehydrogenase (19). It should be remembered that anion-exchange column fractions are in acid pH, and therefore it is necessary to adjust the samples to alkaline pH. On the other hand, other methods of phosphate determination such as acid hydrolysis or the malachite green method do not require this step. However, the acid pH in phosphorus determination is critical and must be carefully checked. The pH of the samples is adjusted to 8.5–9.2 with a small volume of 2 N potassium hydroxide.

Analysis of Inositol Phosphates with Alkaline Phosphatase

Assay Reagents

Sodium carbonate–sodium bicarbonate buffer (0.6 M), pH 9.7
Magnesium chloride solution (18 mM)
Zinc acetate solution (6 μM)
Calf intestinal alkaline phosphatase: the enzyme sample is diluted at least 100-fold with 20 mM of sodium carbonate–bicarbonate buffer with 2 mM magnesium chloride and used as an enzyme source
Sodium hydroxide solution (40 mM) with 0.5% ethylenediaminetetraacetic acid (EDTA) disodium salt
Bio-Rad AG 1-X8 resin column fractions

The procedure described here can accommodate a sample volume of 100 μl of eluates. Sodium carbonate–sodium bicarbonate buffer, magnesium chloride solution, zinc acetate, alkaline phosphatase (50 μl each), and column fractions (100 μl) in a total volume of 0.3 ml are incubated at 37°C for 15 min. The length of incubation depends on the concentration of the phosphate sample in the column fractions. The reaction is stopped by the addition of 1.0 ml of 3 N HCl. The liberated inorganic phosphate is measured by the method using malachite green reagent (18). Potassium dihydrogen phosphate is used to calibrate the standard curve.

TABLE I   Comparison of Extraction Methods[a]

Method	Inositol lipids	Inositol phosphates
Hauser and Eichberg	212,412 (15,730)	851,562 (39,165)
Schacht	107,805 (2414)	1,115,091 (27,886)
p value	<0.0002	<0.0006

[a] Values represent the means of five samples in each group, in units of dpm (S.E.M.)/sample. Analysis statistics used the 2-tailed t-test.

Analysis of Inositol Phosphates by High-Performance Liquid Chromatography

An HPLC (Dionex Corp., Sunnyvale, CA) apparatus is used with a Radiomatic DS flow scintillation counter. A Dionex Carbopac PA1 anion-exchange column is used with authentic tritiated standards, to define the elution times for IP_1, IP_2, IP_3, and IP_4 (New England Nuclear). The following buffers are used: buffer A, deionized water with 5 mM cold *myo*-inositol; buffer B, 2 M ammonium formate (pH 3.7 with phosphoric acid. Elution is carried out as follows: 0–10 min of 100% buffer A; 10.1–15 min of 90% A, 10% B; 15.1–20 min of 80% A, 20% B; 20.1–28 min of 70% A, 30% B; 28.1–33 min of 60% A, 40% B; 33.1–40 min of 30% A, 70% B. Under these conditions, IP_1 elutes at 18 min, IP_2 at 23 min, IP_3 at 30 min, and IP_4 at 36 min. Flo-Scint IV (Packard, Instrs., Meriden, CT) is used as the scintillation fluid at a ratio of 4:1 (v/v).

Acid Extraction of Inositol Phospholipids

In comparing the Hauser and Eichberg method (14) with the Schacht method (11), we found that the Hauser and Eichberg method resulted in higher recovery of total inositol lipids, with the Schacht method yielding a higher recovery of inositol phosphates (Table I). The acidity employed in the Schacht method is greater than that in the Hauser and Eichberg method. The data suggest that hydrolysis of inositol phospholipids occurs with the Schacht method, resulting in loss of inositol phospholipids and gains in water-soluble inositol phosphates (Table II). However, a certain amount of acid is necessary to reverse the strong ionic binding of inositol lipids and phosphates with cellular proteins.

TABLE II   Comparison of Extraction Methods for Individual
Inositol Lipids[a]

Lipid	Hauser and Eichberg ($n = 5$)	Schacht ($n = 5$)	p value
PI	4983 (238)	2532 (78)	<0.0001
PIP	766 (35)	433 (3.6)	<0.0001
PIP$_2$	4240 (130)	1955 (48)	<0.0001
PIP$_3$	836 (53)	592 (39)	<0.0062

[a] Data are expressed as dpm (S.E.M.)/100-μl lipid aliquot spotted. Each aliquot represented 0.56 g wet weight and was dissolved in a 2 ml total volume
of chloroform/methanol (2 : 1, v/v). Analysis statistics used the 2-tailed t-test.

Analysis of Phosphatidylinositol Trisphosphates for Inositol Tetrakisphosphate

For the analysis of PIP$_3$ for IP$_4$, the sample is extracted according to the method of Hauser and Eichberg (14). The approximate number of counts per lane are as follows: PIP$_3$, 400–700; PIP$_2$, 1600–2200; PIP, 300–400; and PI, 1500–2000. To determine the polar head group (except for IP$_4$), the PIP$_3$ sample is concentrated and extracted from several TLC lanes. Later, it is subjected to alkaline hydrolysis. This procedure yields 55% of the counts eluting at 35 min, with a smaller peak (40%) at 28 min, when the above-described HPLC procedure is conducted. The larger peak elutes with the [³H]Ins(1,3,4,5)P$_4$. It is recommended that the small samples be processed for alkaline hydrolysis at a lower temperature or at room temperature for a specified time. However, pilot experiments with samples and authentic radiolabeled compounds are of utmost importance to standardize the HPLC technique. Thus, alkaline hydrolysis of PIP$_3$ yields an inositol 1,3,4,5-tetrakis-phosphate (IP$_4$).

Traynor-Kaplan et al. (7) described the detection of an IP$_4$-containing phospholipid in stimulated neutrophils. This observation showed PIP$_3$ running very close to PIP$_2$, using ³²P as the radiolabel, and the identity of PIP$_3$ was investigated using deacylation and headgroup analysis. The deacylated products in their study are primarily glycero-PIP (51–68%), glycero-PIP$_2$ (13–16%), and glycero-PIP$_3$ (8–21%). In our study HPLC analysis of the headgroup from the last fraction ran parallel with authentic radiolabeled IP$_4$ (New England Nuclear, Boston, MA).

Our radiolabeled technique facilitated the isolation of an IP$_4$-containing lipid in rat brain. A major difference between the method of Traynor-Kaplan et al. (7) and the procedure developed in our laboratory is that PIP$_3$ can be distinctly separated from PIP$_2$ on TLC plates. To characterize PIP$_3$ we tested several TLC solvent systems, including chloroform/methanol/4 N ammonium hydroxide (9:7:2, v/v), chloroform/acetone/methanol/acetic acid/water (80:30:26:24:14, v/v), chloroform/methanol/ammonium hydroxide/water (90:90:7:22, v/v), and chloroform/methanol/ammonium hydroxide/water (70:100:15:25, v/v). The last solvent system, developed by us, proved superior in widening the distance between PIP_2 and the origin and also led to better separation of PIP_2 from PIP_3 by approximatley 1–2 inches. It must be emphasized that the brain tissue is initially extracted with chloroform/methanol (1:1, v/v) to eliminate most of the major phospholipids from the samples; the first acidified extract of the same material is the most concentrated sample of polyphosphoinositides, and that is why we recommend those fractions for PIP_3 analysis.

Fatty Acid Analysis

The fatty acid components of PIP_2 and PIP_3 are quantified by GC, essentially according to Morrison and Smith (20). After conversion to fatty acid methyl esters using boron trifluoride and methanol (Sigma), the samples are injected onto a SP-2330 capillary biscyanopropylphenyl polysiloxane phase column (0.32 × 30 m, Supelco, Bellefonte, PA), with a Perkin-Elmer (Norwalk, CT) Model 8500 gas chromatograph using Omega-2 software for data assessment. Caution is taken to minimize contamination of the samples, and nitrogen is used during all steps to prevent oxidation of unsaturated fatty acids. The same number of TLC bands are used for both PIP_2 and PIP_3. Studies on PIP_3 showed the presence of fatty acids characteristic of other inositol phospholipids, namely, PI, PIP, and PIP_2. Figure 3 depicts the fatty acid composition of the PIP_2 and PIP_3 bands and represents the relative amounts of these lipids in rat cerebrum. GC analysis after deacylation and derivatization clearly shows the presence of archidonic acid, a critical moiety of the inositol phospholipid in the samples of both PIP_2 and PIP_3. Assuming that PIP_3 is a fully acylated lipid, our fatty acid data indicate the molar ratio of PIP_2 to PIP_3 is approximately 40:1. Future research may determine that PIP_3 is linked to specific receptors and, with receptors stimulation, is hydrolyzed to IP_4, which may have second messenger function.

Concluding Remarks

The procedures described here furnish a choice of different methods involving both conventional anion-exchange column chromatographic procedures and TLC and HPLC techniques to suit various laboratory conditions and

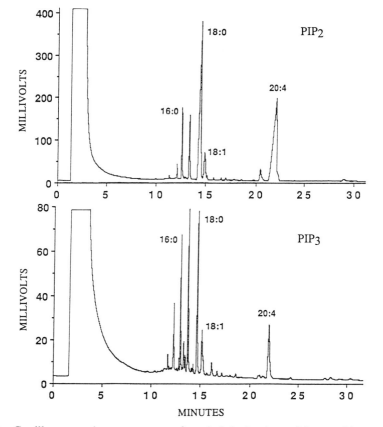

FIG. 3 Capillary gas chromatograms of methyl derivatives of fatty acids extracted from PIP₂ and PIP₃ samples after TLC separation. The top chromatogram shows the pattern obtained from a derivatized extract from PIP₂, and the bottom chromatogram is from PIP₃. Methyl fatty acids are dissolved in GC-grade hexane with the internal standard heptadecanoic acid methyl ester (17:0) which elutes between 16:0 and 18:0 derivatives. Two microliters of PIP₂ or PIP₃ containing 1000 pmol of 17:0 standard is injected into the chromatograph. Arachidonic acid (20:4) is present in both PIP₂ and PIP₃.

needs of investigators for the isolation and analysis of radiolabeled PIP₃ from rat brain.

Acknowledgments

This work was supported by the University of Tennessee, Memphis, and Veteran's Administration Medical Research Funds. L. P. acknowledges the Indian Council of Medical Research, New Delhi, for a J. R. F.

References

1. R. Parthasarathy and F. Eisenberg, Jr., *Biochem. J.* **235,** 313 (1986).
2. R. F. Irvine, *Bioeassays* **13,** 419 (1991).
3. A. Farago and Y. Nishizuka, *FEBS Lett.* **268,** 350 (1990).
4. M. J. Berridge and R. F. Irvine, *Nature (London)* **341,** 197 (1989).
5. T. D. Hill, N. M. Dean, and A. L. Boynton, *Science* **242,** 1176 (1988).
6. M. J. Berridge, *Nature (London)* **361,** 315 (1993).
7. A. E. Traynor-Kaplan, A. L. Harris, B. L. Thompson, P. Taylor, and L. A. Sklar, *Nature (London)* **334,** 353 (1988).
8. C. L. Carpenter and L. C. Cantley, *Biochemistry* **29,** 11147 (1990).
9. H. M. Sarau, M. N. Tzimas, J. J. Foley, J. D. Winkler, M. E. Kennedy, and M. E. Crooke, *in* "Biology of Cellular Transducing Signals," (J. Y. Vanderhoek, ed.), p. 235. Plenum, New York, 1990.
10. P. T. Hawkins, T. R. Jackson, and L. R. Stephens, *Nature (London)* **358,** 157 (1992).
11. J. Schacht, *J. Lipid Res.* **19,** 1063 (1978).
12. R. E. Vadnal and R. Parthasarathy, *Biochem. Biophys. Res. Commun.* **163,** 995 (1989).
13. C. Galli and G. Racagni, *in* "Methods in Enzymology" (W. E. M. Lands and W. L. Smith, eds.), Vol. 86, p. 635. Academic Press, New York, 1982.
14. G. Hauser and J. Eichberg, *Biochim. Biophys. Acta* **326,** 201 (1973).
15. R. Huang, A. Sorisky, W. R. Church, E. R. Simons, and S. E. Rittenhouse, *J. Biol. Chem.* **266,** 18435 (1991).
16. A. N. Carter and C. P. Downes, *J. Biol. Chem.* **267,** 14563 (1992).
17. F. Eisenberg, Jr., and R. Parthasarathy, *in* "Methods of Enzymatic Analysis" (H. U. Bergmeyer, ed.), Vol. 6, p. 371. Verlag Chemie, Weinheim, 1984.
18. F. Eisenberg, Jr., and R. Parthasarathy, *in* "Methods in Enzymology" (P. M. Conn and A. R. Means, eds.), Vol. 141, p. 127. Academic Press, Orlando, Florida, 1987.
19. J. A. Masalanski, L. Leshko, and W. B. Busa, *Science* **256,** 243 (1992).
20. W. R. Morrison and L. M. Smith, *J. Lipid Res.* **5,** 600 (1964).

Section III

Protein Kinase C

[14] Preparation of Protein Kinase C Isozymes and Substrates from Rat Brain

Freesia L. Huang, Kuo-Ping Huang, Fwu-Shan Sheu, and Ken-ichi Osada

Introduction

The potential importance of protein kinase C (PKC) in the regulation of nervous functions has been well recognized. Both the short-term responses associated with neurotransmitter release, modulation of ion channels, regulation of receptor functions, and cellular metabolism as well as long-term responses that are involved in the enhancement of synaptic plasticity and control of growth and differentiation have been linked to the action of PKC. This enzyme family consists of two groups, the Ca^{2+}-dependent group A (α, βI, βII, and γ) and the Ca^{2+}-independent group B (δ, ε, ζ, η, and θ), of phospholipid/diacylglycerol-stimulated serine/threonine protein kinases. These enzymes exhibit distinct cellular and subcellular localizations and show subtle differences in biochemical characteristics and substrate specificities. It is believed that each isoenzyme responds differently to different input signals. However, the detailed mechanism of action of these enzymes *in vivo* is largely unknown. This is in part due to the lack of a specific activator, inhibitor, and substrate for each enzyme to be used for physiological study. Various PKC isoenzymes and several PKC substrates have been isolated from the nervous tissues; these proteins are becoming useful reagents for delineating the role of PKCs in cellular responses.

Reagents

Histone IIIS, protamine sulfate, polylysine-agarose, pepstatin A, and phenylmethylsulfonyl fluoride (PMSF) are from Sigma (St. Louis, MO); leupeptin, chymostatin, histone H1 from Boehringer Mannheim (Mannheim, Germany); phosphatidylserine (PS) and dioleoylglycerol (DAG) from Avanti Polar Lipids (Birmingham, AL); phenyl-Sepharose, Mono Q columns, and Nonidet P-40 (NP-40) from Pharmacia LKB Biotechnology, Inc. (Piscataway, NJ); hydroxylapatite (BioGel HT) and anion-exchange resin AG 1-X8 from Bio-Rad (Richmond, CA); [γ-^{32}P]ATP from Du Pont–New England Nuclear

(Boston, MA); MBP$_{4-14}$ [Gln-Lys-Arg-Pro-Ser(8)-Gln-Arg-Ser-Lys-Tyr-Leu] from Research Genetics (Huntsville, AL); DEAE-cellulose (DE-52) and phosphocellulose paper (P81) from Whatman (Clifton, NJ); and antibodies against PKC α, β, and γ are prepared as previously described (1) and antibody against PKC ε is prepared with a PKC ε-specific peptide.

Assay of Protein Kinase C Activity

The kinase activity is usually monitored by the incorporation of ^{32}P from [γ-^{32}P]ATP into protein or peptide substrates. The Ca^{2+}-dependent enzymes (PKC α, β, and γ) are measured at 30°C in 25 μl of a reaction mixture containing 30 mM Tris-HCl buffer (pH 7.5), 6 mM magnesium chloride, 0.12 mM [γ-^{32}P]ATP, 0.25 mM EGTA, 0.4 mM CaCl$_2$, mixed lipid vesicles containing 40 μg/ml PS and 8 μg/ml DAG or detergent/lipid mixed micelles containing 0.04% NP-40, 100 μg/ml PS, and 20 μg/ml DAG, and 160 μg/ml synthetic peptide MBP$_{4-14}$, 1 mg/ml histone IIIS, or 1 mg/ml protamine sulfate. Mixed lipid vesicles of PS/DAG are prepared by sonication and vortexing of the lipid mixture, with the chloroform previously evaporated off by a stream of N$_2$, suspended in 20 mM Tris-HCl buffer, pH 7.5. Detergent/lipid mixed micelles are prepared by mixing PS/DAG vesicles with NP-40. The Ca^{2+}-independent PKCs are measured under the same conditions without Ca^{2+} but containing 2 mM EGTA.

Incorporation of ^{32}P into peptide substrate is measured by spotting 20 μl of the reaction mixture to a piece of phosphocellulose (Whatman P81) paper (1.2 × 3 cm) numbered with a pencil and dropping it into 75 mM phosphoric acid (5 ml of 85% phosphoric acid/liter). When testing activities in crude tissue and cell homogenates, the endogenously phosphorylated proteins must be removed by the addition of 10 μl of 40% trichloroacetic acid (TCA) and 5 μl of 10 mg/ml bovine serum albumin as carrier. Following standing in ice for at least 10 min, the precipitated protein is removed by centrifugation, and a 20-μl aliquot is spotted to P81 paper and dropped into 75 mM phosphoric acid. The phosphocellulose pieces are washed in a 600-ml beaker fitted at the bottom with a stainless steel screen to allow free rotation of a magnetic bar. The paper pieces are washed 4 times with 200 ml of 75 mM phosphoric acid and dried under a heating lamp. Radioactive ^{32}P-labeled peptide is counted in a scintillation counter after adding 10 ml of scintillant fluid. Measurement of ^{32}P incorporation into protein substrate is done by spotting 20 μl of the reaction mixture to an ITLC (Gelman, Ann Arbor, MI, instant thin-layer chromatography sheet, type SG) strip (1 × 9.5 cm) 1.5 cm from the bottom (previously spotted with 20 μl of 15% TCA containing 50 mM ATP) followed by chromatography for 6 min in a beaker containing 5% TCA and

0.2 M KCl (with protamine sulfate as a substrate, 30% TCA solution is used). After the strips are air dried, the origin (area approximately 1 cm below and 1.5 cm above the line of origin), which contains the phosphorylated protein, is excised for counting in a scintillation counter.

At times, certain small M_r protein substrates are not readily precipitated by 10–20% TCA nor contain enough net basic amino acid residues to allow quantitative binding to phosphocellulose paper; in such cases, the phosphorylated proteins are separated from [γ-^{32}P]ATP by the anion-exchange column method. The kinase reaction is stopped by the addition of 50 μl of glacial acetic acid containing 20 mM ATP, and the entire reaction mixture is transferred to an AG 1-X8/DEAE-cellulose column, packed in a glass wool-plugged disposable glass pipette with DEAE-cellulose (Whatman DE-52) at the bottom to a height of 1 cm and a 4 cm height of AG 1-X8 (100–200 mesh) on top, previously washed with 30% acetic acid. The columns are washed with 0.25 ml of 30% acetic acid and eluted with 0.75 ml of 30% acetic acid. The residual eluate is emptied from the column by blowing a stream of air through the pipette. Radioactivity is determined by scintillation counting after adding 10 ml of scintillant fluid.

To ascertain the phosphorylation of proteins and/or peptide substrates, the kinase reaction is stopped by the addition of sodium dodecyl sulfate–polyacrylamide gel electrophoresis (SDS-PAGE) sample buffer followed by electrophoresis in a 10–20% (w/v) polyacrylamide gradient gel. Radioactive ATP migrates ahead of the bromophenol blue dye and can be cleared from the gel by allowing the dye to migrate off the gel. Phosphorylated proteins and peptides can be detected by autoradiography without staining.

Nonradioactive methods for the assay of PKC have been devised based on the phosphorylation-induced changes in the fluorescent intensity of the substrates. Phosphorylation of a 6-acryloyl-2-dimethylaminonaphthalene-labeled 25-amino acid peptide (2) containing the PKC phosphorylation sites of MARCKS protein (3) and a synthetic peptide derived from the phosphorylation site of the β-subunit of phosphorylase kinase (4) results in a reduction of fluorescence. In our study of the phosphorylation of neurogranin (RC3 protein) from rat brain, we noticed that a 19-amino acid synthetic peptide [AAAKIQAS(36)FRGHMARKKIK] corresponding to the phosphorylation site of this protein was a specific substrate of PKC. Substitution of Phe-37 with tryptophan generated a PKC substrate, and its fluorescence increased over 20% following phosphorylation. The kinase activity can be monitored by the increase in the emission fluorescence at 355 nm when excited at 290 nm. These fluorescent substrates are applicable for kinetics analysis of purified enzymes but are less useful for analyzing the crude enzyme preparations.

Preparation of Protein Kinase C Isozymes and Substrates from Rat Brain

Buffers

Homogenizing buffer: 20 mM Tris-HCl, pH 7.5, containing 1 mM dithiothreitol (DTT), 2 mM EDTA, 5 mM EGTA, 0.5 mM PMSF, and 2 μg/ml each of leupeptin, chymostatin, and pepstatin A

Buffer A: 20 mM Tris-HCl, pH 7.5, containing 1 mM DTT, 0.5 mM EGTA, 0.5 mM EDTA, and 10% glycerol

Buffer B: 20 mM KPO$_4$, pH 7.5, containing 1 mM DTT, 0.5 mM EGTA, 0.5 mM EDTA, and 10% glycerol

Buffer C: 300 mM KPO$_4$, pH 7.5, containing 1 mM DTT, 0.5 mM EGTA, 0.5 mM EDTA, and 10% glycerol

Buffer D: Buffer A plus 0.6 M KCl

Purification of Protein Kinase C Isozymes

PKC α, β, γ, and ε are copurified from the rat brain extract during the early stage of purification, and resolution of each isozyme is achieved at the final step by hydroxylapatite column chromatography. Fresh rat brains (120 g wet weight) from 75 male Sprague-Dawley rats (200–250 g) are homogenized in 600 ml of ice-cold homogenizing buffer using a Polytron (Brinkmann Instruments, Westbury, NY) at setting 5 with four 15-sec bursts. The homogenate is centrifuged at 34,000 rpm at 4°C for 1 hr using Beckman (Fullerton, CA) 35 rotors. The supernatant fluid is decanted carefully to avoid the turbid fluffy layer. The combined fluffy layer and the pellet are extracted once again with 400 ml of the homogenizing buffer.

The combined high-speed supernatant fluid is adjusted to pH 7.5 by adding 2 M Tris base and applied to a DEAE-cellulose column (4.0 × 16 cm) equilibrated with buffer A. The particulate fraction can be extracted twice with homogenization buffer containing 1% NP-40 as starting material for the purification of PKC δ. The column is washed with 1 liter of buffer A, containing 50 mM KCl and PKC is eluted at a flow rate of 120 ml/hr with 0.15 M KCl in buffer A for 7 hr and then an increase of KCl from 0.15 to 0.3 M over 4 hr. PKC α, β, γ, and ε coelute from buffer containing 0.15 M KCl and are pooled (700–800 ml) and concentrated by ultrafiltration to approximately 100–150 ml with two 400-ml Amicon (Beverly, MA) cells fitted with YM10 membranes. Solid KCl is added to a final concentration of 1.5 M, and the sample is applied to a phenyl-Sepharose column (2.5 × 16 cm) equilibrated with buffer A containing 1.5 M KCl. The column is washed with 100 ml of equilibration buffer, and the kinase is eluted with a 1.5–0 M KCl gradient over 5 hr at a flow rate of 100 ml/hr. PKC-containing fractions are pooled and concentrated by ultrafiltration with Amicon cells fitted with YM10 membranes. The concentrated solution (7–10 ml) is applied to Sephacryl S-200 column (2.5 × 95 cm) equilibrated with buffer A. Fractions of 3.5 ml are collected, and the pooled kinase (70–80 ml) is applied to a polylysine-agarose column (2.0 × 14 cm) equilibrated with buffer A. The column is washed with 50 ml of buffer A and eluted with a 0–0.3 M KCl gradient over 3.5 hr and 0.3–0.8 M KCl over 2 hr at a flow rate of 100 ml/hr. Fractions of 5 ml are collected. PKC α, β, and γ are eluted as a broad peak between 0.3 and 0.8 M KCl. PKC ε, which exhibits relatively poor kinase activity toward histone IIIS, does not appear as a separate activity peak by kinase assay and is eluted slightly ahead of the broad PKC activity peak. Positive identification of PKC ε is carried out by immunoblot analysis with a specific antibody.

Fractions containing the major PKC α, β, and γ and those also containing PKC ε are concentrated separately in Amicon cells and exchanged with buffer B by repetitive dilution and concentration. Resolution of PKC, α, β, and γ from the major activity peak by hydroxylapatite column is carried out as previously described (5). The concentrated enzyme (10–15 ml), which contains PKC ε is applied to a hydroxylapatite column packed in a Pharmacia HR 10/10 column (1.0 × 7 cm) and equilibrated with buffer B at a flow rate of 0.5 ml/min controlled by a Pharmacia fast protein liquid chromatography (FPLC) unit. Following washing with 10 ml buffer B, chromatography is carried out by using buffer B and buffer C according to the following program: 0–5 ml, buffer C is maintained at 0%; 5–15 ml, buffer C is increased to 10%; 15–45 ml, buffer C is increased to 20%; 45–65 ml, buffer C is increased to 40%; 65–95 ml, buffer C is increased to 100%; and 95–105 ml, buffer C is kept at 100%. PKC γ, β, ε, and α are eluted at 18, 25, 40, and 65% buffer C, respectively (Fig. 1).

PKC δ is mainly associated with the particulate fraction. The enzyme extracted with homogenization buffer containing 1% NP-40 is purified similarly by column chromatography on DEAE-cellulose, phenyl-Sepharose, and Sephacryl S-200; PKC δ is tailing from the main Ca^{2+}/PS/DAG-dependent histone kinase activity in the last column. This kinase is further purified by poly(lysine)-agarose, Mono Q, and hydroxylapatite column chromatography. PKC ζ has been purified from bovine kidney (6) but not from brain.

Preparation of Protein Kinase C Substrates from Rat Brain

Neuromodulin (B50, F1, GAP43) (for review, see Ref. 7), MARCKS (8), and neurogranin (RC3, p17) (9, 10) are among the most prominent substrates of PKC in the brain. These three proteins share several common properties,

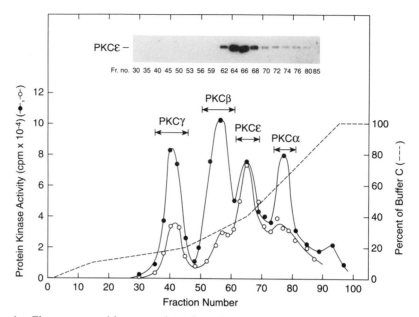

FIG. 1   Chromatographic separation of PKC α, β, γ, and ε from the hydroxylapatite column. Concentrated and dialyzed PKC from the polylysine-agarose column was applied to a hydroxylapatite column packed in a Pharmacia HR10/10 column attached to a Pharmacia FPLC unit at a flow rate of 0.5 ml/min. Fractions of 1 ml were collected for the measurements of histone kinase activity with Ca^{2+}/PS/DAG ($\bullet$) or PS/DAG in the presence of 2 mM EGTA ($\bigcirc$). The increment of buffer C is indicated by the dashed line. Confirmation of the elution position of PKC ε was provided by immunoblot analysis with specific antibodies (inset). Identifications of PKC, α, β, and γ were as previously described [K.-P. Huang, H. Nakabayashi, and F. L. Huang, *Proc. Natl. Acad. Sci. U.S.A.* **83,** 8535 (1986)].

such as stabilities to heat and acid treatments, and exhibit aberrant mobility on SDS-PAGE. Rat brain neurogranin, neuromodulin, and MARCKS have predicted M_r values of 7,500, 24,000, and 29,000, respectively, whereas on SDS-PAGE in the presence of reducing agent, the respective M_r values are 15,000–17,000, 40,000–50,000, and 80,000–87,000, depending on the conditions of electrophoresis. Neuromodulin and neurogranin bind calmodulin in the absence of Ca^{2+} (10, 11), whereas MARCKS is a Ca^{2+}-dependent calmodulin-binding protein (12). These proteins, as a group, can be purified from the same rat brain extract.

Frozen rat brains (250 g), after being thawed at room temperature, are homogenized with a Polytron in 1250 ml of buffer A containing protease inhibitors. The homogenate is centrifuged at 10,000 g in a Sorvall GS-3 rotor for 30 min and the supernatant fluid filtered through glass wool. The resulting pellet is extracted once with 650 ml of the same buffer. To the combined supernatant fluid, 60% $HClO_4$ is added slowly with constant mixing to a final concentration of 2.2%. The precipitated protein is discarded following centrifugation at 10,000 g for 20 min. The supernatant fluid is neutralized with solid KOH and kept at 0°C for at least 10 min to precipitate $KClO_4$. The clarified solution obtained after centrifugation is concentrated and dialyzed in Amicon ultrafiltration cells fitted with YM5 membranes. The resulting pinkish solution (10–20 ml) is applied to a DEAE-cellulose column packed in Pharmacia HR16/10 (1.6 × 10 cm) equilibrated with buffer A. Chromatography is carried out at room temperature with the column attached to a Pharmacia FPLC unit using a KCl gradient made up of buffer A and buffer D (buffer A plus 0.6 M KCl) as follows: 0–25 ml, buffer D is maintained at 0%; 25–375 ml, buffer D is increased to 50%; 375–450 ml, buffer D is increased to 100%. Neurogranin is eluted between 5 and 10%, neuromodulin between 25 and 30%, and MARCKS between 30 and 40% buffer D as identified by SDS-PAGE (10–20% acrylamide gradient) and autoradiography following phosphorylation with PKC β.

Neurogranin is further purified to near homogeneity by chromatography on a hydroxylapatite column with buffer B and C as follows: 0–15 ml, buffer C is kept at 0%; 15–70 ml, buffer C is increased to 100%; 70–85 ml, buffer C is maintained at 100%. Neurogranin is eluted between 15 and 25% of buffer C. Neuromodulin and MARCKS, each pooled separately from the DEAE-cellulose column chromatography step, can be purified by published methods (12, 13). Alternatively, they can be purified by hydroxylapatite column chromatography under the same conditions as used for neurogranin. Neuromodulin is eluted between 25 and 35% and MARCKS between 40 and 60% of buffer C. Homogeneous preparations of neuromodulin and MARCKS are prepared by subsequent purification on a Vydac C_4 reversed-phase column (214-TP510, 1 × 25 cm). Samples from the hydroxylapatite column in 2-ml aliquots are filtered and injected into a C_4 column equilibrated with 0.1% trifluoroacetic acid (TFA) and eluted at 2 ml/min with a CH_3CN (in 0.1% TFA) gradient using a high-performance liquid chromatography (HPLC) unit as follows: 0–10 ml, CH_3CN is maintained at 0%; 10–120 ml, CH_3CN is increased to 60%; 120–122 ml, CH_3CN is increased to 100%; 122–150 ml, CH_3CN is maintained at 100%. Neuromodulin is eluted at 30–33% CH_3CN and MARCKS at 42–44%. Under the same conditions, neurogranin is eluted at 36–39% CH_3CN. SDS-PAGE analysis of the purified proteins is shown in Fig. 2; the apparent M_r values of neurogranin, neuromodulin, and MARCKS estimated under the electrophoresis conditions are 16,000, 40,000, and 80,000, respectively (Fig. 2).

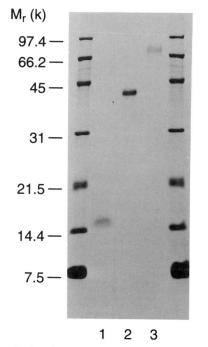

F IG. 2 SDS-PAGE analysis of purified rat brain neurogranin, neuromodulin, and MARCKS. The apparent M_r values of purified neurogranin (M_r 16,000) (lane 1), neuromodulin (M_r 40,000) (lane 2), and MARCKS (M_r 80,000) (lane 3) were estimated using phosphorylase (M_r 97,400), bovine serum albumin (M_r 66,200), ovalbumin (M_r 45,000), carbonate dehydratase (M_r 31,000), soybean trypsin inhibitor (M_r 21,500), lysozyme (M_r 14,400), and rat brain ubiquitin (M_r 7,500) as standard proteins.

Comments

The cofactor requirements of the PKC-catalyzed reaction depend on the substrates used in the assay. With histone H1 as a substrate, PKC α, β, and γ are stimulated by Ca^{2+}, PS, and DAG or phorbol ester, PKC δ and ε are stimulated by PS and DAG, and PKC ζ is stimulated by PS alone. The kinase activity inherent in PKC η and θ has not been well characterized. PKC ε, unlike the other PKCs, phosphorylates histone H1 poorly as compared to myelin basic protein; however, the histone kinase activity is enhanced following proteolysis (15). When assayed with protamine sulfate as a substrate, the activities of all PKCs are independent of the cofactors. Significant variations in the cofactor requirement are related to the interactions among the various components in the assay (16). Synthetic peptides corresponding to the sites of phosphorylation of numerous PKC substrates, with the consensus sequence motifs S/TXK/R, K/RXXS/T, K/RXXS/TXK/R, K/RXS/T, and K/RXS/TXK/R (17), are convenient substrates for measuring cofactor-stimulated PKC activity. Synthetic peptide MBP_{4-14}, containing the PKC phosphorylation site (Ser-8) in myelin basic protein, is a specific peptide substrate of PKC (18).

PKC α, β, γ, and ε are closely related kinases that are copurified by DEAE-cellulose, phenyl-Sepharose, and gel filtration column chromatography. The minor differences in the M_r values of PKC α, β, and γ (80,000–82,000) and PKC ε (90,000–94,000) did not result in the separation of these proteins by Sephacryl S-200 gel filtration chromatography. Partial separation of the enzymes was observed on chromatography on a polylysine-agarose column, from which PKC ε was eluted at a slightly lower salt concentration than PKC α, β, and γ, perhaps owing to a lower affinity of the former toward polylysine than the latter enzymes. Previously, we have unknowingly excluded PKC ε during our purification of PKC α, β, and γ (19) because of the relatively low activity of PKC ε toward histone as a substrate. By including fractions containing PKC ε, as detected by specific antibody, from the polylysine-agarose column chromatography step, PKC α, β, γ, and ε were separated by hydroxylapatite column chromatography. Relying on NP-40 extraction of the particulate fraction, which exclude the bulk of other PKCs, and slight separation of PKC δ from other isozymes on Sephacryl S-200 and polylysine-agarose, this procedure is applicable for the preparation of PKC δ. This kinase can also be prepared according to the recently reported method of Ogita *et al.* (20). Methods for the preparation of PKC ε from rabbit (21) and rat (22) brains have also been described.

Preparation of neuromodulin, neurogranin, and MARCKS is greatly simplified by the perchloric acid precipitation method first described by Baudier *et al.* (23). Development of the current procedures stemmed from our failure to obtain a good yield of rat brain neurogranin and neuromodulin by affinity chromatography on calmodulin-Sepharose, as was also noted by Houbre *et al.* (24). With the procedures described here, several milligrams of neuromodulin and neurogranin could be obtained from 250 g of rat brain; the yield of MARCKS was, however, almost a magnitude less than those of the former two proteins. Identification of these PKC substrates during purification is based on the apparent M_r on SDS-PAGE, immunoreactivities toward specific antibodies, and elution profiles on the C_4 reversed-phase column. It should be noted that these proteins, for yet unknown reasons, are frequently eluted from the C_4 column as cluster of peaks of the same M_r.

PKC activity can be regulated both at the enzyme and the substrate levels. Activators, such as PS, Ca^{2+}, DAG or phorbol esters and related tumor promoters, phosphatidylinositol 4,5-bisphosphate (PIP_2), and unsaturated free fatty acids, and inhibitors, such as sphingosine, alkyllysophospholipid, H-7, staurosporine, and calphostin C, as well as the endogenous PKC inhibitor-1 (25), annexin V (26), and the $M_r = 29,000–33,000$ inhibitor proteins of Toker et al. (27), are believed to target at the kinase. Calmodulin, which binds neuromodulin, neurogranin, and MARCKS at a domain adjacent to the PKC phosphorylation site(s), exerts its inhibitory effect by hindering the access of the kinase to the substrates.

References

1. F. L. Huang, Y. Yoshida, and K.-P. Huang, in "Methods in Enzymology" (T. Hunter and B. M. Sefton, eds.), Vol. 200, p. 454. Academic Press, San Diego, 1991.
2. B. K. McLlroy, J. D. Walters, and J. D. Johnson, Anal. Biochem. **195,** 148 (1991).
3. J. M. Graff, D. J. Stumpo, and P. J. Blackshear, J. Biol. Chem. **264,** 11912 (1989).
4. Z. Zhao, D. A. Malencik, and S. R. Anderson, Biochem. Biophys. Res. Commun. **176,** 1454 (1991).
5. K.-P. Huang and F. L. Huang, in "Methods in Enzymology" (T. Hunter and B. M. Sefton, eds.), Vol. 200, p. 241. Academic Press, San Diego, 1991.
6. H. Nakanishi and J. H. Exton, J. Biol. Chem. **267,** 16347 (1992).
7. P. J. Coggins and H. Zwiers, J. Neurochem. **56,** 1095 (1991).
8. D. J. Stumpo, J. M. Graff, K. A. Albert, P. Greengard, and P. J. Blackshear, Proc. Natl. Acad. Sci. U.S.A. **86,** 4012 (1989).
9. J. B. Watson, E. F. Battenberg, K. K. Wong, F. E. Bloom, and J. G. Sutcliffe, J. Neurosci. Res. **26,** 397 (1990).
10. J. Baudier, J. C. Deloulme, A. VanDorsselaer, D. Black, and H. W. D. Matthes, J. Biol. Chem. **266,** 229 (1991).
11. B. M. Cimler, T. J. Andreasen, K. I. Andreasen, and D. R. Storm, J. Biol. Chem. **260,** 10784 (1985).
12. J. M. Graff, T. N. Young, J. D. Johnson, and P. J. Blackshear, J. Biol. Chem. **264,** 21818 (1989).
13. T. J. Andreasen, C. W. Luetje, W. Heideman, and D. R. Storm, Biochemistry **22,** 4615 (1983).
14. K. A. Albert, A. C. Nairn, and P. Greengard, Proc. Natl. Acad. Sci. U.S.A. **84,** 7046 (1987).
15. D. Schaap, J. Hsuan, N. Totty, and P. J. Parker, Eur. J. Biochem. **191,** 431 (1990).
16. M. D. Bazzi and G. L. Nelsestuen, Biochemistry **26,** 1974 (1987).
17. R. B. Pearson and B. E. Kemp, in "Methods in Enzymology" (T. Hunter and B. M. Sefton, eds.), Vol. 200, p. 62. Academic Press, San Diego, 1991.
18. I. Yasuda, A. Kishimoto, S. Tanaka, M. Tominaga, A. Sakurai, and Y. Nishizuka, Biochem. Biophys. Res. Commun. **166,** 1220 (1990).
19. K.-P. Huang, H. Nakabayashi, and F. L. Huang, Proc. Natl. Acad. Sci. U.S.A. **83,** 8535 (1986).

20. K. Ogita, S. Miyamoto, K. Yamaguchi, H. Koide, N. Fujisawa, U. Kikkawa, S. Sahara, Y. Fukami, and Y. Nishizuka, *Proc. Natl. Acad. Sci. U.S.A.* **89,** 1592 (1992).

21. T.C. Saido, K. Mizuno, Y. Konno, S. Osada, S. Ohno, and K. Suzuki, *Biochemistry* **31,** 482 (1992).

22. H. Koide, K. Ogita, U. Kikkawa, and Y. Nishizuka, *Proc. Natl. Acad. Sci. U.S.A.* **89,** 1149 (1992).

23. J. Baudier, C. Bronner, D. Kligman, and R. D. Cole, *J. Biol. Chem.* **264,** 1824 (1989).

24. D. Houbre, G. Duportail, J. C. Deloulme, and J. Baudier, *J. Biol. Chem.* **266,** 7121 (1991).

25. J. D. Pearson, D. B. De Wold, W. R. Mathews, N. M. Mozier, H. A. Zürcher-Neely, R. L. Heinrikson, M. A. Morris, W. D. McCubbin, J. R. McDonald, E. D. Fraser, H. J. Vogel, C. M. Kay, and M. P. Walsh, *J. Biol. Chem.* **265,** 4583 (1990).

26. D. D. Schlaepfer, J. Jones, and H. T. Haigler, *Biochemistry* **31,** 1886 (1992).

27. A. Toker, L. A. Sellers, B. Amess, Y. Patel, A. Harris, and A. Aitken, *Eur. J. Biochem.* **206,** 453 (1992).

[15] Protein Kinase C, a Zinc Metalloprotein: Quantitation of Zinc by Atomic Absorption Spectrometry

Andrew F. G. Quest, Elaine S. G. Bardes,
John Bloomenthal, Roy A. Borchardt,
and Robert M. Bell

Introduction

Protein kinase C (PKC) is an important enzyme for the control of cellular function and growth. In neuronal tissues it participates in the regulation of processes such as transmitter release, ion channel modulation, receptor down-regulation, neuronal development and regeneration, and long-term potentiation (1–3). Members of the PKC family of serine/threonine protein kinases are divided into two groups based on cDNA-derived protein sequence similarities: calcium-dependent and calcium-independent enzymes. Each type possesses two functionally distinct segments, a COOH-terminal kinase domain and an NH_2-terminal regulatory domain (3, 4). The regulatory domain contains a number of distinct regions that promote interactions of PKC with lipids. One such region, called C1, binds tumor-promoting phorbol esters like phorbol 12,13-dibutyrate (PDBu) and, by inference, is probably also the site of interaction with physiological activators of PKC like sn-1,2-diacyglycerols (DAG). In the calcium-dependent PKC isozymes, PDBu binding sites are located within two cysteine-rich protein regions that show striking similarity to zinc-coordinating sequences identified in transcription factors (4–6). Such regions are also present in calcium-independent enzymes, but not all members of this group bind phorbol esters (7). Initial qualitative evidence for zinc coordination by PKC was provided by the capacity of these cysteine-rich regions expressed as fusion proteins in *Escherichia coli* to bind radioactive zinc (8). Subsequent quantitative analysis of native enzymes and proteolytic fragments derived from them revealed that the lipid-binding regulatory domain of PKC contains four atoms of tightly bound zinc (9).

In some transcription factors, protein structures coordinating zinc are essential for their capacity to recognize and bind to specific DNA sequences (10). Elucidating both the sites of zinc coordination and the resulting protein structure within the regulatory domain should yield insights at the molecular level into the mechanism of PKC activation by lipids. Precise measurements

Methods in Neurosciences, Volume 18

of zinc play a pivotal role in establishing such understanding. Here we describe in detail the methods employed to quantitate zinc by atomic absorption spectrometry in mixtures of PKC isozymes purified from tissue homogenates, individual isozymes expressed in *Spodoptera frugiperda* (Sf9) insect cells, PKCα fragments generated by proteolysis, as well as PKCγ segments expressed in *E. coli* as fusion proteins with glutathione *S*-transferase (GST) (11). Furthermore, we discuss some structural inferences that have been made based on these results.

Methods and Results of Zinc Measurements with Protein Kinase C

Choice of Method of Detection

A wide variety of zinc detection methods are currently available which provide flexibility in terms of the size and number of samples to be measured, the range of zinc concentrations over which measurements are linear, and whether the sample is destroyed by the analysis. The majority of the techniques are spectroscopic with widely varying detection limits (12). At present the most commonly employed methods are based on atomic spectrometry. The amounts of PKC available for such analysis are generally extremely limited (nanogram to microgram range). Electrothermal atomic absorption spectroscopy with its increased sensitivity using small sample volumes (5–50 µl) and a detection limit for zinc of 1.5 pg (13) was the method of choice under these circumstances. Although this method is more sensitive, its precision (5–10%) is less than that obtained with flame atomic absorption spectroscopy (2–5%). The known limitations of electrothermal atomic absorption spectroscopy are due to problems arising when samples are vaporized and atomized under rapidly changing conditions while the analytical measurements is in progress. Anything in the sample medium, such as buffer components, may reduce the accuracy by altering evaporation or the dissociation process. This is discussed later (see Fig. 2).

Preparation of Reagents

Zinc is present everywhere in the environment. Thus, avoiding adventitious sample contamination during analysis is important and represents the major obstacle to experimental success. The steps considered essential for accurate zinc measurements of PKC samples are summarized below. Additional general information concerning any one of these steps is reviewed in Volume 158 of *Methods in Enzymology*.

Water

Ultrapure water is essential. Large volumes of reliably high-quality water are obtained with a HYDRO PICOpure water system (HYDRO, Research Triangle Park, NC). The background zinc readings with water are routinely monitored and must be virtually zero.

Nitric Acid

Nitric acid is required to remove zinc from any surfaces with which buffers and samples might come in contact. It is also used as a diluent of protein samples. The acid is supplied as an approximately 70% concentrated stock solution. Reagent-grade products of most manufacturers are satisfactory (e.g., Mallinckrodt, St. Louis, MO, No. 2704). Note that once a bottle has been verified satisfactory, the entire bottle should be dedicated to this cause and maintained zinc-free by applying the precautions specified below.

Containers and Laboratory Ware

Glass containers or metal surfaces should be avoided. Plastic containers of any kind are generally adequate, but they must be either new or dedicated solely to measuring zinc. Although some pigments used to stain plastic contain metal ions and therefore represent a potential source for zinc contamination, in our experience colored plastic surfaces do not pose an additional threat to the measurements if treated as described. Before each usage containers are washed with 7% (w/v) nitric acid and then rinsed extensively with zinc-free water. For all manipulations gloves should be worn. The gloves are treated externally as described above with acid and zinc-free water. Each pipette tip is rinsed first with 7% (w/v) nitric acid, then with zinc-free water, and finally with 0.2% (w/v) nitric acid immediately before actually pipetting a solution or sample of interest. Metal-free dialysis tubing is prepared as described (14). Sample cups (Perkin-Elmer Cetus, Norwalk, CT, No. BO 119070) are stored inside plastic bags to prevent the accumulation of dust. Cups are only retrieved wearing cleaned gloves. Prior to usage for zinc measurements they are washed with 7% (w/v) nitric acid, rinsed three times with zinc-free water, drained upside down on diaper paper, and left to air-dry.

Buffers and Solutions

Generally reagent-grade chemicals routinely available [i.e., not high-performance liquid chromatography (HPLC) grade] are sufficient, except in the cases specified below (Triton X-100: Surfact-Amps X-100, Pierce Chemical Co., Rockford, IL, No. 28314; dioleylphosphatidylserine: Avanti Polar Lipids Inc., Birmingham, AL). Buffers are made by dissolving the products in zinc-free water in washed plastic containers. If zinc levels are not sufficiently low (i.e., absorption less than 0.08 after 10-fold dilution with diluent), buffers are made zinc-free by either dithizone–chloroform extraction or cation-exchange chromatography (12).

The solution should be pH 7–7.5 for dithizone extraction. One milliliter of 0.01% (w/v) dithizone in pure chloroform is added per 10 ml of solution in a separator funnel. The solutions are mixed by shaking until the green color of the organic phase turns pink. After separation of aqueous and organic phases, the latter is removed. The procedure is repeated until no perceptible color change occurs in the organic phase. Traces of dithizone are removed by back-extraction with 1 ml of chloroform per 10 ml of solution. Residual chloroform is removed under vacuum.

Although very effective in removing zinc, the above method is time-consuming and limited by both pH and the composition of the buffers. Ion-exchange chromatography with a chelating resin, Chelex 100 (Bio-Rad Laboratories, Richmond, CA), is preferentially used following the manufacturer's instructions for conditioning the resin. For large volumes of buffer, the only satisfactory procedure is to make zinc-free concentrated stock solutions and dilute them to the final concentration required with zinc-free water. Storage of such stock solutions is problematic. To ensure that buffers are zinc-free it is simpler, in most cases, to start from fresh reagents using clean labware than to attempt to maintain zinc-free stock solutions.

Chromatographic Columns

The chromatographic columns are washed first with 10 volumes of 10 mM ethylenebis (oxyethylenenitrilo) tetraacetic acid (EGTA) followed by another wash of at least 10 column volumes of zinc-free buffer in which the column is to be equilibrated. Before samples are applied to the column, flow-through fractions are monitored for the presence of zinc.

Purification of Protein Kinase C Samples

Rat Brain Protein Kinase C or Isozymes Expressed in Sf9 Cells

PKC is purified from rat brain or infected Sf9 cells as described (15). Purified enzyme preparations are stored at −70°C in storage buffer [20 mM tris(hydroxymethyl)aminomethane (Tris)-HCl (pH 7.5), 0.5 mM EGTA, 0.5 mM ethylenedinitrilotetraacetic acid (EDTA), 10 mM 2-mercaptoethanol, 10% (v/v) glycerol, and 0.05% (w/v) Triton X-100]. To obtain rat brain PKC of the same quality as the individual isozymes purified from Sf9 cell homogenates, an additional step after phenyl-Superose chromatography on fast protein liquid chromatography (FPLC) HR5/5 Mono Q column (Pharmacia LKB Biotechnology, Piscataway, NJ) is required (9).

Protein Kinase C Domains Expressed as Fusion Proteins in
Escherichia coli

To generate large quantities of PKC subdomains, in particular the cysteine-rich phorbol ester-binding regions, these are expressed in *E. coli* as COOH-terminal fusion proteins with GST from *Schistosoma japonicum* and are purified from *E. coli* extracts by affinity chromatography on a glutathione-agarose matrix (Sigma, St. Louis, MO, No. G-4510). All fusion proteins are stored at $-70°C$ in elution buffer containing 50 mM 4-(2-hydroxyethyl)-1-piperazineethanesulfonic acid (HEPES), pH 8, with 10% (v/v) ethylene glycol. Further details of the procedures involved and particularly the PKC domains characterized in this fashion are presented elsewhere (11, 16). Note, however, that in contrast to rat brain PKC or the individual isozymes, GST fusion proteins with PKC domains are never stored in the presence of chelators, as discussed later (see Fig. 3).

Removal of Adventitious Zinc from Protein Kinase C Samples

PKC samples are prepared from tissue or Sf9 cells in the presence of buffers containing chelators, and GST fusion proteins are prepared in their absence. In any case, contamination of the protein samples by adventitious zinc is to be expected because none of the buffers used during the preparations are zinc-free. Such contaminations can readily exceed the stoichiometric quantities of zinc found in most metalloenzymes and proteins, especially when small amounts of protein are being analyzed. Three methods have been used successfully with PKC and GST fusion proteins to remove such contaminations.

Fast Protein Liquid Chromatography Gel Filtration

To measure zinc, only small amounts of PKC are necessary. Purified enzyme (5–10 μg in 100 μl) is analyzed on an FPLC HR5/5 column packed with 1ml of swollen Sephadex G-50 (Pharmacia LKB Biotechnology Inc.), equilibrated in zinc-free buffer (20 mM Tris-HCl, pH 7.5, 0.5 mM EGTA, 0.5 mM EDTA, 10 mM 2-mercaptoethanol, 0.03% (w/v) Triton X-100, 10% (v/v) ethylene glycol, and 50 mM NaCl), at a flow rate of 1 ml/min. Fractions of 200 μl are collected. The column is calibrated using Triton X-100 to indicate the column void volume and tritiated water to indicate column inclusion volume fractions (Fig. 1A). PKC eluting in void volume fraction 5 (Fig. 1B) is routinely used for zinc stoichiometry determinations.

This procedure has been modified since problems with background zinc levels often arose. These fluctuations are presumably due to the exposure of buffers to metallic and glass surfaces of the FPLC pump, automatic switch

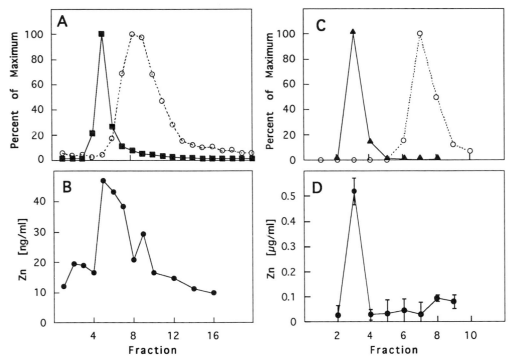

FIG. 1   Removal of adventitious zinc by gel filtration. The void volume calibration
with Triton X-100 micelles (A) or GST (C) and the inclusion volume calibration with
tritiated water (A, C) of a 1-ml Sephadex G-25 FPLC gel filtration column (A, B)
and a 1-ml Ultrogel AcA 202 Bio-Spin gel filtration column (C, D) are illustrated in
A and C, respectively. Absorbance at 280 nm (■), GST activity (▲), and counts/min/
fraction (○) are shown, expressed as percentiles of the maximum values measured.
In B a representative experiment with PKCα shows a major peak of zinc eluting in
void volume fractions (●). Zinc was also present above background levels in the
column inclusion volume, where a similar peak was observed when buffer alone was
analyzed (not shown). In D an experiment with GST–Cys1 fusion protein illustrates
how the peak of zinc (●) coincides with the peak of GST activity in C. Protein
concentrations in peak fractions 5 (A, B) or 3 (C, D) together with zinc measurements
in these fractions provided the basis for most stoichiometry determinations summarized in Table I. Enzyme activities were measured as described [A. F. G. Quest, J.
Bloomenthal, E. S. G. Bardes, and R. M. Bell, *J. Biol. Chem.* **267,** 10193 (1992);
P. C. Simons and D. L. VanderJagt, *Anal. Biochem.* **82,** 334 (1977)].

valve, and column itself. These problems are easily avoided by using larger quantities of protein and conventional gel filtration chromatography or dialysis methods.

Conventional Gel-Filtration Analysis

Polypropylene, 2-ml Bio-Spin tubes (Bio-Rad, Richmond, CA) are treated with nitric acid and zinc-free water as described for plastic ware and packed under gravity flow with 1 ml swollen Ultrogel AcA 202 (LKB-Reactifs IBF, Villeneuve-la-Garenne, France) equilibrated in zinc-free buffer [20 mM Tris-HCl (pH 7.5), 50 mM NaCl, 1 mM dithiotreitol, 0.05% (w/v) Triton X-100, 10% (v/v) ethylene glycol]. Sample volumes of up to 70 μl containing about 1 mg/ml of protein are routinely analyzed. Proteins elute in void volume fractions at a concentration of about 400 μg/ml. Column void volume and inclusion volume fractions are determined with GST and tritiated water, respectively (Fig. 1C). GST fusion proteins eluting in void volume fraction 3 are routinely analyzed for zinc content. The resolution obtained with this column allows efficient separation of protein-associated and nonassociated zinc, as illustrated for a GST–Cys1 fusion protein of M_r 35,000, which is a carboxy-terminal fusion protein of GST with the first cysteine-rich region of PKCγ [amino acids 23–92, as numbered by Knopf *et al.* (17)] (Fig. 1D).

Dialysis

Dialysis is employed primarily in experiments designed to study conditions under which zinc could be removed from PKC enzymes and fusion proteins. Tubing with a molecular weight cut-off of 10,000 (Spectrum Medical Industrials Inc., Los Angeles, CA) is prepared as described earlier. Dialysis buffers (40 mM buffer compound, 50 mM NaCl, 1 mM EGTA, 1 mM dithiothreitol, 10% (v/v) ethylene glycol, 0.03% (w/v) Triton X-100) are adjusted to the pH values indicated as follows: pH 4.3 (40 mM acetate–acetic acid); pH 5.3 [40 mM 3-(N-morpholino)propanesulfonic acid (MOPS)–HCl]; pH 6.6 (40 mM hydrogen phosphate–dihydrogen phosphate); pH 7.5 (40 mM Tris-HCl.

Samples containing at least 100 μg of protein in a volume of 1 ml are dialyzed at a volume ratio of 1 : 100 against zinc-free buffers at 4°C and different pH values for extended periods of time. These small sample volumes are dialyzed in Eppendorf tubes from which the bottom section of the Eppendorf lid had been cut off. By closing the lid with a piece of zinc-free dialysis membrane between lid and tube rim, a semipermeable exchange surface is provided (18). In this manner repetitive sampling is greatly facilitated. Zinc concentrations of the protein solution are monitored periodically after removing sample aliquots at time points of interest (see Fig. 3). Dialysis buffers are replaced every 24 hr by fresh zinc-free buffer solutions. Either when zinc levels remain constant or after 170 hr of dialysis, zinc-free buffers are replaced by pH 7.5 buffer to which zinc is added to a final concentration of 1 mM. Reincorporation of the metal ion is terminated after 24 hr by introducing zinc-free buffer at pH 7.5 again. This buffer is replaced at least twice during the following 48 hr of dialysis, after which zinc concentrations in the protein solutions are determined. By following this procedure, zinc is restored to levels present in fusion proteins before beginning the dialysis experiments (data not shown).

Quantitation of Zinc

Zinc concentrations of solutions are measured using a Perkin-Elmer Zeeman/ 3030 system with an HGA graphite furance (Perkin-Elmer Corp. Analytical Instruments, Norwalk, CT), which performs atomic absorption spectrometer analyses utilizing the Zeeman effect for background correction (see manufacturer's protocol). Samples are prepared for analysis following a rigid standardized protocol. As a general precaution one should work in an area free of air currents and cover the sample cups whenever possible with a sheet of plastic wrap. Every day a fresh solution of sample diluent [0.2% (w/v) nitric acid] is prepared. An aliquot of sample diluent is pipetted into an airdry sample cup and tested for the presence of zinc.

For the analysis, zinc-free, sample diluent (490 μl) is pipetted into each sample cup. Enough sample cups are provided either to allow the analysis of all samples of interest or to reach the sample capacity of the spectrometer. Of this number three are not sample related: one cup is required for the machine calibration curve, and the first as well as the last cup pipetted in a series are measured directly for zinc. If both of the latter cups contain no zinc, it is assumed that none of the cups had become contaminated during the pipetting procedure and the experiment is continued. To each cup containing diluent 10 μl of sample is added. In most initial experiments samples are analyzed at the resulting 1 : 50 dilutions. This dilution factor may vary, however, depending on the amount of zinc present. In current preparations of GST fusion proteins, where protein concentrations are of the order of 1 mg/ ml, we routinely work with final sample dilutions between 1 : 500 and 1 : 1000. Higher dilution factors are preferred because they help eliminate potential distortions of zinc measurements by buffer components (see Fig. 2).

For the machine standard curve, a Perkin-Elmer Cetus zinc calibration standard solution (1000 μg/ml) is diluted to a final concentration of 239 ng/ ml in diluent. The machine uses 5-, 10-, 15-, and 20-μl aliquots thereof to generate a nonlinear internal calibration curve in an automated procedure (see manufacturer's manual). Such calibration curves are considered accurate for

1 day. Zinc concentrations in samples are automatically computed by direct comparison with the standard curve. Machine blank values are reset with diluent after each series of measurements. Numerical values computed by the machine reflect the zinc concentration (in ng/ml) of each sample in diluent. Values illustrated (e.g., Fig. 1) represent the average of at least four measurements. Standard errors for zinc concentrations of individual samples are of the order of 5–10% of the averaged value.

Protein Analysis/Zinc Stoichiometries

A crucial element of any attempt to determine stoichiometry in proteins is the measurement of the protein concentration itself. The Amido Black dye binding assay (19) with fatty acid-free bovine serum albumin (BSA) as a standard has been found to be the most reliable method for quantitation of PKC. Experiments comparing the results obtained in this manner with those of other methods, in particular quantitative amino acid analysis of PKC samples, have been detailed before (9). Standard errors for such protein measurements were 5–10% of the averaged values. In the following paragraph the standard protocol for protein measurements is described.

Each protein sample is diluted to a final volume of 270 μl in a 1.5-ml Eppendorf tube. Then 30 μl of sodium dodecyl sulfate (SDS) sample solution [1 M Tris-HCl (pH 7.5) and 1% (w/v) SDS] is added followed by 60 μl of 60% (w/v) trichloroacetic acid. Samples are vortexed, incubated for at least 2 min at room temperature, and then spotted onto 60-mm, 0.45-μm pore size Millipore HA filters (Millipore, Bedford, MA) under vacuum on a fritted glass filter support. About five samples are spotted per filter. The entire filter is rinsed with 4 ml of 6% (w/v) trichloroacetic acid, immersed in Amido Black staining solution [0.1% (w/v) naphthol blue black (Sigma) in methanol/acetic acid/water (45 : 10 : 45, by volume)] for 1 min, rinsed again for 30 sec in running distilled water, and then washed three times in 20 ml destain solution (methanol/acetic acid/water at a 90 : 2 : 8 volume ratio). Filters are dried by blotting on a paper towel with blue spots facing upward. Staining protein spots are cut out of the filters with a cork borer. Each spot is placed in a 12 $\times$ 15 mm glass tube, to which 600 μl of eluent solution [25 mM NaOH, 0.05 mM EDTA in 50% (v/v) ethanol] is added to extract the dye from filter circles for either 10 min at room temperature for 3 min at 60°C. The absorbance of the dye in solution is measured at a wavelength of 630 nm. Readings are stable for up to 2 hr after dye extraction. The standard curve is measured with 1–10 μg of lipid-free bovine serum albumin (Sigma) delivered from a protein stock solution containing 100 μg/ml.

TABLE I   Zinc Stoichiometries Determined for Protein Kinase C
Isozymes, Subdomains, and Glutathione S-Transferase
Fusion Proteins[a]

PKC (source/isozyme/domain)[b]	Stoichiometry (mol Zn/mol PKC)[c]	Standard Error (% of stoichiometry)[d]
Rat brain	4.2	10
Baculovirus/Sf9 cell culture		
α	4.2	12
γ	4.0	10
α regulatory	4.7	19
α catalytic	Not significant	—
Escherichia coli		
GST	0.16	—
GST–Cys1Cys2	3.9	8

[a] The data shown were taken in part from A. F. G. Quest, J. Bloomenthal, E. S. G. Bardes, and R. M. Bell, J. Biol. Chem. 267, 10193 (1992).

[b] The experimental data summarize zinc stoichiometries (moles of zinc/mole of PKC) determined for PKC isozyme mixtures purified from rat brain, individual PKC isozymes isolated from baculovirus-infected Sf9 cells, and GST fusion proteins affinity purified from transformed E. coli cell extracts. The preparation and characterization of GST–Cys1Cys2 are detailed elsewhere (11).

[c] For most PKC samples, the protein and zinc contents of peak fractions indicated in Fig. 1 were determined. Stoichiometry values for the regulatory domain of PKCα (α regulatory) and the catalytic domain (α catalytic) were measured after association with mixed micelles (PS/Triton X-100) and separation by gel filtration on Ultrogel AcA 44 as described [A. F. G. Quest, J. Bloomenthal, E. S. G. Bardes, and R. M. Bell, J. Biol. Chem. 267, 10193 (1992)]. For each stoichiometry determination, zinc concentrations were measured four times and protein concentrations in duplicate.

[d] The errors indicated for zinc stoichiometries are equivalent to the standard error calculated for averaged stoichiometry determinations expressed as percentiles of the averaged values. Note the larger error for the α regulatory domain which is discussed in Fig. 2 and related sections of the text.

All stoichiometries illustrated in Table I have been calculated based on zinc measurements of fractions indicated in Fig. 1 or, in the case of the PKCα regulatory and catalytic domains, isolated as described earlier (9) and protein measurements by the Amido Black dye binding assay. Molecular masses of 80 kDa for intact PKC, 32 kDa for the lipid-binding regulatory domain, and 42 kDa for GST–Cys1Cys2 [a carboxy-terminal fusion protein of GST with both cysteine-rich regions of PKCγ, containing amino acids 23–171 as numbered by Knopf et al. (17)] and an atomic mass of 65 for zinc were assumed in these calculations. The results presented indicate that four atoms of zinc are coordinated within the two cysteine-rich regions of the PKC regulatory domain. The observed standard error of stoichiometries for samples separated from adventitious zinc by gel filtration reflected the error

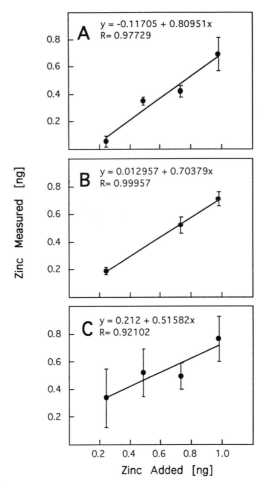

FIG. 2   Buffer effects on zinc measurements and error of stoichiometry determinations. An Ultrogel AcA 44 column equilibrated in zinc-free buffer [20 mM Tris-HCl (pH 7.5), 10 mM 2-mercaptoethanol, 200 μM CaCl$_2$, 20 mM NaCl, 0.02% (w/v) Triton X-100, and 10% (v/v) glycerol] was used to separate proteolytic fragments of PKC in the presence of PS/Triton X-100 mixed micelles as described [A. F. G. Quest, J. Bloomenthal, E. S. G. Bardes, and R. M. Bell, *J. Biol. Chem.* **267,** 10193 (1992)]. Protein-associated zinc was essentially only present at levels significantly above background in the mixed micelle fractions 15–18, which were quantitated directly for zinc stoichiometry determinations. The effects of buffer components on the zinc concentrations detected by atomic absorption spectroscopy are illustrated. PS/Triton X-100 mixed micelles were obtained from an Ultrogel AcA 44 column in the absence of protein, and zinc samples were measured in the presence of buffer components present in fractions 15, 16, 17, and 18. To do so, zinc was initially measured in five samples of

of the measurements involved and lay in the vicinity of 10% of the averaged value. For the regulatory PKCα domain, however, this error was significantly larger (Table I). In this case zinc and protein concentations of proteolytic fragments separated in the presence of mixed micelles (9) were directly assessed. The larger error observed in this case was attributed to effects that the phosphatidylserine (PS)/Triton X-100 mixed micelle components had on zinc measurements.

To verify this, zinc concentrations were recorded in the presence of either buffer components alone or together with PS/Triton X-100 mixed micelles isolated in the same way as described previously (9) except that no protein was included during the separation by gel filtration. Clearly, commonly employed buffer components diluted 1 : 50 with diluent did not alter the calibration curve significantly (compare Fig. 2A, 2B). However, in the presence of PS/Triton X-100 mixed micelles, a substantially larger standard error than usual resulted at the same dilution with diluent (Fig. 2C). This observation provides a likely explanation for the larger error documented for the PKCα regulatory domain in Table I.

Removal of Zinc from Protein Kinase C

Understanding the function of zinc in PKC regulation would be facilitated by methods to remove and reconstitute zinc in the protein. Initial attempts to remove zinc from native full-length PKC by dialysis against EDTA/EGTA

50-fold dilutions of these fractions in diluent. To the four samples in each case with lowest zinc levels a known amount of zinc was added corresponding to 0.25, 1.25, 0.75, or 1 ng total. These values were within the linear range of the assay. After measuring zinc again, background values previously detected were subtracted, and the measured values were plotted as a function of the zinc added. The calibration curve obtained by averaging such determinations will all four fractions from the gel filtration column (C) was compared to a calibration experiment in the presence of buffer alone [20 mM Tris-HCl (pH 7.5), 10 mM 2-mercaptoethanol, 200 μM CaCl$_2$, 20 mM NaCl, 0.02% Triton X-100, and 10% glycerol] diluted 50-fold with diluent (B) or simply in the presence of diluent (A). For each graph the points measured, with the respective standard errors, are shown together with the linear regression plot. The numerical values of each regression analysis expressing zinc measured (y) as a function of zinc added (x) are included together with the regression coefficient (R). The presence of buffer diluted 1 : 50 in diluent did not affect the calibration curve significantly (B), in comparison to the calibration with diluent alone (A). However, zinc measurements in the presence of mixed micelle components (C) had a far greater standard error, which is reflected in the elevated percentage error of the stoichiometry for the PKCα regulatory subunit (Table I).

[0.5 mM of each chelator in either 20 mM Tris-HCl (pH 7) or 50 mM sodium acetate–acetic acid (pH 5)] failed even at low pH values (pH 5) which led to loss of 80% of the kinase activity and 95% of phorbol ester-binding activity in 24 hr (data not shown). Experiments to remove zinc from intact PKC by dialysis against stronger zinc chelators (1,10-phenanthroline) in the presence of denaturing agens (urea) appeared successful, as was predicted from the work of others (8), in that zinc was removed from the enzyme; however, protein recovery was low. In subsequent renaturation steps the protein was always lost (not shown). Thus, in these experiments no correlation could be established between the presence of zinc in the enzyme and its requirement for either catalytic or phorbol ester-binding activity. However, it was established that zinc was very tightly bound to intact PKC and that a loss of zinc by storage in the presence of chelator was not to be expected.

Based on our observations and the reports of others showing that zinc was removed in the presence of denaturing agents, we tested whether zinc could be removed from GST–PKCγ fusion proteins with chelators at low pH under native conditions, as has been described for transcription factors (20). In Fig. 3 results from a dialysis experiment of the GST–Cys1Cys2 fusion protein at different pH values are summarized. The results reveal clearly that zinc can be removed from such soluble fusion proteins containing small regions of PKC, in this case the cysteine-rich Cys1Cys2 region. Furthermore, the rate of removal was strongly dependent on the pH of the chelating solution: at lower pH values removal of zinc from the protein was more rapid. Even at elevated pH values, such as those used for storage (pH 7.5), zinc was removed from the protein at a significant rate, such that after 170 hr of dialysis zinc levels in the protein were reduced to about 25%. Similar results were obtained in dialysis experiments with GST–Cys1, although the rates of zinc removal were more rapid than for GST–Cys1Cys2 (data not shown). For these reasons GST–PKC fusion proteins were stored in the absence of chelators as previously described. These experiments indicated that it is important to establish that both purification and storage do not remove the metal ion from the enzyme.

In contrast to the experiments described for intact PKC enzymes, zinc could be restored to its initial levels in GST–Cys1Cys2 after replacing the chelator with zinc following the protocol described for such dialysis experiments. Although in all cases PDBu binding was reduced to 40% (pH 7.5) or less (5% at pH 4.3) of initial values, recovery of PDBu-binding activity was never detected on restoration of zinc levels in GST–Cys1Cys2 (data not shown). Although zinc removal and replacement by dialysis represent simple methods, current conditions are unsuitable for reconstituting PDBu-binding activity.

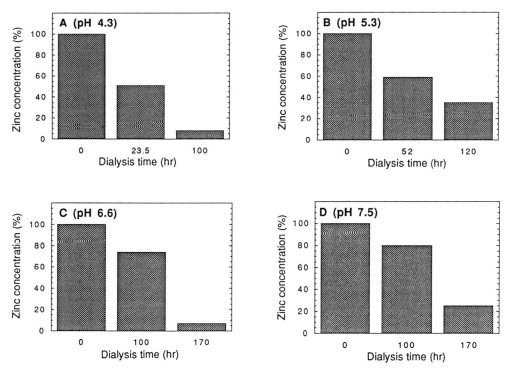

FIG. 3   pH-dependent removal of zinc from the GST–Cys1Cys2 fusion protein by dialysis. Purified GST–Cys1Cys2 samples were dialyzed against zinc-free buffers in the presence of chelator as described at the pH values indicated. Zinc levels in GST–Cys1Cys2 are indicated as a percentile of the initial amount present. At lower pH values removal of zinc was more rapid than at elevated pH values. However, even at pH 7.5, zinc levels were reduced to 20% of the starting value after 170 hr, suggesting that storage at any physiological pH in the presence of chelators could lead to removal of zinc from GST–PKC fusion proteins.

Concluding Remarks

It is possible to quantitate accurately and reproducibly the small amounts of zinc present in proteins by atomic absorption spectrometry. Detailed methods for PKC are described, and the results obtained have been summarized. The limited quantities of PKC available for the initial experiments posed the greatest challenge along with preventing sample contamination. The procedures described are straightforward and overcome these problems.

As the results presented indicate, buffer components did not cause major problems in these measurements if samples were diluted at least 50-fold in diluent [0.2% (w/v) nitric acid]. However, when other components were present, such as detergent/phospholipid mixed micelles, the reproducibility of measurements was strongly affected (Fig. 2). As a general rule, to enhance reproducibility, samples should be analyzed at the highest dilution possible in diluent that will still yield a reading in the linear calibration range. Finally, in situations where stoichiometric determinations are important, our results indicated that purification and storage conditions that do not remove the metal ion must be established (Fig. 3). In this respect intact PKC isozymes and the regulatory domain of PKCα did not present a problem; however, precautions were required for GST fusion proteins with smaller segments of PKCγ.

The sequence similarities between the Cys1 and Cys2 regions of PKC and cysteine-rich, DNA-binding sequences identified in transcription factors have led to the proposal of at least two possible structures by inference for the cysteine-rich phorbol ester-binding regions of PKC, namely, a Cys_4 "zinc finger" and a $Zn(II)_2Cys_6$ binuclear cluster (4). The stoichiometry determinations revealed that four atoms of zinc were coordinated within the two cysteine-rich regions of the lipid-binding domain (Table I), favoring the possible existence of a binuclear cluster-like structure. However, the underlying assumption that only cysteine residues were involved in the coordination of zinc may not be true. Alternatively, indirect evidence obtained by extended X-ray absorption fine structure (EXAFS) analysis favors a model of zinc coordination between one nitrogen and three sulfur atoms in nonbridged sites (21). The strong dependence of the rate or zinc removal from the GST–Cys1Cys2 fusion protein on the pH of dialysis solutions in the range indicated (Fig. 3) also suggests that one or more histidines may play a crucial role in the coordination of zinc. This was demonstrated more conclusively by deletion analysis within the Cys2 region, where His-101 was found to be essential for both phorbol ester binding and zinc coordination (16). Clearly, further studies are necessary to resolve the coordination sphere of zinc, and they should shed light on the molecular mechanisms of lipid-dependent regulation of this important intracellular protein kinase and perhaps on its many roles in the control of neuronal processes.

Acknowledgment

This research was supported by National Institutes of Health Grant GM 38737.

References

1. Y. Nishizuka, *Science* **225,** 1365 (1984).
2. Y. Nishizuka, *Science* **233,** 305 (1986).
3. Y. Nishizuka, *Nature* (*London*) **334,** 661 (1988).
4. R. M. Bell and D. J. Burns, *J. Biol. Chem.* **266,** 4661 (1991).
5. Y. Ono, T. Fujii, K. Igarashi, T. Kuno, C. Tanaka, U. Kikkawa, and Y. Nishizuka, *Proc. Natl. Acad. Sci. U.S.A.* **86,** 4868 (1989).
6. D. J. Burns and R. M. Bell, *J. Biol. Chem.* **266,** 18330 (1991).
7. Y. Ono, T. Fujii, K. Ogita, U. Kikkawa, K. Igarashi, and Y. Nishizuka, *Proc. Natl. Acad. Sci. U.S.A.* **86,** 3099 (1989).
8. S. Ahmed, R. Kozma, J. Lee, C. Monfries, N. Harden, and L. Lim, *Biochem. J.* **280,** 233 (1991).
9. A. F. G. Quest, J. Bloomenthal, E. S. G. Bardes, and R. M. Bell, *J. Biol. Chem.* **267,** 10193 (1992).
10. J. E. Coleman, *Annu. Rev. Biochem.* **61,** 897 (1992).
11. A. F. G. Quest, R. A. Borchardt, E. S. G. Bardes, and R. M. Bell, "Functional characterization of lipid interaction sites in the regulatory domain of protein kinase Cγ," manuscript in preparation.
12. K. H. Falchuk, K. L. Hilt, and B. L. Vallee, *in* "Methods in Enzymology" (J. F. Riordan and B. L. Vallee, eds.), Vol. 158, p. 422. Academic Press, San Diego, 1988.
13. T. Kumamaru, J. F. Jordan, and B. L. Vallee, *Anal. Biochem.* **126,** 214 (1982).
14. D. S. Auld, *in* "Methods in Enzymology" (J. F. Riordan and B. L. Vallee, eds.), Vol. 158, p. 13. Academic Press, San Diego, 1988.
15. D. J. Burns, J. Bloomenthal, M.-H. Lee, and R. M. Bell *J. Biol. Chem.* **265,** 12044 (1990).
16. A. F. G. Quest, E. S. G. Bardes, and R. M. Bell, "A phorbol ester binding domain of protein kinase Cγ: high affinity binding to a glutathione-S-transferase/Cys2 fusion protein" and "A phorbol ester binding domain of protein kinase Cγ: deletion analysis of the Cys2 domain defines a minimal 45 amino acid peptide," manuscripts submitted.
17. J. L. Knopf, M.-H. Lee, L. A. Sultzman, R. W. Kris, C. R. Loomis, R. M. Hewick, and R. M. Bell, *Cell* (*Cambridge, Mass.*) **46,** 491 (1986).
18. P. Falson, *BioTechniques* **13,** 21 (1992).
19. W. Schaffner and C. Weissmann, *Anal. Biochem.* **56,** 502 (1973).
20. T. Pan and J. E. Coleman, *Proc. Natl. Acad. Sci. U.S.A.* **86,** 3145 (1989).
21. S. R. Hubbard, W. R. Bishop, P. Kirschmeier, S. J. George, S. P. Cramer, and W. A. Hendrickson *Science* **254,** 1776 (1992).

[16] Expression of Protein Kinase C Isozymes in Insect Cells and Isolation of Recombinant Proteins

Silvia Stabel, Marek Liyanage, and David Frith

Introduction

The transduction of extracellular signals by increased metabolism of specific cellular lipids constitutes a mechanism that is apparently employed in many types of cells and in many different physiological situations (1–3). The breakdown of phospholipid in response to extracellular signals results in an increased local concentration of the neutral lipid diacylglycerol (DAG), which is able to activate protein kinase C (PKC) *in vitro* and *in vivo*. In the presence of an acidic phospholipid such as phosphatidylserine, PKC acts as a receptor for the lipid second messenger DAG and thus constitutes a crucial component of this signal transduction mechanism (4). The apparent universality of the signal transduction pathway involving PKC and the activation of this enzyme by tumor-promoting phorbol esters have led to intense investigations on the role of PKC in such diverse processes as mitogenesis, differentiation, secretion, development, gene expression, and carcinogenesis, to name a few. However, much remains unclear about the regulation and role of this enzyme in particular physiological or pathological situations.

The isolation of the first cDNA clones for PKC in 1986 (5, 6) revealed the existence of a family of structurally related proteins in mammals, including PKC-α, -βI, -βII, and -γ, which called for a reinvestigation of previously established enzymatic properties of PKC preparations from brain with regard to the possible presence of additional related enzymes in these preparations. Although separation of the α, β, and γ subtypes from brain extracts was subsequently achieved by chromatography on hydroxyapatite columns (7–9), analysis of the subtypes was still hampered by the possibility of contamination by yet unidentified subtypes or by the failure to separate PKC-βI and PKC-βII, which are very similar in sequence (10).

The first report that expression of PKC from a baculovirus expression vector in insect cells yields an active and functional enzyme instigated the use of this expression system to assess the biochemical and pharmacological properties of the PKC enzyme family, which has expanded so rapidly through cDNA cloning (11). This expression system has been employed in several

Methods in Neurosciences, Volume 18

laboratories to produce active PKC isozymes as well as engineered PKC mutants, and it promises to be relevant for structural studies on PKC enzymes, which require large amounts of functional protein (12–19).

Although it has become common practice to express a novel cDNA clone in a mammalian expression system by means of transient or stable transfection in order to identify the gene product, the use of mammalian expression systems has limitations for the biochemical analysis of PKC enzymes. Up to now there are no mammalian cells described that are devoid of PKC and that would therefore be suitable for the analysis of exogenously expressed PKC enzymes. Unlike mammalian cells, the insect cell line Sf9 (derived from *Spodoptera frugiperda*) does not show measurable phorbol ester-binding activity, and there is no endogenous kinase activity detectable even in crude extracts stimulated under the assay conditions used to measure mammalian PKCs. Even activity measurements using less specific conditions as applies for the assays of some of the novel PKCs can be carried out in high-speed supernatants from crude cytoplasmic extracts as discussed below. Apart from providing milligram amounts of recombinant protein that are easy to purify, the insect cell system may also prove to be useful for screening pharmacological compounds designed to interact with individual PKC isozymes. For the measurement of phorbol ester binding and kinase activity, the recombinant proteins need not be purified from the extracts. As far as we can determine high-speed supernatants from crude extracts behave the same way as the purified recombinant proteins.

Insect Cell Culture Techniques

The use of baculoviruses for the expression of foreign proteins was initiated and developed in the laboratory of Summers (20). This group supplied the Sf9 insect cells and the wild-type baculovirus *Autographa californica* nuclear polyhedrosis virus (AcNPV) as well as a very detailed and easy to follow manual (21), which serves as a useful guide for establishing the system. For routine insect cell culture we follow the published procedures using either commercial Grace's insect cell medium (GIBCO BRL, Gaithersburg, MD) supplemented with lactalbumin hydrolyzate, yeastolate, and 10% (v/v) fetal calf serum (FCS) or the less expensive version of medium (TNM-FH) prepared according to the manual (21).

For the expression of secreted proteins, the serum-free medium Excel 400 sold by J. R. Scientific (Woodland, CA) greatly facilitates the purification of secreted proteins from the cell culture medium (22). Although we have also used Excel 400 for expression of PKCs, we prefer the classic TNM-FH medium supplemented with FSC because protein yields appear to be higher.

When grown as monolayer cultures cells are usually passaged every 3 to 4 days when they reach confluence. However, we routinely grow cells in suspension cultures which saves plastic material used for tissue culture and avoids the loss of cells that occurs when detaching the cells from the plastic tissue culture flask. This loss can amount to 30–50%.

For setting up suspension cultures 10^7 cells are either thawed directly into 100 ml of medium in a 500-ml stirring flask (Techne, Princeton, NJ), or 100 ml of TNM-FH medium is inoculated with the same number of cells detached from a monolayer culture. The cultures are continuously stirred at 60 rpm at 27°C either in a water bath (Techne) or on a stirrer (Techne) fitted inside an incubator. Stirring at 80 rpm considerably increases the growth rate and the maximum number of cells obtained, but this speed is too high for infected cells, which are more fragile. To reach high cell densities and good doubling times only 200 ml of suspension cell cultures is grown in 1.5-liter flasks to ensure optimal aeration. When the cells have reached a density of $1–1.5 \times 10^6$ cells/ml, they are diluted $1:10$ or $1:20$ with fresh medium or used for infections.

Infection of 200 ml of cell suspension is done by centrifuging the cells at 500 g for 5 to 10 min at ambient temperature. The cell pellet is resuspended in 40 ml virus stock corresponding to a multiplicity of infection of 10 and left at 27°C for 60 min with occasional swirling. Then the cells are centrifuged as above and resuspended at 1×10^6 cells/ml in medium with antibiotics (21). After 2 to 3 days of stirring at 27°C the infected cells are harvested by centrifugation as above and can be stored frozen as pellets at $-20°$ or $-70°C$ for several months.

Every 2 to 3 months new cultures are started from frozen cells. For transfection and infection of monolayer cultures, cells are removed from the suspension, seeded onto 25-, 75-, or 175-cm^2 plastic flasks, and left to attach for 1 hr. For all transfections and infections we found it essential to use cells that had been diluted the day before and/or were dividing at the maximum rate.

Construction and Isolation of Recombinant Viruses

For expression of recombinant PKC proteins we have used the expression vectors pAcC3, pAcC4, pAcC5, and pAcYM1. The first three were constructed and kindly provided by Robin Clark (CETUS, Emeryville, CA), the latter one by Dr. David Bishop (NERC Institute of Virology, Oxford, UK). The general features of these vectors are described by Luckow and Summers (23). In brief, the pAcC series of expression vectors requires the presence of an NcoI restriction site at the 5' end of the cDNA surrounding the start codon ATG. The advantage of this series of expression vectors is that the

5'-untranslated sequences upstream of the initiating ATG of the mammalian cDNA are removed, which can otherwise interfere with high level expression (especially if the sequences are GC-rich). The pAcC vector series also takes into account that the 5'-untranslated region of the polyhedrin message has to be conserved up to the start ATG in order to achieve high levels of expression (24). There are also other nonfusion vectors available with these properties: e.g., pVL941, pVL985, pVL945, and pAcYM1 (24, 25).

The cDNAs for PKC-α, -γ, and -ε contain an *NcoI* site surrounding the start ATG and can be directly cloned into the pAcC vectors. A baculovirus expressing PKC-α is constructed by excising the coding sequence of bovine PKC-α plus an additional 250 base pairs of 3'-untranslated sequence from the clone λbPKCα (5) with *Eco*RI. The fragment is eluted, digested with *Nco*I to yield two fragments (owing to the presence of an internal *Nco*I site), and subsequently ligated with the vector pAcC4 cut with *Nco*I and *Eco*RI. The construction of a baculovirus expressing PKC-γ has been described (11), and the cDNA for PKC-ε is transferred in two sequential ligations as an *Nco*I/*Bam*HI and a *Bam*HI fragment into the expression plasmid pAcC5. To insert the coding sequences for PKC-βI and -βII into the expression vector, an *Nco*I site surrounding the initiating ATG codon of the PKC-β sequences has to be created. A *Sma*I/*Pst*I fragment containing the initiator ATG is excised from clone λhPKCβ$_2$ (6, but note that the nomenclature in Ref. 6 is reversed, i.e., β$_2$ is β1) and subcloned into M13mp18, and the sequence surrounding the first methionine codon (AGATGG) is mutagenized to an *Nco*I restriction site (CCATGG) using an oligonucleotide-directed site-specific mutagenesis kit from Amersham (Bucks, UK). The coding sequence of PKC-β is not changed by this procedure. The mutated fragment is then ligated as an *Nco*I/*Pst*I fragment together with a partially *Pst*I-digested *Sma*I fragment eluted from pSP65-β1 into the vector pAcC3, which had been linearized with *Nco*I and *Sma*I. For the construction of the PKC-βII expression vector, a C-terminal *Pst*I/*Sma*I fragment is exchanged in pAcC3–PKC-βI which contains the sequence divergence between PKC-βI and PKC-βII. Therefore, the pAcC3–PKC-βI construct is digested with *Pst*I and *Sma*I, and the vector plus adhering PKC-βI sequences is eluted and ligated to a C-terminal *Pst*I partial fragment generated from pSP65–PKC-βII excised at the 3' end with *Sma*I. The construction of baculoviruses expressing PKC-δ, -ζ, and -η has also been described (19).

For the isolation of recombinant viruses the expression vector plasmid construct is transfected together with wild-type baculovirus DNA into Sf9 cells following precisely the published protocol using the transfection method I in Ref. 21. The wild-type virus DNA is also isolated as described in Ref. 21. Recombinant viruses are identified after performing several rounds of plaque assays as described (21) and hybridizing the plaques with the respective cDNA probes. In the last round of plaque assays recombinant plaques are always picked under the microscope from plates where the agarose has not been "flopped" in order to avoid contamination with residual wild-type virus plaques on the same dish. For each virus construct several final plaques (5 to 6) are picked to test for expression, although they usually all express the recombinant protein. A potential improvement of this step is discussed under Comments below.

A single plaque is used to infect 1×10^6 insect cells on a 25-cm^2 flask. After 4 days 50 μl of the medium is used to infect 2.3×10^7 cells in a 175-cm^2 flask to expand the virus. After this round of amplification the virus stock is used to infect a 200-ml suspension culture at a density of 1×10^6 cells/ml with a multiplicity of infection (m.o.i.) of 10 as described above.

Detection of Recombinant Protein Kinase C Proteins, Solubility, and Phorbol Ester Binding

For freshly isolated virus the time course of infection and total protein production is monitored by immunoblotting whole cell lysates. To this purpose 10^7 cells are infected in 75-cm^2 flasks with 2 ml virus. At 1, 2, 3, and 4 days postinfection the cells are detached from the flasks by tapping and sedimented at 500 g at room temperature for 5 to 10 min. The pellet is washed once with 5 ml phosphate-buffered saline (PBS) and centrifuged again. The cell pellet is then loosened by tapping the centrifuge tube vigorously, and whole cells are lysed by the addition of 300–400 μl boiling hot sodium dodecyl sulfate (SDS) sample buffer (26). The lysate is heated at 95°C for 5 min and can be stored at this stage at -20°C for several weeks.

In general the presence of insect cell DNA in the whole cell lysates does not present a problem at this concentration. If larger numbers of cells are used, however, it may be necessary to shear the cellular DNA by passing the solution up and down a syringe before electrophoresis.

For immunodetection of PKC the whole cell lysates corresponding to about 5×10^5 cells are loaded on 8% SDS–polyacrylamide gels, and the gel is blotted onto a nitrocellulose filter. Nonspecific binding of the filter is blocked by incubation for a minimum of 1 hr with 0.02% (v/v) Tween 20 in either PBS or 5% (w/v) skimmed milk powder solution. Immunodetection with ^{125}I-labeled protein A is performed as described (27) or using the enhanced chemoluminescence (ECL) kit (Amersham) as recommended by the manufacturer. With all PKC types the highest levels of protein expression are usually seen between 2 and 3 days postinfection. An additional means of visualizing the recombinant PKC proteins is by metabolic labeling either with [35S]methionine or ortho[32P]phosphate (see Figs. 8 and 9).

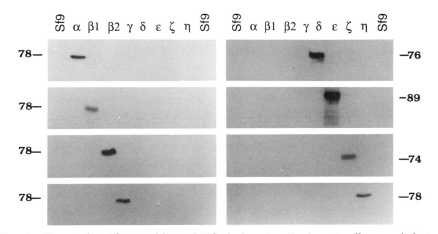

Fig. 1 Expression of recombinant PKCs in insect cells. Insect cells were infected with the recombinant baculoviruses as indicated, lysed in 20 mM Tris-HCl (pH 7.5), 10 mM EGTA, 2 mM EDTA, 2 mM dithiothreitol, and fractionated by centrifugation. Aliquots of 20 µg soluble protein were separated on 8% SDS–polyacrylamide gels, which were then immunoblotted with isozyme-specific antisera. Only the area of interest of the gel is shown. PKC-α was detected with the monoclonal antibody MC5 (Amersham). PKC-β1- and -β2-specific antibodies were kindly provided by Susan Jaken, W. Alton Jones Cell Science Center (Lake Placid, NY). The antibody against PKC-γ was from Seikagaku Kogyo Co., Tokyo, Japan, and antibodies against PKC-δ, -ε, -η and -ζ were polyclonal antisera against synthetic C-terminal peptides (D. Fabbro, Ciba-Geigy, Basel, Switzerland, unpublished 1992). Numbers indicate apparent sizes ($\times 10^{-3}$) of the recombinant polypeptides.

The solubility of the recombinant PKC proteins is investigated as follows: At 2 days postinfection 2×10^6 cells are lysed on ice in 400 µl buffer A (20 mM Tris-HCl, pH 7.5; 10 mM EGTA; 2 mM EDTA; 0.3% 2-mercaptoethanol) containing 1% Triton X-100 and 50 µg/ml phenylmethylsulfonyl fluoride (PMSF). Soluble and detergent-insoluble fractions are separated by centrifugation at 4°C for 20 min and 15,000 g, and aliquots of pellet and supernatant corresponding to 2×10^5 cells each are immunoblotted with a 1:10,000 dilution of the respective antisera.

Figure 1 shows an example of soluble fractions of insect cells infected with recombinant PKC baculoviruses and immunodetected with the respective antisera. For the various PKC enzymes the fraction of the recombinant protein that is detergent-insoluble varies from 20 to 50% of the total PKC protein expressed. We have not systematically analyzed the factors influencing the solubility of the recombinant proteins, and thus the reasons for the different solubilities are not known. Because it is not clear if denaturation and renaturation of the insoluble fraction would yield functional protein, we discard the insoluble fraction and only work with the soluble protein. The soluble fraction can be used to immunoprecipitate native PKC polypeptides according to standard techniques. Antisera directed against synthetic peptides corresponding to the C-terminal sequences of PKC-δ (Phe-Val-Asn-Pro-Lys-Tyr-Glu-Gln-Phe-Leu-Glu-Leu) or PKC-ζ (Ile-Asn-Pro-Leu-Leu-Leu-Ser-Ala-Glu-Glu-Ser-Val) (19) are able to immunoprecipitate native PKC from infected insect cells.

Phorbol ester binding of PKC expressed in insect cells can be carried out in either of two ways using live infected insect cells or cytoplasmic extracts from infected cells. For phorbol ester binding on live insect cells 2.5 $\times$ 10^6 cells are seeded on 60-mm dishes and infected with the recombinant baculovirus. At about 40 hr postinfection cells are incubated with 1 ml of fresh medium containing 0.5 μCi/ml (11 nM) [^{3}H]phorbol dibutyrate (PDBu) (Amersham) for 30 min at room temperature. After incubation cells are washed gently three times with 1 ml PBS and scraped into 500 μl PBS, and the total suspension is counted in a liquid scintillation counter after addition of 10 ml scintillation cocktail. Although this method does not allow kinetic and quantitative analyses, it is a fast and simple method if only comparative values are needed. This type of binding assay obviously does not require the addition of phospholipids. Figure 2A shows an example of phorbol ester binding on whole insect cells.

Phorbol ester binding on cytoplasmic extracts *in vitro* is carried out as follows: 2 $\times$ 10^6 cells are lysed by vortexing in buffer A (see above) containing 0.1% Triton X-100 and 50 μg/ml PMSF and centrifuged at 15,000 g at 4°C for 20 min. Twenty microliters of the supernatant is incubated at 30°C for 30 min in a volume of 300 μl in 50 mM Tris-HCl (pH 7.5), 4 mg/ml bovine serum albumin (BSA), 0.05 μCi ^{3}[H]phorbol dibutyrate (Amersham) in the presence or absence of 250 μg/ml sonicated phosphatidylserine in 50 mM Tris-HCl (pH 7.5). Proteins are then collected by filtration through a GF/C glass fiber filter and rapidly washed three times each with 1 ml ice-cold PBS. Filter-bound radioactivity is counted in a liquid scintillation counter. Under these conditions phorbol ester binding is strictly dependent on the presence of phosphatidylserine, as shown in Fig. 2B. All PKC isozymes, apart from PKC-ζ, bind phorbol ester in both types of assays. PKC-ζ does not bind phorbol ester in either of the two assays.

Expression and Purification of Classic Protein Kinase C Enzymes α, βI, βII, and γ

Based on previous purification schemes (28, 29) we have developed a rapid and simple purification procedure for the classic group A PKCs that allows substantial purification of the recombinant proteins within 12 hr. Suspension

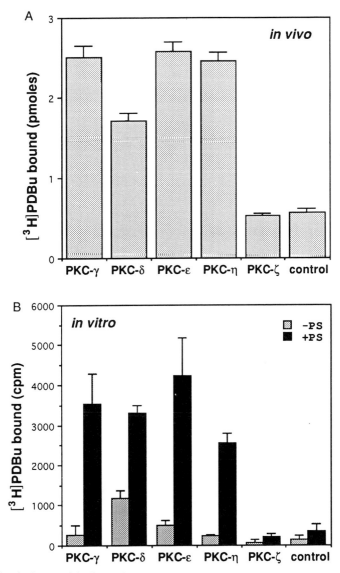

FIG. 2 Phorbol ester binding of recombinant PKCs. (A) Phorbol ester binding on whole infected insect cells. Insect cells (3×10^6) were infected with recombinant PKC-encoding baculoviruses as indicated or with an unrelated virus (control) and incubated with [^{3}H]phorbol dibutyrate (PDBu) at 40 hr postinfection as described in the text. Shown is the cell-associated radioactivity determined in three experiments. (B) Phorbol ester binding *in vitro* on crude cytoplasmic extracts. Insect cells (2×10^6) were infected with the recombinant viruses as indicated, harvested after 2 days, and lysed in extraction buffer. Aliquots of the cytoplasmic fractions were incubated with ^{3}H-labeled PDBu in the absence (stippled bars) or presence (solid bars) of phosphatidylserine (PS) as described in the text. Control cells were infected with a baculovirus expressing an unrelated protein.

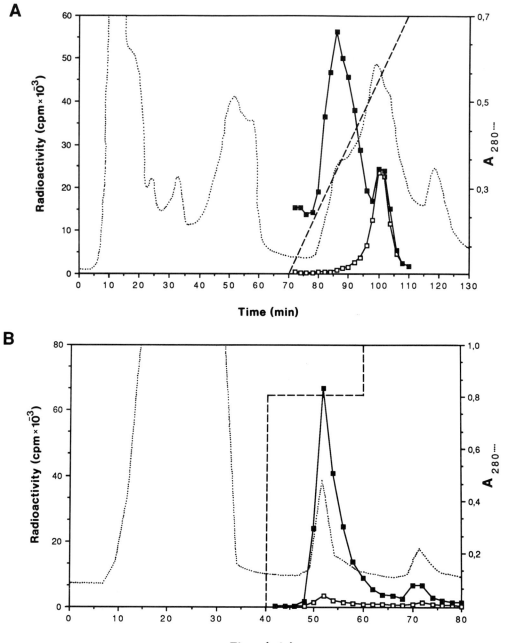

cultures (800 ml) of insect cells are infected with 160 ml recombinant virus, and infected cells are harvested by centrifugation at 500 g on day 2 or 3 after infection. The cell pellet is resuspended in 50 ml buffer A (20 mM Tris-HCl, pH 7.5; 2 mM EDTA; 10 mM EGTA; 0.3% 2-mercaptoethanol) containing 10 mM benzamidine and 50 μg/ml PMSF and disrupted with 10 to 15 strokes on ice in a Dounce homogenizer. The particulate fraction is removed by centrifugation at 4°C and 15,000 g for 20 min, and the supernatant is loaded onto a 50-ml (1.6 × 25 cm) DEAE-Sepharose fast flow (Pharmacia, Freiburg, Germany) column equilibrated in buffer A and connected to a fast protein liquid chromatography (FPLC) system (Pharmacia). The column is washed with buffer A at 5 ml/min, and bound protein is eluted by applying a continuous gradient from 0 to 0.3 M NaCl in buffer A also at 5 ml/min.

Fractions are assayed for PKC activity in the absence and presence of phosphatidylserine/phorbol 12-myristate 13-acetate (PMA) at 30°C in a volume of 40 μl as described (11) using Triton X-100 mixed micelles (30). The reaction mixture contains 50 mM Tris-HCl (pH 7.5), 1.25 mg/ml histone IIIS (Sigma, St. Louis, MO), 12.5 mM MgCl$_2$, 0.75 mM CaCl$_2$, 125 μM [δ − ^{32}P]ATP at 50–100 counts/min (cpm)/pmol, and 0.25% Triton X-100 with or without 625 μg/ml phosphatidylserine (5.75 mol%)/2 mM PMA (0.01 mol%). Phosphatidylserine is purchased from Lipid Products (Surrey, UK), and PMA is from Sigma. Figure 3A shows a typical DEAE-Sepharose profile of a human PKC-βII preparation. PKC activity elutes at about 150 mM NaCl and can be separated into two peaks displaying phospholipid-dependent and phospholipid-independent activity (Fig. 3A). The phospholipid-independent activity by chromatography on DEAE-Sepharose is seen with all group A PKCs and is clearly related to the recombinant PKC polypeptide and not due to some cellular or viral kinase activity induced by the infection. Uninfected cells or cells infected with unrelated recombinant baculoviruses do not show PKC-related kinase activity under these assay conditions. The activator-independent kinase activity always elutes after the peak of activator-dependent PKC activity and can be separated from the latter. The size of the peak of independent activity varies from one preparation to the next;

Fig. 3 Purification of recombinant human PKC-βII. (A) Elution profile of PKC-βII on DEAE-Sepharose fast flow. Kinase activity of the recombinant protein was assayed on histone using the mixed micellar assay in the absence (□) and presence (■) of phosphatidylserine/PMA as described in the text. (B) Elution profile of PKC-βII from the phenyl-Sepharose fast flow column. The kinase activity was determined as above. The dashed line indicates the salt gradient, the dotted line the absorption at 280 nm.

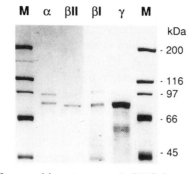

FIG. 4   Purification of recombinant group A PKC isozymes. Recombinant PKC isozymes as indicated were purified on DEAE-Sepharose and phenyl-Sepharose fast flow columns as shown in Fig. 3 and visualized on an 8% SDS–polyacrylamide gel by Coomassie blue staining. Sizes of marker proteins (M) are given in kilodaltons (kDa).

this activator-independent activity may be due to a proteolytic fragment generated during the extraction.

Active fractions of the DEAE-Sepharose column are pooled, adjusted to 1.5 M NaCl, and loaded onto a 50 ml phenyl-Sepharose fast flow (Pharmacia) column (1.6 × 25 cm) equilibrated in buffer B (20 mM Tris-HCl, pH 7.5; 2 mM EDTA; 0.3% 2-mercaptoethanol; 1.5 M NaCl). The column is washed with the same buffer, and bound protein is eluted by stepping the salt concentration from 1.5 to 0.3 M NaCl and then to 0 M NaCl at a flow rate of 5 ml/min. Active fractions are dialyzed into 20 mM Tris-HCl (pH 7.5), 2 mM EDTA, 1 mM dithiothreitol, 0.02% Triton X-100, 50% glycerol and can be stored at −70°C for several months. The phenyl-Sepharose column profile of human PKC-βII is shown in Fig. 3B. All group A isozymes behave in a similar manner on these columns and yield preparations of 50 to 80% purity as judged by Coomassie blue staining.

Figure 4 shows a Coomassie blue-stained SDS–polyacrylamide gel of PKC-α, -βI, -βII, and -γ purified by the procedure described above. By immunoblotting with antisera directed against C-terminal sequences it was confirmed that the preparations do not contain potentially active kinase domain fragments generated by proteolysis (not shown). The PKC-α, -βI, and -βII subtypes purify as apparently single polypeptides of approximately 86, 82, and 81 kDa, respectively, according to the migration in 8% (w/v) SDS–polyacrylamide gels (Fig. 4). In contrast, purification of PKC-γ reproducibly yields a doublet of 82 and 84 kDa apparent molecular mass that has been shown to consist of differentially phosphorylated forms of the protein (11).

All four group A mammalian PKC isozymes expressed in insect cells are dependent on phospholipid for their histone kinase activity and are activated by the phorbol ester PMA. For activity assays with the purified enzymes, they are diluted in 20 mM Tris-HCl (pH 7.5), 2 mM EDTA, 0.3% (v/v) 2-mercaptoethanol, 0.02% (v/v) Triton X-100.

Expression and Properties of Novel Protein Kinase C Enzymes

For the novel PKCs δ, ε, ζ, η and θ (31; reviewed in Refs. 32 and 33), which were first identified as cDNAs with no appropriate assay or purification conditions available to investigate the natural enzymes, the availability of an expression system will help in developing specific assay conditions for these enzymes (12, 19). Of the group B PKC enzymes mouse PKC-ε has been purified and analyzed in more detail using the baculovirus system (12, 34). We have expressed rat PKC-δ, -ε, -ζ, and human PKC-η from baculovirus expression vectors and have begun to investigate their specific properties (19). For kinase activity assays 2×10^6 infected cells are usually lysed in 500 μl buffer A (20 mM Tris-HCl, pH 7.5; 10 mM EGTA; 2 mM EDTA; 0.3% 2-mercaptoethanol) with 50 μg/ml PMSF and 0.1% Triton X-100 and centrifuged at 4°C for 20 min at 15,000 g. Five microliters of the supernatant is then analyzed in a kinase assay using the mixed micelle assay as described above. Assay mixtures are incubated at 37°C for 5 min, and then 30 μl is spotted on phosphocellulose paper (P81, Whatman, Clifton, NJ) and washed twice for 10 min with 30% acetic acid. After drying the filters are counted in a liquid scintillation counter.

Figure 5 shows PKC kinase activity assays on histone IIIS (Sigma) using crude cytoplasmic supernatants from baculovirus-infected cells. Unlike the group A enzymes (e.g., PKC-γ in Fig. 5), for which histone is a traditional substrate, all novel PKCs fail to phosphorylate this substrate to a significant extent (Fig. 5A). This has been noted earlier for recombinant PKC-ε (12) and has been confirmed (19), suggesting distinct substrate specificities of the group B enzymes. However, if the lipid activators are present in the sonicated form and not as detergent-mixed micelles, PKC-δ shows highly efficient and stimulatable phosphorylation of histone (Fig. 5B). This is in contrast to the behavior of all group A enzymes, which are activated to the same or very similar extent by either sonicated PS/PMA or PS/PMA offered as detergent-mixed micelles (30, and M. Liyanage, D. Frith, and S. Stabel, manuscript in preparation, 1993). This may explain the apparent discrepancy between our previous report that PKC-δ is not active on histone (19) and the properties described for a presumably PKC-δ enzyme purified from spleen which is active on histone (35). We have confirmed this unexpected behavior of recombinant PKC-δ after partial purification of the enzyme by DEAE-Sepharose chromatography.

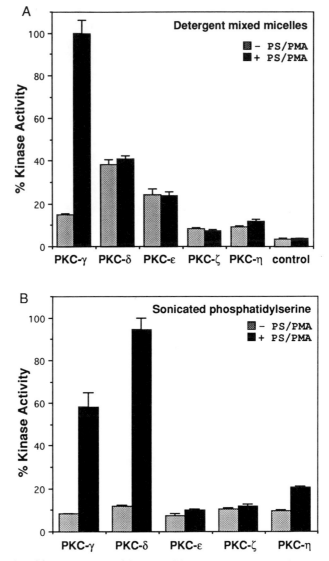

FIG. 5 *In vitro* kinase assays with recombinant group B PKC isozymes. Infected insect cells were lysed and cytoplasmic supernatants were assayed for kinase activity on histone IIIS as described in the text, either using detergent-mixed micelles (A) or sonicated phospholipid (B). Assays were performed in the absence (stippled bars) or presence (solid bars) of activators (PS/PMA).

This observation suggests that the regulatory domain of PKC-δ does not permit activation by the mixed micellar structures; however, when phospholipid/PMA is offered in the sonicated form without the addition of detergent activation can occur. The apparent difference in substrate specificity between the PKC isozymes may largely depend on the structure of the regulatory domain and its activation requirements. This interpretation is supported by previously published results on a chimeric construct between PKC ε and PKC-γ. After replacement of the regulatory domain of PKC-γ by the regulatory domain of PKC-ε, the chimeric enzyme was unable to phosphorylate histone, even though the catalytic domain was derived from PKC-γ (36). Although these observations hint at distinct and specific activation mechanisms for the novel group B enzymes compared to the classic isozymes α, β, and γ, this phenomenon requires further investigation.

In our hands PKC-ζ shows the highest expression levels of the group B enzymes. Therefore, we devised a two-step purification procedure for PKC-ζ that takes advantage of the high level of expression of this protein. Whether this procedure will be useful for the purification of other group B subtypes from infected insect cells remains to be seen. For the purification of PKC-ζ, 5×10^7 cells are lysed in a Dounce homogenizer in 20 ml buffer A (see above) containing 50 μg/ml PMSF and 10 mM benzamidine, then centrifuged at 4°C with 15,000 g for 20 min; the supernatant is precipitated at 4°C with increasing concentrations of ammonium sulfate. The precipitates corresponding to 30, 40, 50, 60, and 85% saturation with ammonium sulfate are collected by centrifugation at 4°C and 15,000 g for 10 min, resuspended in SDS sample buffer, and analyzed on a Coomassie blue-stained polyacrylamide gel. Figure 6 shows that the major protein in the soluble fraction (sn) is the PKC-ζ polypeptide. For purification purposes, a 50-ml suspension culture of infected insect cells (5×10^7 cells) is lysed as above and precipitated with 45% ammonium sulfate. The 45% ammonium sulfate precipitate is dissolved in 1 ml buffer A, 10 mM benzamidine, 0.5 M NaCl and applied onto a 16/60 Superdex S-200 column (Pharmacia) and connected to an FPLC system (Pharmacia). The column is run at 1 ml/min, and 1-ml fractions are collected.

PKC-ζ activity is measured by assaying 5 μl of each fraction in 40 μl of 50 mM Tris-HCl (pH 7.5), 12.5 mM $MgCl_2$, 1.25 mg/ml protamine sulfate, and 125 μM [δ − ^{32}P]ATP with a specific activity of about 100–150 cpm/pmol for 5 min at 37°C. Then 30 μl of the reaction mixture is spotted on a 1×1 cm phosphocellulose paper square (P81, Whatman), washed twice for 10 min with 30% acetic acid, and counted in a liquid scintillation counter. Figure 7 shows that this two-step procedure yields an appropriately purified protein for enzymatic studies. The specific activity of the Superdex S-200 pool is around 100–150 units/min/mg, whereby 1 unit incorporates 1 nmol

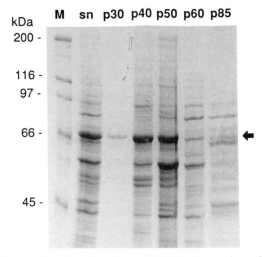

FIG. 6   Ammonium sulfate fractionation of PKC-ζ. Approximately 5×10^7 cells were infected with the PKC-ζ baculovirus, lysed after 2 days in 20 ml buffer A with 50 μg/ml PMSF, 0.1% Triton X-100, and centrifuged. The supernatant (sn) was fractionated by ammonium sulfate precipitation as described in the text, and the precipitates corresponding to 30, 40, 50, 60, and 85% saturation with ammonium sulfate were resolved on an SDS–polyacrylamide gel and stained with Coomassie blue. The arrow marks the position of the prominent PKC-ζ band in the supernatant, the 30%, the 40%, and the 50% ammonium sulfate pellet.

of phosphate into the ζ-substrate peptide (Gly-Glu-Asp-Lys-Ser-Ile-Tyr-Arg-Arg-Gly-Ser-Arg-Arg-Trp-Arg-Lys-Leu-Tyr-Arg-Ala) derived from the pseudosubstrate sequence of the PKC-ζ polypeptide (37, 38). Obviously, the assay employed here for the activity measurement of PKC-ζ cannot be applied as a PKC-ζ-specific assay in mammalian cells since all PKCs accept protamine sulfate as a substrate as well as the ζ-substrate peptide. However, the availability of purified PKC-ζ should help in identifying specific activators and/or specific assay conditions for this subtype.

Posttranslational Modifications of Classic Group A Enzymes in Insect Cells

Posttranslational modification as identified by decreased electrophoretic mobility of the protein in SDS–polyacrylamide gels has been described for PKC in mammalian cells (39–42). Moreover, it appears that insect cells carry out the modifications required to generate PKC proteins, which are silent when

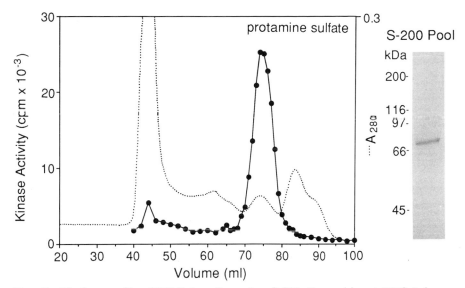

FIG. 7   Elution profile of PKC-ζ on Superdex S-200. Recombinant PKC-ζ from a 50-ml suspension culture was precipitated with 45% ammonium sulfate, and the precipitate was dissolved in 1 ml buffer A and resolved by gel filtration on Superdex S-200. Kinase activity (●) was assayed in the absence of activators on protamine sulfate as a substrate. Addition of activators (PS/PMA) gave the same profile. The size of the native PKC-ζ protein on this column was determined to be 80 kDa. Active fractions were pooled, separated by SDS–polyacrylamide gel electrophoresis, and stained with Coomassie blue (S-200 pool).

isolated from the cells but can be activated on the addition of the standard activators on the appropriate substrates *in vitro*.

By pulse–chase labeling of recombinant proteins posttranslational modifications can be identified and analyzed. For pulse–chase labeling of PKCs with [^{35}S]methionine, 3×10^6 insect cells in 60-mm dishes are infected with the recombinant virus. After 2 days the cells are preincubated in 2 ml methionine-free TNM-FH medium [prepared according to Summers and Smith (21) or obtained from GIBCO] with 5% FCS at 27°C for 1 hr. The cells are then pulse-labeled in 1 ml for 15 min with 120 μCi [^{35}S]methionine (Amersham), washed with PBS, and chased in ordinary TNM-FH for increasing times. At the appropriate time points the cells are washed with PBS and lysed for immunoprecipitation of the labeled polypeptide.

Figure 8 shows results from a pulse–chase [^{35}S]methionine-labeling experiment with insect cells expressing bovine PKC-α and human PKC-βI and PKC-βII. All group A enzymes are synthesized as (unphosphorylated?) pre-

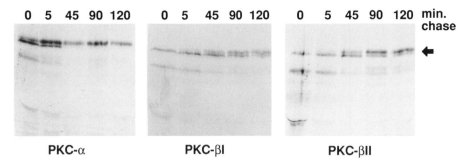

FIG. 8   Posttranslational modification of PKC-α, -βI, and -βII in insect cells. Infected insect cells were pulse labeled with [^{35}S]methionine and chased with unlabeled methionine for the indicated times as described in the text. PKC proteins were immunoprecipitated, resolved on an 8% SDS–polyacrylamide gel, and autoradiographed. The arrow marks the position of the PKC polypeptides.

cursor molecules which are shifted in molecular weight with time. In the case of mammalian PKC-α, -δ, -ε, and insect cell-expressed PKC-γ, the molecular weight shift has been shown to be due to phosphorylation (11, 41–43).

By means of *in vivo* labeling with ortho[^{32}P]phosphate, it is clear that all PKC subtypes including group B enzymes are produced as phosphoproteins in insect cells and can autophosphorylate after addition of activator (PMA) either directly to the infected cells or in an *in vitro* autophosphorylation assay. Metabolic labeling with ortho[^{32}P]phosphate is most conveniently done in 35-mm plastic tissue culture dishes. For this purpose 1×10^6 cells are infected with recombinant baculovirus and incubated in a wet box at 27°C in order to minimize evaporation of the medium (21). At 2 days postinfection, when cells are still well attached, the cells are washed once with Tris–saline and labeled for 4 hr with ortho[^{32}P]phosphate (100–250 μCi/ml) in 1 ml of phosphate-free TMN-FH medium prepared according to Summers and Smith (21) or obtained from GIBCO. After the labeling period the cells are carefully washed once with 2 ml Tris–saline, lysed in buffer A containing 50 μg/ml PMSF, 0.1% Triton X-100, and processed for immunoprecipitation.

Figure 9 shows the immunoprecipitates from 1×10^6 cells infected with PKC-γ or a kinase-negative mutant PKC-γ_{M380} (15) and labeled with [^{32}P]phosphate for 4 hr as described above. PKC-γ is produced as a phosphoprotein in insect cells; a considerable part of this phosphorylation is due to autophosphorylation since it is absent in the kinase-deficient mutant (Fig. 9). It should be noted, however, that this *in vivo* autophosphorylation activity does not continue in the presence of ATP once the protein is extracted from the

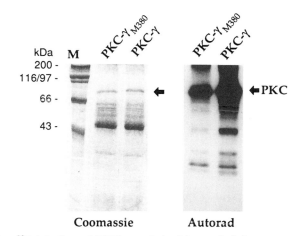

FIG. 9   *In vivo* ^{32}P-labeling of PKC-γ and the kinase-deficient mutant PKC-γ_{M380} in insect cells. Insect cells expressing PKC-γ or the kinase-negative mutant PKC-γ_{M380} (15) were labeled with ortho[^{32}P]phosphate as described in the text, and the PKC polypeptides were immunoprecipitated. The arrows indicate the positions of the Coomassie blue-stained PKC polypeptides in the immunoprecipitate and the ^{32}P-labeled PKC proteins, respectively.

cells. *In vitro* autophosphorylation of recombinant as well as authentic PKC requires the addition of activators.

Comments

A kit has been introduced (BaculoGold by Invitrogen, San Diego, CA) that employs a novel strategy to isolate recombinant baculoviruses, avoiding the generation of wild-type virus and thereby eliminating the need to screen for recombinant viruses. Although we have not tested the kit with any of the PKC cDNAs, we have used it successfully with the pAcYM1 vector to isolate several unrelated recombinant baculoviruses. The kit can be used for five transfections; the speed and ease of isolation of recombinant viruses make the kit the present system of choice for the expression of novel cDNAs. By performing the transfection in a 35-mm plate, it is possible to use only one-fifth of the recommended material from the kit per transfection, which makes the kit suitable for 25 transfections.

Analysis of the properties of the recombinant PKCs indicate that the recombinant proteins are authentic in size, posttranslational modification (as far as analyzed), and enzymatic characteristics (phorbol ester binding, stimulation by activators, specific activity). For the group of novel PKCs δ, ε, ζ, η, and θ, the properties of the recombinant proteins still have to be confirmed. This will have to await the isolation of the respective enzymes from natural sources, as has already been reported for PKC-δ, -ε, and -ζ (41, 42, 44). At present there is no indication that the recombinant PKCs differ in enzymatic properties from the subtypes that have been purified from natural sources.

Acknowledgments

We gratefully acknowledge the crucial technical and scientific contributions of Gunvanti Patel, Nic Jones, and Peter J. Parker for initiating the baculovirus expression of PKC. We also thank Doriano Fabbro for sharing unpublished results and for providing the immunoblot shown in Fig. 1. Work in the author's laboratory was supported by a grant from the Ministry for Research and Technology (BMFT).

References

1. R. Michell, *Trends Biochem Sci.* **17,** 274 (1992).
2. M. J. Berridge and R. F. Irvine, *Nature* (*London*) **312,** 315 (1984).
3. Y. Nishizuka, *Nature* (*London*) **308,** 693 (1984).
4. Y. Nishizuka, *Science* **233,** 305 (1986).
5. P. J. Parker, L. Coussens, N. Totty, L. Rhee, S. Young, E. Chen, S. Stabel, M. D. Waterfield, and A. Ullrich, *Science* **233,** 853 (1986).
6. L. Coussens, P. J. Parker, L. Rhee, T. L. Yang-Feng, T. L. Chen. M. D. Waterfield, U. Francke, and A. Ullrich, *Science* **233,** 859 (1986).
7. K.-P. Huang, H. Nakabayashi, and F. Huang, *Proc. Natl. Acad. Sci. U.S.A.* **83,** 8535 (1986).
8. U. Kikkawa, Y. Ono, K. Ogita, T. Fujii, Y. Asaoka, K. Sekiguchi, Y. Kosaka, K. Igarashi, and Y. Nishizuka, *FEBS Lett.* **217,** 227 (1987).
9. R. M. Marais and P. J. Parker, *Eur. J. Biochem.* **182,** 129 (1989).
10. L. Coussens, L. Rhee, P. J. Parker, and A. Ullrich, *DNA* **6,** 389 (1987).
11. G. Patel and S. Stabel, *Cell. Signalling* **1,** 227 (1989).
12. D. Schaap and P. J. Parker, *J. Biol. Chem.* **265,** 7301 (1990).
13. D. J. Burns and R. M. Bell, *J. Biol. Chem.* **266,** 18330 (1991).
14. D. J. Burns, J. Bloomenthal, M.-H. Lee, and R. M. Bell, *J. Biol. Chem.* **265,** 12044 (1990).
15. I. Freisewinkel, D. Riethmacher, and S. Stabel, *FEBS Lett.* **280,** 262 (1991).
16. A. J. Flint, R. D. Paladini, and D. E. Koshland, Jr., *Science* **249,** 408 (1990).
17. B. Fiebich, H. Hug, and D. Marmé, *FEBS Lett.* **277,** 15 (1990).
18. S. R. Hubbard, W. R. Bishop, P. Kirschmeier, S. J. George, S. P. Cramer, and W. A. Hendrickson, *Science* **254,** 1776 (1991).

19. M. Liyanage, D. Frith, E. Livneh, and S. Stabel, *Biochem J.* **283,** 781 (1992).
20. G. E. Smith, M. D. Summers, and M. J. Fraser, *Mol. Cell. Biol.* **3,** 2156 (1983).
21. M. D. Summers and G. E. Smith, *Texas Agric. Exp. Stn. Bull.* No. 1555 (1987).
22. J. Krieger, K. Raming, G. D. Prestwich, D. Frith, S. Stabel, and H. Breer, *Eur. J. Biochem.* **203,** 161 (1992).
23. V. A. Luckow and M. D. Summers, *Bio/Technology* **6,** 47 (1988).
24. Y. Matsuura, R. D. Possee, H. A. Overton, and D. H. L. Bishop, *J. Gen. Virol.* **68,** 1233 (1987).
25. V. A. Luckow and M. D. Summers, *Virology* **170,** 31 (1989).
26. U. K. Laemmli, *Nature (London)* **227,** 680 (1970).
27. S. Stabel, A. Rodriguez-Pena, S. Young, E. Rozengurt, and P. J. Parker, *J. Cell. Physiol.* **130,** 111 (1987).
28. P. J. Parker, S. Stabel, and M. D. Waterfield, *EMBO J.* **3,** 953 (1984).
29. S. Stabel, D. Schaap, and P. J. Parker, *in* "Methods in Enzymology" (T. Hunter and B. M. Sefton, eds.), Vol. 200, p. 670. Academic Press, San Diego, 1991.
30. Y. A. Hannun, C. Loomis, and R. M. Bell, *J. Biol. Chem.* **260,** 10039 (1985).
31. S.-I. Osada, K. Mizuno, T. C. Saido, K. Suzuki, T. Kuroki, and S. Ohno, *Mol. Cell. Biol.* **12,** 3930 (1992).
32. Y. Nishizuka, *JAMA, J. Am. Med. Assoc.* **262,** 1826 (1989).
33. S. Stabel and P. J. Parker, *Pharmacol. Ther.* **51,** 71 (1991).
34. D. Schaap, J. Hsuan, and P. J. Parker, *Eur. J. Biochem.* **191,** 431 (1990).
35. H. Leibersperger, M. Gschwendt, and F. Marks, *J. Biol. Chem.* **265,** 16108 (1990).
36. C. Pears, D. Schaap, and P. J. Parker, *Biochem. J.* **276,** 257 (1991).
37. C. House and B. E. Kemp, *Science* **238,** 1726 (1987).
38. S. Stabel, *in* "Growth Factors, Differentiation Factors and Cytokines" (A. Habenicht, ed.), p. 414. Springer-Verlag, Berlin, 1990.
39. C. Borner, I. Filipuzzi, M. Wartmann, U. Eppenberger, and D. Fabbro, *J. Biol. Chem.* **264,** 13902 (1989).
40. P. J. Parker, F. Mitchell, S. Stabel, R. Marais, A. Ullrich, and J. Goris, *Adv. Protein Phosphatases* **4,** 363 (1987).
41. K. Ogita, S. Miyamoto, K. Yamaguchi, H. Koide, N. Fujisawa, U. Kikkawa, S. Sahara, Y. Fukami, and Y. Nishizuka, *Proc. Natl. Acad. Sci. U.S.A.* **89,** 1592 (1992).
42. H. Koide, K. Ogita, U. Kikkawa, and Y. Nishizuka, *Proc. Natl. Acad. Sci. U.S.A.* **89,** 1149 (1992).
43. C. Pears, S. Stabel, S. Cazaubon, and P. J. Parker, *Biochem J.* **283,** 515 (1992).
44. H. Nakanishi and J. H. Exton, *J. Biol. Chem.* **267,** 16347 (1992).

[17] Immunochemical Localization of Protein Kinase C and Phosphoinositide-Specific Phospholipase C

Susan Jaken and Karen Leach

Introduction

Several phosphoinositide-specific phospholipase (PI–PLC) and protein kinase C (PKC) isoforms have been identified (1). A given tissue or cell type may contain multiple isoforms of each enzyme; however, the specific functions of individual isoforms remain undefined. One approach toward gaining a better understanding of the purpose of PLC and PKC heterogeneity is to compare the regulation, activation, and localization of the PI–PLCs and PKCs in well-defined cellular systems.

In general, agonist stimulation of PI–PLC activity is rapid and transient. Rapid activation can be attributed to ligand binding to G-protein-linked receptors or receptor tyrosine kinases (1). The dependence of PKC activation on diacylglycerol derived from PI–PLCs indicates a potential requirement for close proximity of the two enzymes in the cell. Although DAG is readily diffusible it is also rapidly metabolized. Thus, spatial organization of the PI–PLCs and the PKCs may be an important modulator of the signal transduction pathway.

Ligand-dependent activation of PI–PLC is transient, indicating that inactivation pathways exist to strictly limit this catalytic activity. Inactivation mechanisms are less clear, but several lines of evidence suggest that PKCs are involved (1). PI–PLC-β has been shown to be directly phosphorylated by PKC (2). Direct effects of PI–PLC-β phosphorylation on catalytic activity were not observed (2); however, pretreatment of cells with phorbol esters or overexpression of PKCs has been shown to down-modulate agonist-stimulated PI–PLC hydrolysis in some (see references cited in Ref. 2) but not all cases (3). These results suggest that PKC is a negative regulator of PI–PLC activity but that the effect is indirectly mediated, perhaps by modulating the coupling of the PI–PLCs to effector G proteins (2). Inhibition of PI–PLC-γ may be indirectly mediated through PKC phosphorylation and inhibition of receptor tyrosine kinases (4). Immunohistochemical localization studies have demonstrated that PI–PLC-γ and the epidermal growth factor (EGF) receptor colocalize in epidermis and mammary epithelium (5, 6).

Methods in Neurosciences, Volume 18

Compartmentalization of PI–PLCs and PKCs may be essential for regulated activation of PKC and inactivation of PI–PLC. Although little is known about the localization of the PI–PLCs and the PKCs at present, some evidence suggesting that the cytoskeleton may provide the appropriate scaffolding for the organization of signal-transducing molecules has accumulated. This model is supported by the direct regulation of the functions of several cytoskeletal-associated proteins by PKC phosphorylation (7). The following is a report of useful methods for studying the interactive relationships between PI–PLCs and PKCs.

Diacylglycerol Production and Protein Kinase Activation

The first step in considering the relationship between PI–PLCs and PKCs is to compare the time courses for PLC activation and PKC isozyme activation. The recognition that both PLCs and PKCs are gene families raises the obvious question: Could activation of specific PLCs be linked to activation of specific PKCs? It should be noted that each of the PKCs identified to date (except PKC-ζ which is not a phorbol ester receptor) can be activated *in vitro* by diacylglycerols (DAGs) (8–10). Thus, DAGs could potentially regulate the cellular activity of each of these PKCs, although other lipid activators may also be important. It should also be emphasized that PI–PLCs are not the only source of agonist-stimulated DAG accumulation. Agonist-stimulated phosphatidylcholine hydrolysis by PLC and phospholipase D (PLD) activities also contribute to cellular DAG levels (11).

GH_4C_1 rat pituitary cells are a hormonally responsive cell line that express immunoreactive α-, β-, δ-, ε- and ζ-PKCs. Thus, they are a useful model system for studying the regulation of several PKCs simultaneously in response to a variety of agonists. Treatment of GH_4C_1 cells with activating phorbol esters causes redistribution of immunoreactive PKCs (except PKC-ζ) from the soluble to the particulate fractions (12–16). Thus, in these as in most cells, chelator-stable association of PKCs with the particulate fraction is a good indicator of enzyme activation. The use of chelators is essential because calcium alone will also promote association of the calcium-dependent (group A) isozymes (α, β, γ) with the particulate fraction. The calcium-independent PKCs (group B) are refractory to calcium-promoted association with the particulate fraction, and, in fact, calcium-dependent particulate association can be used to separate group A and group B PKCs (15).

The link between hormone-stimulated PI hydrolysis and PKC activation has been explored in GH_4C_1 cells. Thyrotropin-releasing hormone (TRH), which regulates the synthesis and secretion of prolactin by these cells, is known to stimulate PI–PLC through a G-protein-dependent pathway

(17, 18). However, TRH must stimulate additional lipid metabolic pathways since TRH was shown to induce three distinct phases of DAG production in the cells (12). The effect of each of the three TRH-induced DAG pools on PKC isozymes was analyzed by determining the distribution of PKCs between soluble and particulate fractions at different times after TRH treatment (12). First, TRH causes a rapid rise in DAG (within 15 sec), which declines within 3 to 5 min. This time course correlates with the rapid and transient increase in inositol 1,4,5-trisphosphate (IP_3) and cytosolic calcium levels, and, therefore, phase 1 DAG appears to be derived from PI–PLC. The type of G-protein-sensitive PI–PLC stimulated by TRH has not yet been determined.

Attempts to identify immunoreactive PLC-β in these cells have not been successful, which may indicate that a different G-protein-sensitive PLC exists in these cells. Phase 1 DAG caused redistribution of each of the isozymes (except ζ). Time courses for redistribution for each PKC were similar and closely paralleled DAG production. Thus, there was no selectivity for the combined calcium and DAG signal characteristic of phase 1 for activating group A rather than group B PKCs.

A second phase of DAG production peaks around 10 min and declines by 20 min. Comparison of the fatty acid composition of these DAGs with cellular phospholipids indicated that phosphatidylcholine or phosphatidylethanolamine were the likely sources of this second phase DAG (13). In contrast, phase 2 DAG did not correlate with redistribution of any of the isozymes. In other words, the DAG derived from this source did not appear to activate (redistribute) any of the PKCs. Phase 3 DAG also did not influence PKC isozyme distribution between soluble and particulate compartments.

To account for the possibility that redistribution may not always be the best marker for PKC activation, a second marker for PKC activation was also studied. Activation of PKCs is associated with increased phosphate incorporation into the PKCs themselves (19). To study PKC phosphorylation, cells were prelabeled with $^{32}PO_4$. Cell lysates were collected various times after TRH treatment, and PKCs were immunoprecipitated with isozyme-specific antibodies. PKC-α and PKC-ε were analyzed as representatives of group A and B PKCs, respectively. Phorbol 12,13-dibutyrate (PDBu) caused increased phosphate incorporation into both PKC-α and -ε, indicative of its activating ability (12). TRH also increased phosphate incorporation into both PKC-α and -ε within 15 sec. However, the increased phosphate was no longer apparent 10 min after TRH addition. Thus, according to both criteria for PKC activation, redistribution and phosphorylation, no evidence for isozyme activation during phase 2 DAG could be found (12).

Methods

Measurement of Cellular Diacylglycerol Mass

Culture conditions can markedly affect DAG mass values. For example, basal DAG mass values are 2- to 3-fold higher in cells maintained in serum-containing versus serum-free medium. For consistency, it is best to maintain cells in serum-free medium for 24 to 48 hr prior to agonist treatment. DAG mass is quantitated using the DAG kinase method of Preiss et al. (20).

Redistribution of Protein Kinase C Isozymes

Lysates are prepared from cells grown in 100-mm dishes. Monolayers are washed twice with 50 mM Tris-Cl (pH 7.4) containing 2.5 mM magnesium chloride and 0.25 M sucrose (buffer A). All procedures are performed at 4°C. Cells are then scraped into buffer A containing 2.5 mM EDTA, 1 mM phenylmethylsulfonyl fluoride (PMSF), 1 mM dithiothreitol (DTT), 10 μg/ml leupeptin, and 1 μg/ml aprotinin. Cells are lysed by sonication, and soluble and particulate fractions are collected by centrifugation at 100,000 g for 60 min. Typically, 100 μg of soluble and particulate fractions is analyzed for PKC isozyme content on immunoblots using isozyme-specific antibodies. Redistribution of catalytic activity may also be monitored by measuring kinase activity; however, differences in optimal substrates and assay conditions among the isozymes makes this approach less reliable. Monitoring redistribution of phorbol ester binding activity with [³H]PDBu may also be useful in some circumstances (21).

Radiolabeling and Sample Preparation for Immunoprecipitation

Maximal $^{32}PO_4$ labeling of PKCs is achieved by growing cells to high density in 35- or 60-mm dishes under optimal conditions, then serum-starving the cells for 48 hr. In our experience, reducing the serum to 0.2% works well for most cultured cells. Cultures are washed 3 times in phosphate-free Dulbecco's modified Eagle's medium (DMEM) buffered with 10 mM HEPES (pH 7.4) and then incubated in 2 ml of the same medium supplemented with 0.2% serum for 60 min in a 37°C CO_2 incubator. Cells are then labeled in phosphate-free DMEM containing 0.2% serum and 0.1 mCi $^{32}PO_4$/ml medium for 4 hr. Agonists are added during the end of the labeling period. Cell lysates are collected in RIPA [1% sodium deoxycholic acid, 1% Triton X-100, 0.1% sodium dodecyl sulfate (SDS), 50 mM Tris-Cl (pH 7.4), 150 mM sodium chloride, 1 mM EDTA, 2 μM leupeptin, 1.5 μM aprotinin, and 1 mM PMSF] containing phosphatase inhibitors (50 mM sodium fluoride and 100 μM sodium vanadate). To avoid radioactive contamination of the sonicator, cells are lysed by drawing the samples through a narrow-gauge needle. Alternatively, soluble and cytoskeletal fractions (see below) are prepared in the presence of phosphatase inhibitors. For immunoprecipitation, samples are brought to 1× RIPA by the addition of 5× concentrated stock. Standard immunoprecipitation procedures are used to collect the immune complexes on protein A-Sepharose.

Diacylglycerol Production and Protein Kinase Down-Modulation

The distribution of the PKCs before and after the sustained TRH treatment corresponding to phase 3 DAG was not significantly different. However, the sustained TRH treatment caused a significant decrease in the amount of immunoreactive PKC-ε (12). Levels of the other isozymes were not affected. To determine the mechanism for this TRH effect, PKC-ε was immunoprecipitated from cells metabolically labeled with [^{35}S]methionine in appropriate pulse–chase protocols. TRH did not influence the rate of PKC-ε synthesis but did increase the rate of PKC-ε degradation by approximately 2-fold. Results from several laboratories have established the relationship between increased PKC activity and increased degradation rate (22, 23). Catalytically active PKCs are more susceptible to proteolysis than are the inactive conformers. Taken together, these results indicate that TRH specifically influences the activity of PKC-ε, although this effect cannot be monitored as a redistribution or increased phosphorylation of PKC-ε.

Methods

Measuring Rates of Protein Kinase C Synthesis and Degradation

Dense cultures in 60-mm dishes are washed twice with phosphate-buffered saline and then incubated in 4 ml of methionine-free DMEM containing 1% serum and buffered with 10 mM HEPES, pH 7.4, for 1 hr in a 37°C CO$_2$ incubator. To determine the rate of synthesis, cells are pretreated with agonist for the appropriate times, after which they are pulse-labeled with [^{35}S]methionine-containing medium (0.5 mCi) for 10 to 15 min. To determine the rate of degradation, cultures are prelabeled with [^{35}S]methionine (0.1 mCi) for at least 4 hr; 18 to 24 hr is often convenient. Cultures are then washed and switched to nonradioactive methionine-containing medium for chase times from 1 to 24 hr in the presence or absence of agonist. For both procedures, cell lysates are collected in 0.5 ml RIPA [1% deoxycholate, 1% Triton X-100, 0.1% SDS, 50 mM Tris-Cl (pH 7.4), 150 mM sodium chloride, and 1 mM EDTA with 2 μM leupeptin, 1.5 μM aprotinin, and 1 mM PMSF added as protease inhibitors]. Phosphatase inhibitors (50 mM sodium fluoride and 100

μM sodium vanadate) can also be added. The dish is washed with a second 0.5 ml of RIPA. The combined lysates are homogenized with several passes through a 26-gauge needle. Typically, 0.5 ml of the RIPA lysate is used for immunoprecipitation of each PKC isozyme.

Cytoskeletal Association of Protein Kinase C Isozymes

To analyze the properties of the subcellular compartments to which the PKCs redistribute, both subcellular fractionation and immunocytofluorescence techniques should be employed to cross-check and verify results. In GH_4C_1 cells, particulate PKCs were not readily solubilized by Triton X-100 in the presence of chelators (14, 16). These results suggested that the redistributed PKCs associated with the cytoskeletal fraction, which is operationally defined as the detergent-insoluble particulate fraction. Immunocytofluorescence studies supported the biochemical analyses. Immunoreactive PKC-α, -δ, and -ε were localized in detergent-insoluble preparations by immunofluorescence (12, 14, 16). Agonist stimulation, with either TRH or phorbol ester, increased the amount of each antigen in the cytoskeletal preparations. Cytoskeletons are prepared by removing soluble components by incubating the cells in detergent before fixing and immunostaining. Only the detergent-insoluble components, namely, the cytoskeleton and cytoskeletal-associated proteins and the nucleus, remain in these preparations.

In the rat fibroblast cell line REF52, PKC-α was shown to be associated with the cytoskeleton in the absence of an activating stimulus. Immunocytofluorescence studies demonstrated that PKC-α was concentrated in certain areas and in fact colocalized with the focal contact protein talin (24). Focal contacts are sites of cell–substratum attachment in which the microfilaments are indirectly linked to the extracellular matrix receptor integrin via several proteins including talin, vinculin, and α-actinin (25, 26). Focal contacts are important mediators of cell attachment and migration. In transformed cells, less stable and more dynamic structures known as close contacts mediate cell–substratum attachment. Interestingly, PKC-α was not concentrated in close contacts of SV40-transformed REF52 cells (27).

The discrete and transformation-sensitive distribution of PKC-α in these cells provided an interesting background on which to compare PLC and PKC localizations. Immunoblot and immunoprecipitation studies demonstrated that a small percentage of the total cellular PKC-α and PLC-γ were recovered in cytoskeletal fractions (28). Immunocytofluorescence studies demonstrated that PLC-γ colocalized with phalloidin, which specifically stains filamentous actin. PLC-γ colocalized with talin at the tips of the microfilaments, but, unlike talin, PLC-γ was distributed along the entire length of the actin cables.

These results demonstrate that PLC-γ and PKC-α are both present in the focal contacts; however, PLC-γ has a more general cytoskeletal location than PKC-α.

Platelet-derived growth factor (PDGF) increased the total amount of cytoskeletal-associated PLC-γ recovered by immunoprecipitation (28). Immunoblots of the precipitated cytoskeletal PLC-γ demonstrated that it contained phosphotyrosine. What might be the link between cytoskeletal-associated PLC-γ and signal transduction? The substrate for PLC-γ, phosphatidylinositol 4,5-bisphosphate (PIP$_2$), tightly associates with several actin-binding proteins including profilin. In fact, profilin inhibits PLC-γ activity *in vitro* owing to its ability to sequester PIP$_2$ (29–31). Whereas PIP$_2$ bound to profilin was not a good substrate for unphosphorylated PLC-γ, it has been shown to be the preferred substrate for tyrosine-phosphorylated PLC-γ (32). The accumulated data suggest that activation of receptor tyrosine kinases which are linked to phosphorylation of PLC-γ can promote hydrolysis of PIP$_2$ bound to profilin. The free profilin could then bind to monomeric actin and thereby inhibit nucleation and elongation of actin polymers. These conditions, which favor actin depolymerization, may be related to the rapid effect of growth factors that activate receptor tyrosine kinases on membrane ruffling and morphological changes. This model is attractive in view of evidence demonstrating that activation of PI–PLC-γ by PDGF and fibroblast growth factor (FGF) is not necessary for the mitogenic activity of these factors (33–36).

Methods

Extraction of Particulate-Associated Protein Kinase C Isozymes

Soluble and particulate fractions (100,000 g, see above) are prepared. Particulate fractions (4 mg) from control and stimulated cultures are resuspended by sonicating in buffer A as described above for redistribution of PKCs. EGTA-soluble and particulate fractions are collected after centrifuging at 10,000 g for 15 min. The particulate fraction is washed once more in TE [20 mM Tris-Cl (pH 7.4), containing 1 mM EDTA, 1 mM DTT and 10 μg/ml leupeptin] and recentrifuged. The pellet is resuspended by pipetting in 100 μl TE containing 1% Triton X-100 and is incubated for 15 min at 4°C. The sample is diluted with TE to 500 μl and recentrifuged. The Triton X-100 soluble fraction is collected. The Triton X-100 insoluble fraction is directly resuspended in electrophoresis sample preparation buffer or RIPA.

Preparation of Soluble and Cytoskeletal Fractions

Cells are grown in 100-mm dishes. To prepare cytoskeletons, cultures are washed twice in 0.1 M PIPES (pH 6.9), 2 M glycerol, 1 mM EDTA, and 1 mM magnesium acetate (MSB) as described (37). Soluble proteins are then extracted during a 4-min incubation in 1.0 ml MSB containing 0.2% Triton X-100, 10 μg/ml aprotinin, and 10 μg/ml leupeptin. Phosphatase inhibitors (50 mM sodium fluoride and 1 mM sodium vanadate) can be included when appropriate. Cytoskeletons can be directly scraped into RIPA for immunoprecipitation. Soluble fractions are brought to 1× RIPA by the addition of 5× concentrated RIPA.

In some cases with loosely adherent cells, we have found that Triton X-100 removes the cells from the dish. Substituting 0.5% digitonin for the Triton X-100 overcomes this difficulty (14).

Immunocytofluorescence

Cells are grown on 12-mm round glass coverslips in 35-mm dishes. For loosely adherent cells, it may be necessary to precoat the coverslips with polylysine or extracellular matrix components. Cells are washed twice in phosphate-buffered saline (PBS), then fixed for 10 min at room temperature in 3.7% formaldehyde (prepared from paraformaldehyde) in PBS. Coverslips are washed twice in PBS and then incubated at −20°C for 6 min in methanol. For phalloidin staining, acetone rather than methanol must be used. The samples are washed twice more in PBS, then blocked by incubating for 30 min in PBS containing 1% (w/v) bovine serum albumin (PBA). Coverslips are incubated for 1 hr with first antibody diluted in PBA, washed 3 times with PBA, and then incubated with second antibody diluted in PBA for 30 min.

Cytoskeletons can be prepared from cells grown on coverslips using the detergent extraction in MSB outlined above. After washing in MSB, cells are fixed and processed as described for the whole cell preparations above.

Protein Kinase C-Binding Proteins Target Protein Kinase C to Cytoskeleton

Immunocytofluorescence studies have demonstrated that PKC-α is concentrated in focal contacts of REF52 cells and in cell–cell contacts of rat primary renal proximal tubule epithelial cells (24, 38). The discrete localization of PKC-α to specific cytoskeletal structures suggested that PKC was targeted to these locations via interactions with cytoskeletal-associated proteins (27). A biochemical assay to detect PKC-binding proteins was used to investigate this possibility. In this method, cellular proteins are separated by denaturing polyacrylamide gel electrophoresis (SDS-PAGE) and then blotted to nitrocellulose. The immobilized proteins are "overlayed" with partially purified PKC, which under appropriate conditions binds to target proteins. Overlay assays have been widely used to study the interactions of cytoskeletal components and were first introduced to the PKC field in 1986 by Wolf and Sahyoun (39).

Two lines of evidence demonstrate the utility of the overlay assay. First, the two major binding proteins detected in REF52 cells, p71 and p>200 kDa, were not detected in SV40 transformed REF52 cells (27). Thus, there is a correlation between loss of cytoskeletal-associated PKC-α and loss of PKC-α-binding proteins. Second, the properties of the two major binding proteins correlate with the properties of the two major PKC substrates in these cells. These properties include molecular weight, isoelectric point, heat stability, and retention on calmodulin-Sepharose affinity columns (39a). Furthermore, the two substrates were not detected in extracts of the SV40-transformed cells. These data indicate that the overlay assay is a useful method for identifying PKC substrates.

Methods

Overlay Assay

Protein samples may be prepared as cell lysates, 100,000 g soluble and particulate fractions, or soluble and cytoskeletal fractions as described above. Samples (≤ 100 μg) are separated by SDS-PAGE and blotted to nitrocellulose. Nitrocellulose sheets are blocked with 5% (w/v) nonfat instant milk (we find Carnation brand dissolves easily) in 50 mM Tris-Cl (pH 7.4) containing 0.5 M NaCl (TBS), then washed twice with TBS. Blocked nitrocellulose sheets can be stored for several months.

In the standard assay, the nitrocellulose sheets are incubated for 1 hr at room temperature in TBS containing 10 μg/ml partially purified rabbit brain PKC, 10 μg/ml bovine serum albumin, 20 μg/ml phosphatidylserine (PS), 1 mM EGTA, 1.2 mM calcium, 10 μg/ml leupeptin, and 10 μg/ml aprotinin. Because binding is reversible, PS and calcium must be retained throughout all the washes and incubations with first and second antibodies. However, we have found that fixing the PKC to the binding proteins eliminates this requirement. Therefore, after incubating with PKC, samples are washed twice for 5 min each time in PBS containing PS, EGTA, and calcium. Proteins are fixed by incubating in 0.5% formaldehyde in PBS for 20 min at room temperature. Unreacted aldehydes are blocked in a subsequent incubation with 2% glycine in PBS for 20 min. After washing 3 times in TBS, samples are incubated with isozyme-specific PKC antibodies, washed, and finally incubated with alkaline phosphatase-conjugated second antibodies. Both the endogenous PKC contained in the sample and the PKC-binding proteins are detected with appropriate color development.

Nuclear Phosphoinositide-Specific Phospholipase C and Protein Kinase C

A central problem in defining signal transduction pathways is understanding how signals generated at the cell surface can be transmitted to the nucleus. Preliminary evidence suggesting that both PI–PLC and PKC activities are present in highly purified nuclear preparations (40, 41) indicates that agonist-stimulated nuclear phosphoinositide metabolism may directly regulate the phosphorylation of target proteins, such as lamin B and DNA topoisomerase II (45–47). A major component of these experiments is demonstrating the purity of the nuclear preparations used for biochemical analyses. Immunocytofluorescence experiments should be used in conjunction with the biochemical analyses to cross-check and verify results.

A series of studies has demonstrated the existence of nuclear PI–PLC activity. In 3T3 cells, insulin-like growth factor-1 (IGF-1) rapidly stimulated nuclear PI–PLC activity. In these experiments, nuclei were prepared from control and IGF-1-treated cells and the masses of DAG and polyphosphoinositides were measured (44). The sensitive mass assays used avoid problems in interpretation of radiolabeling experiments, including the very slow labeling of nuclear phosphoinositides with [^{3}H]inositol as a precursor. The rapid rise in nuclear but not total cellular DAG by IGF-1 suggested that the PI–PLC activity involved is compartmentalized in the nucleus. Corollary experiments indicated that the nuclear DAG may mediate translocation of PKCs to the nucleus, thus providing evidence for a functional nuclear PI–PLC/PKC signaling pathway. Immunoblotting and immunocytofluorescence experiments indicated that the β isoform of PI–PLC and not the δ or γ isoforms is associated with the increased nuclear catalytic activity (42, 43). Immunoblot analysis of subcellular fractions indicated that PLC-β was specifically recovered in purified nuclear fractions. Calpain inhibitors (N-acetyl/leucyl/leucyl/norleucinal and N-acetyl/leucyl/leucyl/normethioninal) were essential for recovery of the 150-kDa form of the enzyme; in their absence, only a lower M_r form of 100,000 was detected (42). Although IGF-1 did not increase the amount of nuclear PLC-β, the amount of PI–PLC catalytic activity was increased (42). Immunocytofluorescence studies confirmed the nuclear localization (42, 43). Because PLC-β activity is known to be regulated by G-protein-linked membrane receptors, it seems likely that the nuclear form described in these experiments is only one of several PLC-β isoforms and that this form is preferentially recognized by the antibodies used. In other words, distinct PLC-β isoforms may be compartmentalized in different subcellular locations.

Using immunological and biochemical analysis, we and others have demonstrated the presence of PKC in the nuclei of hepatocytes (48), HL-60 cells (49), 3T3 cells (40, 44, 50), and IIC9 cells (51). In some systems, PKC appears to be constitutively expessed in the nucleus. For example, in liver, PKC-β is present in nuclei from unstimulated tissues (48). PKC-ζ was detected by immunofluorescence in nuclei from resting Purkinje cells (52). In contrast, in a number of other cell models, such as 3T3 cells, IIC9 cells, and HL-60 cells, PKC is present in nuclei prepared from stimulated but not unstimulated cells. Stimuli resulting in PKC nuclear localization include phorbol 12-myristate 13-acetate (PMA), bryostatin, IGF-1, and α-thrombin (40, 44, 50, 51, 53). PMA and bryostatin may be able to activate PKC directly, leading to nuclear localization, but the mechanisms by which mitogens such as α-thrombin result in increased levels of nuclear PKC are not known.

To address this question, we have utilized IIC9 cell fibroblasts. α-Thrombin treatment of these cells increases cellular DAG levels and activates PKC (54). Using nuclei isolated from α-thrombin-treated cells, we have showed that increases in nuclear DAG levels contribute to the α-thrombin-stimulated increase in cellular DAG levels (51). The time course of nuclear DAG elevation was quite rapid, with maximal values occurring at approximately 2–5 min following treatment with agonist. Results from whole cell experiments demonstrated that simulated PLD activity does not account for the increased DAG levels (55), suggesting that increased nuclear PLC activity is responsible for the elevated DAG levels. We do not yet know, however, the phospholipid source of the α-thrombin-stimulated nuclear DAGs. In cells that were prelabeled with [^{3}H]myristic acid, nuclear DAGs were labeled, suggesting that they are derived, at least in part, from stimulated phosphatidylcholine (PC) hydrolysis. Further work is required to determine whether stimulation of both PI–PLC and PC–PLC account for the stimulated DAG levels.

Increases in nuclear PKC-α levels accompanied the increased nuclear DAG levels in the IIC9 cells (51). The presence of PKC was detected both immunologically, using Western blot analysis, as well as by kinase activity assays. The localization of PKC to the nucleus occurred very rapidly following α-thrombin treatment, suggesting that nuclear localization is an early step in PKC activation.

Mitogen-stimulated nuclear PKC and DAG levels have also been demonstrated by Divecha *et al.* (44). They showed that increased DAG levels and decreased mass levels of intranuclear phosphoinositides are induced by IGF-1 treatment of 3T3 cells. The time course of DAG elevation was quite rapid, and DAG levels increased approximately 2-fold relative to the control level. In addition, a rise in nuclear PKC, as demonstrated by Western blot analysis, occurred following IGF-1 treatment. Taken together, the results of the IIC9 cell and 3T3 cell studies are consistent with the hypothesis that changes in nuclear DAG levels may be a determinant of PKC nuclear localization.

Although nuclear localization of PKC has been demonstrated by activity measurements as well as by immunofluorescence and Western blot experiments, the presence of nuclear PLC has been shown primarily by changes in DAG and phosphoinositide levels, as described above. As PLC antibodies are now commercially available, immunological evidence for nuclear PLC localization will undoubtedly increase.

Methods

Isolation of Nuclei

Several different isolation methods have been reported (44, 51, 53). For our IIC9 cell studies, lysis in the complete absence of detergent is carried out in order to avoid possible extraction of nuclear phospholipids and DAGs (51). Following treatment with agonist, cells grown on 150-mm plates are quickly rinsed with ice-cold saline and scraped into buffer B [10 M Tris (pH 7.5) containing 10 mM NaCl, 1 mM EDTA, and 0.5 mM EGTA]. The cells are homogenized 15 times in a Potter–Elvehjem homogenizer and spun at 500 g for 7 min. The nuclear pellet is resuspended in buffer B and homogenized 10 times in a Dounce homogenizer with an A pestle. The suspension is layered over 45% (w/w) sucrose (in buffer B) and centrifuged at 1660 g for 30 min. The pellet is resuspended in buffer C [10 mM Tris (pH 7.5) containing 10 mM NaCl, 10% sucrose, and 1 mM MgCl$_2$], homogenized 7 times in a Dounce homogenizer with an A pestle, and spun at 500 g for 5 min. The final nuclear pellet is resuspended in buffer D [25 mM Tris (pH 7.5) containing 2 mM EDTA, 0.5 mM EGTA, and 5 mM DTT] and sonicated to lyse the nuclei.

To assess potential changes in nuclear PLC and PKC levels, it is absolutely essential to establish the purity of the isolated nuclei. The major contaminants of the nuclei are usually plasma membrane and cytoskeletal elements. Electron microscopy provides a good indication of the purity of the nuclei, since contaminating organelles are readily apparent. Plasma membrane contamination can be assessed biochemically, using adenylate cyclase or 5'-nucleotidase assays. Specific activities and percentages of total PLC and PKC activities recovered in the nuclear fraction should be reported and, furthermore, should be compared with similar quantitative measurements of nonnuclear proteins such as plasma membrane-associated adenylate cyclase and cytosolic glucose-6-phosphatase. Immunofluorescence experiments and Western blot analysis using antibodies to cytoskeletal proteins such as tubulin, actin, and vimentin can be utilized to estimate cytoskeletal contamination.

Enzyme Activity Measurements

As with plasma membrane-associated PKC, it is necessary to extract PKC from the nucleus with detergent prior to measuring activity. Triton X-100 (1% final concentration) is added to the nuclear lysates followed by incubation for 1 hr at 4°C and centrifugation at 100,000 g for 60 min at 4°C (51). Following DEAE chromatography, PKC activity can be measured using protein substrates. In addition, phosphorylation of endogenous nuclear proteins can be assessed by adding radiolabeled ATP and activating phorbol esters to the nuclear preparation (41).

PI–PLC can be assayed directly in nuclear extracts using [^{3}H]PIP$_2$ as exogenous substrate (56). Changes in mass levels of polyphosphoinositide lipids can also be assayed as an indicator of PLC activity (44). Radiolabeling of inositides by [^{3}H]inositol in the nucleus is quite low (57), however, and thus this method is not recommended. In addition, the aqueous inositol phosphates such as IP$_3$ are too short lived to be measured reliably, relative to the time required to isolate nuclei. Changes in nuclear DAG levels can be readily quantified using a DAG kinase assay (51), although, as discussed above, the phospholipid sources and enzymes involved in the DAG generation must be identified to assess the contribution of PI–PLC activity.

Immunocytofluorescence

Immunolocalization can be performed on whole cells, cytoskeletons, or nuclear preparations. For nuclear preparations, we wash the nuclear pellet in buffer C, resuspend the nuclei in PBA (PBS containing 1% bovine serum albumin), and spin them at 250 rmp for 5 min onto glass slides (40). The nuclei are fixed by dipping in −20°C methanol and then incubated with primary and secondary antibodies as described for whole cells.

Useful controls, which should be investigated wherever possible, include comparison of the staining observed with different antibody preparations to the same antigen and staining of cells that do not express the antigen of interest. These controls are essential for verifying that the staining pattern observed can actually be attributed to PKC or PLC. For example, we have observed nuclear PI–PLC-β by immunocytofluorescence in a variety of epithelial and fibroblast cell lines; however, in only one cell line could we demonstrate immunoreactive PI–PLC-β by immunoblotting and immunoprecipitation (S. Jaken, unpublished). Possibly, the antibody used cross-reacts with nuclear proteins and complicates interpretation of the data. It should also be noted, however, that specific calpain inhibitors, which were noted in Ref. 42 as essential for recovering intact PI–PLC-β, were not included in these early studies.

References

1. S. G. Rhee and K. D. Choi, *J. Biol. Chem.* **267,** 12393 (1992).
2. S. H. Ryu, U. H. Kim, M. I. Wahl, A. B. Brown, G. Carpenter, K.-P. Huang, and S. G. Rhee, *J. Biol. Chem.* **265,** 17941 (1990).
3. H. M. Lee and J. N. Fain, *J. Neurochem.* **56,** 1471 (1991).
4. S. J. Decker, C. Ellis, T. Pawson, and T. Velu, *J. Biol. Chem.* **265,** 7009 (1990).
5. L. B. Nanney, R. E. Gates, G. Todderud, L. E. King, and G. Carpenter, *Cell Growth Differ.* **3,** 233 (1992).
6. C. L. Arteaga, M. D. Johnson, G. Todderud, R. J. Coffey, G. Carpenter, and D. L. Page, *Proc. Natl. Acad. Sci. U.S.A.* **88,** 10435 (1990).
7. S. Jaken, *in* "Protein Kinase C: Current Concepts and Future Perspectives" (R. Epand and D. Lester, eds.), p. 237. Ellis Horwood, Chichester, 1992.
8. Y. Nishizuka, *JAMA, J. Am. Med. Assoc.* **262,** 1826 (1989).
9. S. Jaken, *Curr. Opin. Cell Biol.* **2,** 192 (1990).
10. S. Stabel and P. J. Parker, *Pharmacol. Ther.* **51,** 71 (1991).
11. J. H. Exton, S. J. Taylor, G. Augert, and S. B. Bocckino, *Mol. Cell. Biochem.* **104,** 81 (1991).
12. S. C. Kiley, P. J. Parker, D. Fabbro, and S. Jaken, *J. Biol. Chem.* **266,** 23761 (1991).
13. T. F. J. Martin, K.-P. Hsieh, and B. W. Porter, *J. Biol. Chem.* **265,** 7623 (1990).
14. S. C. Kiley and S. Jaken, *Mol. Endocrinol.* **4,** 59 (1990).
15. S. Kiley, D. Schaap, P. Parker, L. L. Hsieh, and S. Jaken, *J. Biol. Chem.* **265,** 15704 (1990).
16. S. C. Kiley, P. J. Parker, D. Fabbro, and S. Jaken, *Mol. Endocrinol.* **6,** 120 (1992).
17. R. E. Straub, G. C. Frech, R. H. Joho, and M. C. Gershengorn, *Proc. Natl. Acad. Sci. U.S.A.* **24,** 9514 (1990).
18. T. F. J. Martin, *in* "Inositol Lipids in Cell Signaling" (R. H. Michell, A. H. Drummond, and C. P. Downes, eds.), p. 113. Academic Press, London, 1989.
19. F. E. Mitchell, R. M. Marais, and P. J. Parker, *Biochem. J.* **261,** 131 (1989).
20. J. Preiss, C. R. Loomis, W. R. Bishop, R. Stein, J. E. Niedel, and R. Bell, *J. Biol. Chem.* **261,** 8597 (1986).
21. S. Jaken, *in* "Measurement of Phorbol Ester Receptors in Intact Cells and Subcellular Fractions" (A. R. Means and P. M. Conn, eds.), p. 275. Academic Press, New York, 1987.
22. F. L. Huang, Y. Yoshida, J. R. Cunha-Melo, M. A. Beaven, and K.-P. Huang, *J. Biol. Chem.* **264,** 4238 (1990).
23. A. Kishimoto, K. Mikawa, K. Hashimoto, I. Yasuda, S. Tanaka, M. Tominaga, T. Kuroda, and Y. Nishizuka, *J. Biol. Chem.* **264,** 4088 (1990).
24. S. Jaken, K. Leach, and T. Klauck, *J. Cell Biol.* **109,** 697 (1989).
25. B. T. Geiger, T. Volk, T. Volberg, and R. Bendori, *J. Cell Sci.* **8,** 252 (1987).
26. K. Burridge, K. Fath, T. Kelly, G. Nuckolls, and C. Turner, *Annu. Rev. Cell Biol.* **4,** 487 (1988).

27. S. L. Hyatt, T. Klauck, and S. Jaken, *Mol. Carcinog.* **3,** 45 (1990).

28. K. McBride, S. G. Rhee, and S. Jaken, *Proc. Natl. Acad. Sci. U.S.A.* **88,** 7111 (1991).

29. P. J. Goldschmidt-Clermont, L. M. Machesky, J. J. Baldassare, and T. D. Pollard, *Science* **247,** 1575 (1990).

30. A. Vojtek, B. Haarer, J. Field, J. Gerst, T. D. Pollard, S. Brown, and M. Wigler, *Cell (Cambridge, Mass.)* **66,** 497 (1991).

31. P. J. Goldschmidt-Clermont and P. A. Janmey, *Cell (Cambridge, Mass.)* **66,** 419 (1991).

32. P. J. Goldschmidt-Clermont, J. W. Kim, L. M. Machesky, S. G. Rhee, and T. D. Pollard, *Science* **251,** 1231 (1991).

33. T. D. Hill, N. M. Dean, L. J. Mordan, A. F. Lau, M. Y. Kanemitsu, and A. L. Boynton, *Science* **248,** 1660 (1990).

34. B. Margolis, A. Zilberstein, C. Franks, S. Felder, S. Kremer, A. Ullrich, S. G. Rhee, K. S. Korecki, and J. Schlessinger, *Science* **248,** 607 (1990).

35. M. Mohammadi, C. A. Dionne, W. Li, T. Spivak, A. M. Honegger, M. Jaye, and J. Schlessinger, *Nature (London)* **358,** 681 (1992).

36. K. G. Peters, J. Marie, E. Wilson, H. E. Ives, J. Escobedo, M. DelRosario, and D. Mirda, *Nature (London)* **358,** 678 (1992).

37. M. Osborn and K. Weber, *Methods Cell Biol.* **24,** 97 (1992).

38. L. Dong, J. L. Stevens, and S. Jaken, *Am. J. Physiol.* **2610,** F679 (1991).

39. M. Wolf and N. Sahyoun, *J. Biol. Chem.* **261,** 13327 (1986).

39a. S. Hyatt and S. Jaken, in preparation.

40. K. L. Leach, E. A. Powers, V. A. Ruff, S. Jaken, and S. Kaufmann, *J. Cell Biol.* **109,** 685 (1989).

41. A. P. Fields, G. R. Pettit, and W. S. May, *J. Biol. Chem.* **263,** 8253 (1988).

42. A. M. Martelli, R. S. Gilmour, V. Bertagnolo, L. M. Neri, L. Manzoli, and L. Cocco, *Nature (London)* **358,** 242 (1992).

43. M. Mazzoni, V. Bertagnolo, L. M. Neri, C. Carini, M. Marchisio, D. Milani, F. A. Manzoli, and S. Capitani, *Biochem. Biophys. Res. Commun.* **187,** 114 (1992).

44. N. Divecha, H. Banfic, and R. F. Irvine, *EMBO J.* **10,** 3207 (1991).

45. P. Hornbeck, K. P. Huang, and W. E. Paul, *Proc. Natl. Acad. Sci. U.S.A.* **85,** 2279 (1988).

46. D. S. Samuels, Y. Shimizu, and N. Shimizu, *FEBS Lett.* **259,** 57 (1989).

47. D. E. Macfarlane, *J. Biol. Chem.* **261,** 6947 (1986).

48. A. Masmoudi, G. Labourdette, M. Mersel, F. L. Huang, K.-P. Huang, G. Vincendon, and A. N. Malviya, *J. Biol. Chem.* **264,** 1172 (1989).

49. B. A. Hocevar and A. P. Fields, *J. Biol. Chem.* **266,** 28 (1991).

50. T. P. Thomas, H. V. Talwar, and W. B. Anderson, *Cancer Res.* **48,** 1910 (1988).

51. K. L. Leach, V. A. Ruff, M. B. Jarpe, S. L. D. Ada, D. Fabbro, and D. M. Raben, *J. Biol. Chem.* **267,** 21816 (1992).

52. M. Hagiwara, C. Uchida, N. Usuda, T. Nagata, and H. Hidaka, *Biochem. Biophys. Res. Commun.* **168,** 161 (1990).

53. A. P. Fields, S. M. Pincus, A. S. Kraft, and W. S. May, *J. Biol. Chem.* **264,** 21896 (1989).

54. K. L. Leach, V. A. Ruff, T. M. Wright, M. S. Pessin, and D. M. Raben, *J. Biol. Chem.* **266,** 3215 (1991).
55. T. M. Wright, S. Willenberger, and D. M. Raben, *Biochem. J.* **285,** 395 (1992).
56. B. Payrastre, M. Nievers, J. Boonstra, M. Breton, S. Verkleij, and P. M. P. VanBergen en Henegouwen, *J. Biol. Chem.* **267,** 5078 (1992).
57. L. Cocco, A. Martelli, R. S. Gilmour, A. Ognibene, F. A. Manzoli, and R. F. Irvine, *Biochem. Biophys. Res. Commun.* **159,** 720 (1989).

NOTE ADDED IN PROOF: Although most (98%) of turkey erythrocyte PLC is cytosolic, a small amount was recovered in cytoskeletons prepared from erythrocyte ghosts. Disruption of ghost cytoskeletons attenuated agonist and GTP-stimulated PI–PLC responses in ghosts. These results indicate that the integrity of the actin cytoskeleton is important for localization and regulation of PI–PLC activity [C. Vaziri and C. P. Downes, *J. Biol. Chem.* **267,** 22973 (1992)].

[18]   Quantitative Analysis of Molecular Species of Diacylglycerol in Biological Samples

Chunghee Lee and Amiya K. Hajra

Introduction

Diacylglycerol (1,2-diacyl-*sn*-glycerol, DAG) has multiple roles in cellular metabolism. DAG has long been known as an important intermediate in the biosynthesis of glycerolipids in eukaryotic cells (1), and it has also been shown to be an important effector in the process of signal transduction across cellular membranes (2). It has been postulated that DAG acts as a second messenger by activating protein kinase C, which catalyzes the phosphorylation of specific cellular proteins (3).

Originally it was believed that the signal DAG is formed by the hydrolysis of phosphoinositides [especially phosphatidylinositol 4,5-bisphosphate (PIP_2)] by phosphoinositide-specific phospholipase C. However, reports from several laboratories indicate that during the signal transduction process other lipids [especially phosphatidylcholine (PC)] also break down to generate a relatively large amount of DAG (4, 5). The exact physiological significance of the formation of DAG from different sources during signal transduction is not clear, but the presence of DAG from different sources makes it difficult to study the mechanism of formation and metabolism (deactivation) of signal DAG. One way to differentiate between the different cellular pools of DAG is to analyze quantitatively the molecular species and composition of DAG and compare that with the molecular species profile of different glycerolipids. Because the fatty acid composition (and hence the molecular species) is unique for each precursor lipid and remains constant under specific nutritional (for whole animals) or cultural (for tissues) conditions, it is possible to deduce a precursor–product relationship between different lipids by analyzing the molecular species profile. This approach has been successfully used by different laboratories, including ours, to quantify the amount of DAG formed from different sources and also its metabolism to various other lipids (6–9).

Different methods have been used to analyze the molecular species composition of DAG and other glycerides (6–15). Our method is a modification and combination of the methods described from several laboratories (10–14) in which DAG is first derivatized with a chromophoric group (benzoyl) and different molecular species are then separated according to hydrophobicity

Methods in Neurosciences, Volume 18

by chromatography in a reversed-phase column (15). This method is described below.

Methods

Extraction of Diacylglycerol from Tissues and Cultured Cells

A modified neutral Folch extraction method is used to extract DAG from tissues, and a neutral Bligh and Dyer extraction method is used to extract DAG from cell suspensions. The tissues are homogenized (Polytron, Brinkmann Instruments, Westbury, NY) in 12 volumes of $CHCl_3$–methanol (1 : 1, v/v), and a known amount of (10–30 nmol/g tissue) of an internal standard DAG (1,2-distearoyl-sn-glycerol) is added during homogenization. The homogenate is centrifuged (1000 g, 10 min) at room temperature, and the supernatant is saved. The residue is dispersed in water (0.5 ml/g tissue) and then reextracted with 12 volumes of $CHCl_3$–methanol as above. The two supernatants are combined (18 vol/g of tissue), and 9 volumes of $CHCl_3$ (per gram of original tissue) is added, followed by 5.5 volumes of 0.9% (w/v) aqueous NaCl. The phases are mixed well (vortex mixer) and centrifuged at 1000 g for 10 min at room temperature. The upper layer and the interfacial materials are discarded and the solvents evaporated from the lower layer either by blowing a stream of N_2 or by using a rotary evaporator.

The lipids from cell suspensions or incubation mixtures are extracted by adding 3 volumes of $CHCl_3$–methanol (1 : 2, v/v). After adding the internal standard DAG (0.1–0.2 nmol/mg protein), the mixture is sonicated three times in an ultrasonic bath (Laboratory Supply Co., Hicksville, NY) for 20 sec each and then centrifuged (1000 g, 10 min). The supernatant is saved, and the pellet is extracted with 2 volumes of $CHCl_3$–methanol (1 : 1, v/v), the sample centrifuged as above, and the supernatants combined. One volume of $CHCl_3$ and 2.4 volumes of 0.9% (w/v) aqueous NaCl are added to the combined supernatant, mixed well (vortex mixer), and centrifuged at 1000 g for 10 min. The upper layer and the interfacial material are discarded, and the lower layer is evaporated to dryness as described above. The DAG from the lipid extracts is isolated by thin-layer chromatography (TLC) as follows.

Purification of Diacylglycerol

The lipid extracts are spotted as a band (<0.5 mg lipid/cm) on a 20 × 20 cm thin-layer plate (Merck, silica gel 60, 0.25 mm thick), and the plate is developed with toluene–diethyl ether–methanol (80 : 10 : 10, v/v) up to 12 cm from the origin. After air-drying, the plate is lightly sprayed with primuline (16) and the lipid bands localized by viewing under long-wavelength UV light. The DAG band (R_f 0.6), which runs above cholesterol, is identified by running standard DAG (diolein) on the same plate. In this system, 1,3-diacyl-*sn*-glycerol (R_f 0.68) separates out from the 1,2-isomer. The DAG band is scraped out with a razor blade, and the DAG is extracted from the TLC powder by suspending in 2 ml diethyl ether, sonicating in an ultrasonic bath to aid dispersal, and then centrifuging at low speed (600 g, 10 min). The extraction process is repeated twice, and the combined ether extracts are evaporated dry at room temperature by blowing a stream of N_2. The purified DAG is immediatley benzoylated as described below.

Benzoylation of Diacylglycerol

Reagents

Benzene: Dry benzene by distilling it from CaH_2 and store in a desiccator over Drierite

4-Pyrrolidinopyridine (Sigma Chemical Co., St. Louis, MO): Store in a desiccator over Drierite

Benzoic anhydride (Sigma): Store as above

Protocol

The TLC-purified DAG is transferred to a Reacti-Vial (Pierce, Rockford, IL) with anhydrous ether which is then removed by blowing dry N_2. To the dried DAG (<40 nmol), 0.1 ml of dry benzene and 0.04 ml of a mixture containing 6.8 μmol 4-pyrrolidinopyridine and 5.5 μmol of benzoic anhydride in dry benzene are added. The mixture is capped and stirred by means of a triangular Teflon-coated magnet (Pierce) for 1 hr at room temperature. The reaction is stopped by adding 0.1 ml methanol. The benzoyl-DAG is purified by TLC, followed (if necessary) by normal-phase high-performance liquid chromatography (HPLC).

Purification of Benzoyldiacylglycerol

The reaction mixture, after benzoylation, is spotted as a band on a thin-layer plate, and the plate is developed in a solvent mixture containing benzene–hexane–ether–17 N NH_4OH (50 : 45 : 5 : 1, v/v) up to 12 cm from the origin. The plate is air dried and sprayed with primuline, and the lipid bands are located under UV light. The benzoyl-DAG bands (R_f 0.53) are scraped from the plate, and the benzoyl-DAG is isolated from the TLC powder by extracting the powder three times with 2 ml diethyl ether as described above.

If necessary, the benzoyl-DAG is further purified by normal-phase polytetrafluoroethylene (HPLC).* The ether extracts containing the benzoyl-DAG are filtered through a PTFE filter (0.45-μm pore size), the ether is removed by blowing a stream of N_2, and the dry residue is dissolved in a minimal volume of cyclohexane. A 20-μl aliquot is injected into a silica gel HPLC column (25 × 0.46 cm, particle size 5 μm) and the column is eluted, isocratically with cyclohexane containing 3.7% diethyl ether, at a flow rate of 1 ml/min at room temperature. The elution is monitored at 228 nm, and the benzoyl DAG peak, having a retention time of 14–16 min, is collected. In this system benzoylated 1-alkyl-2-acyl (R_f 6.7 min) and 1-alkenyl-2-acyl (R_f 5.6 min) glycerol species separate well from the diacyl species.

Reversed-Phase High-Performance Liquid Chromatography of Benzoyldiacylglycerol

The solvent is removed from the purified benzoyl-DAG by blowing a stream of N_2. The residue is dissolved in a small volume of acetonitrile, and a 20-μl aliquot is injected into a reversed-phase (octadecyl silica gel, Beckman, Fullerton, CA) column (25 × 0.46 cm, 5 μm) and eluted isocratically with acetonitrile containing 30% 2-propanol. The effluent is monitored at 228 nm (Spectroflow), and the peak areas are integrated using an electronic integrator (Nelson Analytical) attached to the monitoring system. A typical result obtained with total adult rat brain DAG is shown in Fig. 1.

Characterization of Molecular Species of Diacylglycerol in Reversed-Phase Chromatography Peaks

The HPLC peaks are tentatively identified by comparing the retention time of the unknowns with that of standard DAG of known composition. Because separation in this system is based on hydrophobicity of the molecule, increasing the chain length will increase retention time, and the presence of a double

---

* This step is necessary to remove large amounts of impurities absorbing at 228 nm, which are eluted quickly (<5 min) from the HPLC column. If the absorbance peaks from the impurities do not overlap those of any of the benzoyl-DAG species, then this normal-phase HPLC purification is not necessary. By using the modified TLC system mentioned above to purify the benzoyl-DAG, most UV-absorbing impurities (benzoic anhydride, methyl benzoate) are eliminated.

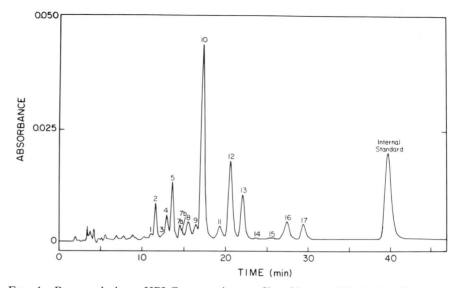

FIG. 1   Reversed-phase HPLC separation profile of benzoyl-DAG. DAG isolated from rat brain (1 min postmortem) was benzoylated and subjected to HPLC separation as described in the text. The detector output ($A_{228\ nm}$) versus time is plotted. The composition of each numbered peak is given in Table I. 1,2-Distearoyl-*sn*-glycerol was used as the internal standard DAG. [Reproduced with permission from *Neurochem*. C. Lee and A. K. Hajra, *J. Neurochem*. **56,** 374 (1991).]

bond will decrease retention time. From the separation profile, we can see that the acyl group at the C-1 position interacts more with the stationary phase than the group at the C-2 position (10). The position of the double bond(s) in the chain also affects the interaction of the molecule with the nonpolar phase. Patton *et al.* (13) described a useful method of plotting the carbon number of the acyl chain at C-1 versus the logarithm of retention time. This yields a series of parallel lines which depend on the carbon number and the degree of unsaturation of the acyl chain at C-2. This kind of plot is useful for tentative identification of the species present in the HPLC peaks. One such plot obtained for the rat brain DAG is shown in Fig. 2.

The molecular species present in each peak can be accurately identified by analyzing the fatty acid composition of each peak. After collection from the HPLC column, the peaks are subjected to methanolysis (BF$_3$–methanol), and the methyl ester of the fatty acids are separated from each other by capillary gas–liquid chromatography (GLC) (15). The identity and the amount of each molecular species present in that peak can be deduced from the number and relative amounts of each fatty acid present as analyzed by GLC. A 1 : 1 molar ratio of any two fatty acids is indicative of a particular molecular

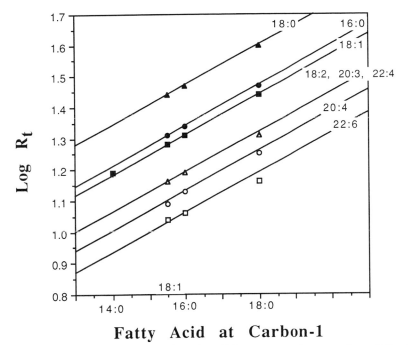

FIG. 2   Plot of logarithm of retention time (R_t) versus carbon number of the fatty acid at position 1 for different molecular species of rat brain DAG. The nature of the fatty acid at C-2 of the molecule is shown for each straight line.

species of DAG. The position of the fatty acid in the glycerol moiety cannot be ascertained by this method, but, in most cases, it may be assumed that the more saturated fatty acid is at C-1 and the more unsaturated fatty acid at the C-2 position of the DAG. An analysis of the molecular species composition of each peak in Fig. 1 is given in Table I.

Quantitation of Each Molecular Species of Diacylglycerol

The amount of DAG present in each peak can be quantified by integrating the area under the HPLC peak and comparing that with the area under the internal standard peak. Because the amount of the internal standard added during lipid extraction is known, the amount of DAG present under any peak can be calculated. The calculation should be done on a molar basis because the absorbance at 228 nm is due to the benzoyl group, which is present at 1 mol per mole of DAG. Therefore, the amount (nmol/total lipid extract) of

TABLE I   Molecular Species Composition of Rat Brain Diacylglycerol[a]

Peak	Retention time (min)	Concentration (nmol/g of brain)	mol%	DAG species
1	10.95	0.54	0.55	18:1-22:6 (n-3)
2	11.42	4.43	4.52	16:0-22:6 (n-3)
3	12.26	0.26	0.26	18:1-22:5 (n-3)
4	12.77	3.69	3.76	18:1-20:4 (n-6)
		0.23	0.23	16:0-22:5 (n-3)
5	13.40	7.29	7.44	16:0-20:4 (n-6)
6	13.90	Trace	Trace	18:0-20:5 (n-3)
7a	14.37	1.51	1.54	18:0-22:6 (n-3)
7b	14.61	0.10	0.11	16:1-18:1
		0.06	0.06	18:1-18:2 (n-6)
		0.34	0.35	18:1-22:4 (n-6)
		0.09	0.09	18:1-20:3 (n-6)
8	15.35	0.22	0.22	14:0-18:1
		0.88	0.90	16:0-16:1
		0.96	0.98	16:0-18:2 (n-6)
		1.01	1.03	16:0-22:4 (n-6)
		0.47	0.48	16:0-20:3 (n-6)
9	16.30	2.34	2.39	18:0-22:5 (n-3)
10	17.78	35.30	36.04	18:0-20:4 (n-6)
11	19.18	2.61	2.67	18:1-18:1
12	20.38	16.00	16.31	16:0-18:1
		0.58	0.59	18:0-18:2 (n-6)
		0.84	0.85	18:0-22:4 (n-6)
		0.73	0.75	18:0-20:3 (n-6)
13	21.87	9.03	9.22	16:0-16:0
14	23.52	Trace	Trace	18:0-20:3 (n-9)
15	25.15	0.43	0.44	18:1-20:1
16	27.25	4.31	4.40	18:0-18:1
17	29.25	3.71	3.79	16:0-18:0
18	35.50	Trace	Trace	18:0-20:1
19	40.00	Internal standard	—	18:0-18:0

[a] The peak numbers correspond to the separation profile presented in Fig. 1. Each peak from the HPLC column was collected, and its fatty acid composition was determined by GLC analysis. When more than one species of DAG was present in the peak (more than two fatty acids), the assignment of species was done from the ratio of each fatty acid and the hydrophobicity of each species as described in the text. In the identified peaks the first number indicates the length of the carbon chain and the second the number of double bonds in the chain. Reproduced with permission from C. Lee and A. K. Hajra, *J. Neurochem.* **56,** 375 (1991).

DAG of any species a equals the product of the area under peak a times the nanomoles of internal standard added to the lipid extract divided by the area under the internal standard peak. The total amount of DAG present in the sample is obtained by adding up the amount of DAG present in each peak.

When the HPLC peaks are not fully resolved, the area under each peak can be electronically integrated by assigning proper baselines from the peaks. The best way to quantify such species, of course, is to collect each peak and quantitatively analyze the fatty acid composition by GLC. Fortunately, in most systems, such as in brain, the major molecular species are well resolved from one another on reversed-phase HPLC (Table I).

Analysis of Molecular Species of Phosphoglycerides

The above method can also be used to analyze the molecular species composition of other membrane glycerolipids. The phosphoglycerides are enzymatically hydrolyzed to DAG which, after benzoylation, is subjected to reversed-phase HPLC as described above. Details of the hydrolytic conversion of different glycerolipids to DAG are described elsewhere (9, 15).

Comments

The method is sensitive enough to analyze samples containing 2–3 nmol of total DAG ($\geq$50 pmol of individual component). One advantage of the method is that samples can be recovered after HPLC separation for further analysis. Therefore, DAG of unknown composition can be characterized very definitively. For example, in the SK-N-SH neuroblastoma cell line, we identified some unknown peaks after HPLC separation as DAG species containing n-9 polyunsaturated acid (9).

One precaution has to be taken to ensure that acyl migration during processing of DAG is minimized, because such intramolecular acyl migration will result in the formation of 1,3-diacyl-sn-glycerol from the corresponding 1,2-isomer. One should process the sample from the extraction to the benzoylation step as quickly as possible before storing it for a long period of time. We found that, under these conditions, very little (<10%) acyl migration occurs, and any 1,3-isomer that is formed will mostly be removed during the purification of DAG by TLC as described above. If samples need to be stored before benzoylation, they should be stored at low temperature under neutral or acidic conditions to slow the rate of acyl migration.

We used 1,2-distearoyl-*sn*-glycerol (18:0-18:0) as the internal standard because we found that very little of it is present in DAG (or phosphoglycerides) or most tissues, and its benzoyl derivative does not comigrate with any other known species. However, the absence of 18:0-18:0 in the system to be studied should be verified before it is used as the internal standard. We did find 18:0-18:0 species present in a considerable amount in the cellular DAG and in PC in one system [i.e., Madin Darby canine kidney (MDCK) cells] we studied (C. Lee, A. K. Hajra, and J. Shayman, unpublished work, 1992). Therefore, other appropriate internal standards should be used for the purpose of quantification. The internal standard DAG, having known molecular composition, can be generated from the corresponding PC by phospholipase C hydrolysis (9). PC of known fatty acid compositions are available commercially (Avanti Polar Biochemicals, Birmingham, AL; Sigma Chemical Co.). The internal standard should be purified by TLC from time to time using the toluene–methanol–ether solvent system (see above) to remove any 1,3-species. The amount of internal standard in the stock solution should also be quantified before use. This can be done by gas–liquid chromatography after methanolysis and using known amounts of 17:0 methyl ester as the GLC internal standard.

References

1. E. P. Kennedy, *in* "Lipids and Membranes" (J. A. F. op den Kamp, B. Roelofsen, and K. W. A. Wirtz, eds.), p. 171. Elsevier, Amsterdam, 1986.
2. Y. Nishizuka, *Nature (London)* **308,** 693 (1984).
3. Y. Nishizuka, *Science* **258,** 607 (1992).
4. J. H. Exton, *J. Biol. Chem.* **265,** 1 (1990).
5. M. M. Billah and J. C. Anthes, *Biochem. J.* **269,** 281 (1991).
6. D. A. Kennerly, *J. Biol. Chem.* **262,** 16305 (1987).
7. M. S. Pessin and D. M. Raben, *J. Biol. Chem.* **264,** 8729 (1989).
8. G. Augert, S. B. Bocckino, P. F. Blackmore, and J. H. Exton, *J. Biol. Chem.* **264,** 21689 (1989).
9. C. Lee, S. K. Fisher, B. W. Agranoff, and A. K. Hajra, *J. Biol. Chem.* **266,** 22837 (1991).
10. Y. Nakagawa and L. A. Horrocks, *J. Lipid Res.* **24,** 1268 (1983).
11. M. Batley, N. H. Packer, and J. W. Redmond, *J. Chromatogr.* **198,** 520 (1980).
12. M. L. Blank, M. Robinson, V. Fitzgerald, and F. Snyder, *J. Chromatogr.* **298,** 473 (1984).
13. G. M. Patton, J. M. Fasulo, and S. J. Robins, *J. Lipid Res.* **23,** 190 (1982).
14. R. H. McCluer, M. D. Ullman, and F. B. Jungalwala, *in* "Methods in Enzymology" (S. Fleischer and B. Fleischer, eds.), Vol. 172, p. 538. Academic Press, San Diego, 1989.
15. C. Lee and A. K. Hajra, *J. Neurochem.* **56,** 370 (1991).
16. R. S. Wright, *J. Chromatogr.* **59,** 220 (1971).

Section IV

Measurement of Inositol Phosphates and Enzymes Regulating Inositol Phosphate Metabolism

[19] Measurement of Inositol Trisphosphate by Gas Chromatography/Mass Spectrometry: Femtomole Sensitivity Provided by Negative-Ion Chemical Ionization Mass Spectrometry in Submilligram Quantities of Tissue

Leona J. Rubin, Fong-Fu Hsu, and William R. Sherman

Introduction

D-*myo*-Inositol 1,4,5-trisphosphate (IP_3) is a ubiquitous intracellular second messenger produced following enzymatic hydrolysis of the membrane lipid precursor, phosphatidylinositol 4,5-bisphosphate. Increases in cellular levels of IP_3 are known to signify (1) receptor activation and (2) release of Ca^{2+} from intracellular stores. Traditionally, receptor-stimulated production of IP_3 has been assessed from cells or tissues incubated in the presence of radiolabeled precursors ([^{3}H]inositol or $^{32}PO_4$). Although the radiotracer studies are extremely sensitive, only qualitative information can be obtained concerning IP_3 signaling. Furthermore, in situations where the radiolabel does not have access to *in vivo* tissues, or if the tissue or cells are not viable for the duration required for radiolabeling, even qualitative assessments of IP_3 signaling are not possible. Thus, methods for analysis of IP_3 mass have evolved and include gas chromatography (GC) (1, 2), radioimmunoassay, high-performance liquid chromatography (HPLC) postcolumn detection, and ion chromatography/HPLC (3–5). The sensitivity of most of these methods is such, however, that picomole amounts of IP_3 are required, necessitating relatively large quantities of tissue. Direct quantitation of inositol polyphosphates by gas chromatography/mass spectroscopy (GC/MS) (6), fast-atom bombardment mass spectroscopy (6), or thermospray-liquid chromatography/mass spectroscopy (7), although promising, has failed to improve on sensitivity or has suffered the limitation of a lack of specificity (8).

Thus far, the most sensitive (0.2 pmol/injection) GC/MS method (9) for quantitation of IP_3 evolved from procedures designed to measure the dephosphorylated cyclitol inositol (1, 10). By necessity, therefore, this method requires prior separation of the inositol polyphosphate species, dephosphorylation of the compounds to free inositol, and then quantitation of a derivatized product by GC/MS. Utilizing a modification of the basic procedure, we describe here a method for femtomole quantitation of IP$_3$ from submilligram quantities of tissue. This procedure utilizes a novel dephosphorylation method, a high molecular weight fluoroacyl derivative of inositol, and high mass GC/MS analysis.

Procedures

Required Chemicals and Sources

Heptafluorobutyric anhydride (HFBA), acetonitrile, and the BCA reagent kit are from Pierce (Rockford, IL); AG 1-X8 resin (100–200 mesh, formate form) is from Bio-Rad (Richmond, CA); dichlorodimethylsilane is from Aldrich Chemical Co. (Milwaukee, WI); Dowex 50-X8 resin (200–400 mesh, hydrogen form), trichloroacetic acid (TCA), bovine serum albumin (BSA), ammonium formate, and formic acid are from Sigma Chemical Co. (St. Louis, MO); and ammonium hydroxide, diethyl ether, toluene, and methanol are from Fisher Scientific (St. Louis, MO). *myo*-Inositol and deuterium-labeled *myo*-inositol (*myo*-inositol-c-d_6), referred to as d6-*myo*-inositol in this chapter, are from MSD Isotopes (Montreal, Quebec, Canada).

Extraction of Inositol Phosphates from Small Tissue Samples

We routinely extract inositol phosphates from 0.30–2 mg quantities of freshly dispersed porcine coronary artery smooth muscle cells or substrate-attached, adult rat cardiac ventricular myocytes in primary culture with ice-cold 10% TCA (1–1.5 ml). TCA extracts are then transferred to 2.0-ml Eppendorf tubes, and the protein is pelleted by centrifugation (4°C, 16,000 g, 10 min). All glassware for inositol phosphate analysis is silanized by coating with a solution of 7% (v/v) dichlorodimethylsilane in toluene. Supernatants from TCA extracts are transferred to 50-ml conical polypropylene tubes and the TCA extracted with water-saturated diethyl ether (4 × 5 ml); residual ether is removed by vaporization at 60°C for 30 min. Samples can then be stored frozen at −20°C. The precipitated protein from the extracts is solubilized in 400 μl of 0.1 N NaOH with 1% sodium dodecyl sulfate (SDS), refrigerated overnight, and quantitated by the Pierce BCA assay using BSA as standard.

Separation of Inositol Phosphates

Inositol phosphate separation by anion-exchange chromatography on AG 1 X8 columns is a well-characterized and reliable method for separation of the major classes of inositol phosphates (11). There are, however, inherent problems in anion-exchange separations as used in this study. First, baseline resolu-

TABLE I   Recovery of [^{3}H] Inositol
1,4,5-Trisphosphate^a

Treatment	Recovery (%)
Extraction with TCA/ether	92 ± 6
Dowex 1 chromatography	85 ± 4
Dowex 50 desalting	78 ± 2
Lyophilization	51 ± 6

^{a} Recovery of [^{3}H]IP$_3$ following each step in the protocol is listed. Approximately 50,000 cpm [^{3}H]IP$_3$ was
added to each well of a 6-well plate containing adult
ventricular myocytes (~150 μg protein) and 1.5 ml
of 10% TCA. Recovery was assessed at each step
by counting an aliquot of the sample and correcting
for volume. The yield at each step is expressed as a
percentage of the original. Values represent mean ±
SEM for six samples.

tion of inositol bisphosphate (IP$_2$), IP$_3$, and inositol tetrakisphosphate (IP$_4$) is
not possible, and therefore some IP$_2$ or IP$_4$ may exist in the IP$_3$ fractions. Second, separation of IP$_3$ isomers is also not possible, and therefore information
concerning inositol polyphosphate metabolism is lost. Nevertheless, to facilitate the development of our high sensitivity method, and as a first approxima-
tion to more high-resolution chromatography, an AG 1-X8 anion-exchange
column is used in the study.

Extracts containing the separated inositol phosphates are diluted in
10–20 ml double-distilled water and applied to an AG 1-X8 column
(1 ml, formate form) equilibrated with double-distilled water. Inositol
phosphates are then eluted from the column according to the procedure
of Downes and Michell (11). Recovery of IP$_3$ is assessed by spiking every
cell extract with [^{3}H]IP$_3$ (Amersham, Arlington Heights, IL) immediately
after adding TCA. We routinely add 30,000 counts/min (cpm) [^{3}H]IP$_3$, and
recovery from anion-exchange columns is typically 80–90% (Table I). In
contrast to the mentioned disadvantages of anion-exchange separations,
a distinct advantage of this particular procedure is the ease with which
the ammonium formate salt can be removed from the samples. Desalting
is accomplished either by repeated lyophilization (2–3 days) or by elution
over a 3.0-ml Dowex 50 (H$^+$ form) column followed by lyophilization
(1–2 days). Dried samples can be stored at −20°C for up to 3 months
without appreciable loss of [^{3}H]IP$_3$, as verified by rechromatography. Loss
of [^{3}H]IP$_3$ following desalting by either procedure is due primarily to
adsorption to polypropylene tubes during lyophilization. Adsorptive loses
are, however, much higher if extracts are lyophilized in glass tubes, even

if the tubes are silanized. The desalting procedure used here is far less labor intensive than other desalting procedures reported (1, 2, 9), is easier to perform, and is readily applicable to many laboratories.

Dephosphorylation of Inositol 1,4,5-Trisphosphate Samples

Quantitation of inositol trisphosphates by quantitative analysis of inositol obviously requires removal of the phosphate moieties from the cyclitol ring. Dephosphorylation of IP_3 can be accomplished by enzymatic dephosphorylation with alkaline phosphatase (2, 9, 12). This procedure, however, requires resolubilizing samples in a salt solution conducive for alkaline phosphatase activity. Unfortunately, these solutions frequently interfere with derivatization of inositol for GC and must therefore be removed by further desalting chromatography. Hsu *et al.* (7) noted that during thermospray mass spectrometry aqueous solutions of inositol monophosphates and inositol polyphosphates were rapidly dephosphorylated on short exposure to temperatures of the order of 200°C. We have therefore employed this approach as a novel, nonenzymatic dephosphorylation method, which involves heating aqueous samples to 200°C in a sealed glass tube.

Exhaustive silanization of the glass tubes in which dephosphorylation is carried out is necessary to avoid severe losses of the analyte. Tubes are therefore silanized as follows: 7-cm sections of 4–5 mm inner diameter borosilicate glass tubing are heat-sealed at one end, washed with 2–3 changes of methanol, and air dried. Silanization is performed by soaking tubes in 7% (v/v) dichlorodimethylsilane in toluene for 10 min at room temperature, decanting, heating the tubes at 200°C until dry (5–10 min), and then cooling. This procedure, when repeated 2–3 times, ensures adequate coating of the reactive glass surface such that inositol recoveries of 80–90% are achieved.

For dephosphorylation, the lyophilized, desalted extracts are resolubilized in 500 μl of doubly distilled water; 50-μl aliquots are counted to assess recovery, and 50- to 100-μl aliquots are transferred to the silanized tubes for hydrolysis. In addition, 10 μl of d6-*myo*-inositol (1 pmol/μl) is added to each tube, which serves as an internal standard for GC/MS quantitation. The tops of the tubes are then heat-sealed and the samples heated at 200°C for 3 min in a sand bath in an oven equilibrated to 200°C. After cooling, tubes are opened and the samples evaporated to dryness in a Savant (Farmingdale, NY) centrifugal evaporator. Under these conditions IP_3 is completely dephosphorylated to inositol, as demonstrated by rechromatography of a heated sample containing [^{3}H]IP_3 (Fig. 1). Furthermore, commercially prepared IP_3 (Sigma) is quantitatively recovered as *myo*-inositol. The phosphate remaining in the sample appears to have no effect on derivatization or quantitation of inositol. In fact, addition of 100 pmol of phosphate or 10 pmol of ATP (the most likely contaminant from tissue samples) to inositol standards has no effect on quantitation.

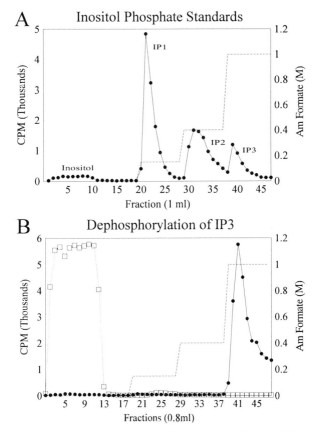

FIG. 1   Anion-exchange chromatography of inositol phosphates. (A) Typical elution profile of radiolabeled inositol phosphates from an AG 1-X8 column. A sample of [³H]IP₁, [³H]IP₂, and [³H]IP₃ was applied to a 1-ml AG 1-X8 column, eluted with increasing concentrations of ammonium formate buffered to pH 5.0 with ammonium hydroxide (dotted line), and collected as 1-ml fractions. One molar ammonium formate was used to elute IP₃ as there was no IP₄ in the samples. (B) Elution profile of 10 pmol of IP₃ containing [³H]IP₃ (100,000 cpm) before (●) and after (□) dephosphorylation by heating samples to 200°C as described. [³H]IP₃ was not detected in the IP₃ fraction following dephosphorylation. Furthermore, IP₃ was quantitatively recovered as *myo*-inositol from fractions 2–12. For graphical purposes, values as shown are not corrected for quench.

Preparation of Standard Curve

Each set of tissue samples is analyzed with reference to a newly prepared set of *myo*-inositol standards. To more closely approximate the conditions of tissue extract analysis, standards are not prepared by dilution of a prederivatized *myo*-inositol sample, but rather are made from a series of individual standards containing a total of 0.2, 0.4, 1.0, 2.0, 4.0, 10, 20, or 40 pmol each of *myo*-inositol. Each standard solution is prepared by dilution from an aqueous frozen stock (1×10^{-8} mol/μl) to ensure consistency between curves. Each standard and sample also contains 10 pmol of the internal standard (d6-*myo*-inositol), which is also prepared by dilution from a frozen stock solution (1×10^{-8} mol/μl). Sample blanks are prepared each time by drying and derivatizing 200–300 μl of the doubly distilled water used for preparation of the samples. Any *myo*-inositol in the blank must be subtracted from both the standard and sample mass values. We detected no inositol, however, in our water blanks.

Derivatization

The inositols in the samples are esterified with heptafluorobutyric anhydride (HFBA) to produce perheptafluorobutyrylinositol (HFB_6-inositol) which is detected with high sensitivity by negative-ion chemical ionization (NICI) mass spectrometry. The derivative is formed by adding 20 μl each of anhydrous acetonitrile and HFBA to the tubes containing dried samples. The tubes are then heat-sealed and the derivatization allowed to proceed at room temperature at least overnight. GC/MS analyses of known quantities of either free *myo*-inositol or dephosphorylated *myo*-IP_3 indicated that derivatization was 100% using this procedure. Tubes should remain sealed until immediately before analysis by GC/MS. No deterioration of the sample or derivative has been observed under these conditions for at least 2 months. A precautionary note with respect to the derivatization step is that some lots of HFBA are not miscible with acetonitrile, on a 1 : 1 (v/v) basis, at room temperature. Sometimes, a single phase can be obtained by slight warming of the sample just prior to injection. This problem is minimized by using HFBA from 1-ml ampoules and discarding any remainder. In any case, testing the miscibility prior to adding reagent to the samples is advisable.

Gas Chromatography/Mass Spectrometry Conditions

NICI analyses are carried out on a HP Model 5988A GC/MS system (Hewlett-Packard, Palo Alto, CA), with a 2000 dalton upper mass limit, operating with a Vector/One Data System (Teknivent Corp., St. Louis, MO) using methane as the reagent gas. The instrument is mass calibrated using m/z 194 (an ion derived from HFBA that is always resident in the instrument) and m/z 633, derived from perfluorotributylamine (Scientific Instruments Services, Inc., Ringoes, NJ) and introduced via the instrument calibrant valve. The intensities of both ions are maximized by mass spectrometer lens tuning while maintaining unit-mass resolution. The sensitivity, resolution, and mass calibration are then checked by injecting HFB_6-sorbitol (2 pmol/μl, Sigma), a six-carbon sugar alcohol not present in the IP_3 fractions, and monitoring at m/z 1338.

Gas chromatography is performed on a 15-m fused silica capillary column (DB-210, 0.5-μm film thickness, 0.32 mm I.D.; J&W Scientific, Folsom, CA) in split mode (10 : 1 to 20 : 1) using a silanized glass injection port liner and Teflon-faced septa. Difficulties with sample carryover (ghosting) can be encountered when using splitless mode injection. Chromatographic conditions are as follows: injection port 220°C, He carrier gas pressure 5 p.s.i., column temperature program 120–220°C at 10°C/min.

Measurement of *myo*-Inositol and Validation of Analysis

The NICI partial spectra of HFB$_6$-*myo*-inositol and HFB$_6$-d6-*myo*-inositol are shown in Fig. 2. Quantitative analysis is carried out using selected ion monitoring of *m/z* 1336, for the endogenous inositol, and *m/z* 1341 for the internal standard HFB$_6$-d6-*myo*-inositol. Integrated areas of the ion profiles, obtained as the inositols elute from the chromatograhic column, are used for quantitation. The origin of *m/z* 1336 and other ions is shown in Fig. 3. The ion originating from the internal standard (HFB$_6$-d6-*myo*-inositol) which corresponds to *m/z* 1336, is *m/z* 1341 which arises from the loss of ^{2}HF from the internal standard. A standard curve is prepared as described above, and the intensity ratio of *m/z* 1336 to that of *m/z* 1341 is plotted against the total amount of inositol per sample (Fig. 4).

The identity of the measured inositol is determined by retention time (always corresponds to that of the internal standard within experimental error) and by the ratios of ions in the spectrum of the inositol. The ratio of intensities of a pair of ions in the mass spectrum is a highly unique parameter, and thus there should be correspondence between the ratio in the standards and that of the sample. In a typical experiment the intensity ratio (*m/z* 1159) : (*m/z* 1336) in authentic HFB$_6$-*myo*-inositol is 0.142 ± 0.029 (SD, *n* = 3), whereas that of the HFB$_6$-inositol in cardiac myocytes is 0.138 ± 0.052 (SD, *n* = 3). The correspondence of both this ratio and the peak retention time is a strong case for identity of the analyte and the standard. This protocol can just as effectively be used with any of the other naturally occurring inositols, namely, *chiro-*, *neo-* and *scyllo-*inositol, all of which are separated by the chromatographic procedure.

Gas Chromatography/Mass Spectrometry Quantitation of Inositol in Tissue Samples

The above-described procedures have been applied in the analysis of IP$_3$ levels from two preparations that do not readily lend themselves to mass analysis by other procedures: (1) substrate-attached isolated adult ventricular

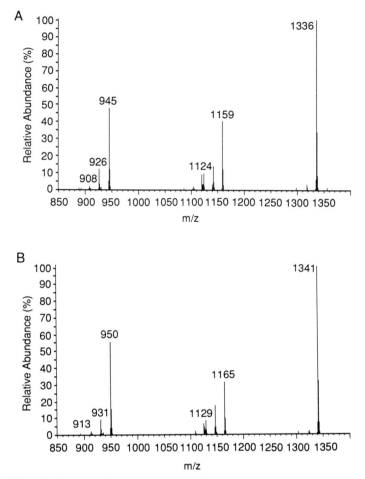

FIG. 2 Negative-ion methane chemical ionization mass spectrum of HFB$_6$-*myo*-inositol (A) and HFB$_6$-d6-*myo*-inositol (B). The principal ion in the spectrum of unlabeled HFB$_6$-*myo*-inositol is *m/z* 1336, which results from the loss of HF from the molecular ion *m/z* 1356; the latter is visable as a trace ion in the spectrum. The deuterium-labeled HFB$_6$-*myo*-inositol has, as principal ion, *m/z* 1341, which results from the loss of ^{2}HF from *m/z* 1362, the molecular ion of the labeled molecule present as a trace abundance ion.

myocytes and (2) freshly dispersed coronary artery smooth muscle. Isolated adult ventricular myocytes are dissociated from 8 to 12-week-old Wistar Kyoto rats (~250 g) by retrograde perfusion of the intact heart with a collagenase solution according to published procedures (13). Myocytes are prepared so as to be Ca^{2+} tolerant and are then plated at high density on laminin-

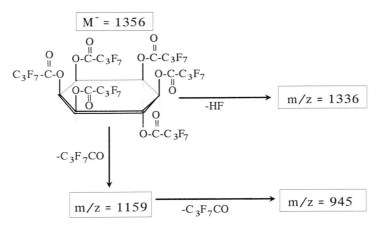

Fig. 3 Diagram of ion losses from HFB$_6$-*myo*-inositol.

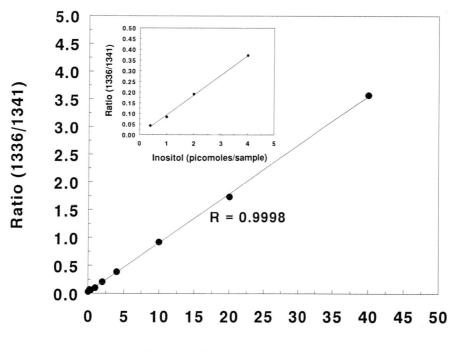

Fig. 4 Standard curve of HFB$_6$-*myo*-inositol measured by negative-ion chemical ionization monitoring using *m/z* 1336 for HFB$_6$-*myo*-inositol and *m/z* 1341 for HFB$_6$-d6-*myo*-inositol. Ratios reflect integrated peak areas. The measured amount of *myo*-inositol was linear from 10 fmol (0.4 pmol/40 μl sample, see inset) to 1 pmol per microliter injected onto the column.

coated glass coverslips. Rod-shaped, Ca^{2+}-tolerant myocytes adhere preferentially to laminin. Damaged cells are removed, and cultures are therefore enriched for viable myocytes by replacing the medium 1–2 hr after plating. Experiments described here are performed on cells within 2–3 hr of isolation. These preparations typically contain 30–200 μg protein. Cell density constraints on myocyte attachment and viability prohibit increasing cell numbers to levels sufficient for mass analysis by other procedures (5, 9).

Freshly dispersed porcine (Yucatan miniature swine) coronary smooth muscle is obtained by enzymatic dissociation of the left anterior descending coronary artery (14). Each vessel typically yields 8–10 samples with 75–250 μg protein each. Myocytes are maintained in an enzyme-free solution and are utilized within 1 hr of isolation. Visual examination of preparations routinely reveals 90–95% isolated, elongated smooth muscle cells. Fura-2 analysis of cells from similarly digested preparations demonstrates unchanged internal Ca^{2+} levels for several hours after digestion (14).

Basal levels of IP_3 in substrate-attached ventricular myocytes and isolated porcine coronary smooth muscle (Fig. 5) are 235 $\pm$ 55 (mean $\pm$ SEM for 3 preparations with 6 determinations/preparation) and 144 $\pm$ 37 (mean $\pm$ SEM for 4 preparations with 8 determinations/preparation) pmol/mg protein, respectively. These IP_3 levels are within the range reported for other tissues analyzed with a variety of quantitative methods (for review, see Ref. 3). However, IP_3 levels of adult cardiac myocytes are an order of magnitude higher than the IP_3 levels reported for isolated canine ventricular myocytes using GC (2) or GC/MS (9). Although these differences may be due to subtle variations in methods, more likely explanations include (1) species variations, (2) the enrichment procedures utilized here for rod-shaped myocytes, or (3) the use of substrate-attached versus unloaded myocytes.

Summary

Using NICI GC/MS with selected ion monitoring, we have extended the limit of detection for inositol to the femtomole level with a high degree of chemical specificity. The high sensitivity of the method and the simplified procedures for tissue extraction and dephosphorylation allow us to measure quantitatively levels of any of the inositol polyphosphates from submilligram quantities of tissue. With the recent developments of ion chromatography HPLC (which provides good separation of inositol polyphosphate isomers) and ion suppression procedures in which the inositol phosphates elute in water it should be possible, with our method, to measure the amounts of many of the individual inositol polyphosphates in small amounts of tissue.

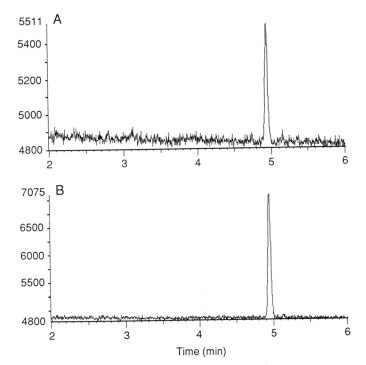

FIG. 5   Selected ion monitoring analysis of isolated porcine coronary artery smooth
muscle. An aliquot (1/10) of the dephosphorylated IP$_3$ fraction was derivatized to the
fluoroacyl derivative with HFBA, and 1/40 of the volume (1 μl) was injected onto
the GC column. (A) Trace of *m/z* 1336 arising from endogenous *myo*-inositol (at 4.95
min); (B) trace of *m/z* 1341 from the internal standard, HFB$_6$-d6-*myo*-inositol, which
has a slightly longer retention time than does unlabeled HFB$_6$-*myo*-inositol. The
amount of derivatized tissue extract injected corersponds to 8–10 μg of original
tissue, and the amount of HFB$_6$-*myo*-inositol detected is 250 fmol.

Acknowledgments

The authors thank M. H. Laughlin for providing the invaluable porcine coronary
artery tissue. This research was supported by an American Heart Association Grant-
in-Aid (L. J. Rubin) and by a grant from the National Heart, Lung, and Blood Institute
to M. H. Laughlin (HL-36531, University of Missouri, Columbia). The GC/MS analysis was performed at the Washington University Mass Spectrometry Facility, St.
Louis, Missouri (supported by grants RR00954 and AM20579 from the National
Institutes of Health).

References

1. S. E. Rittenhouse and J. P. Sasson, *J. Biol. Chem.* **260,** 8657 (1985).
2. G. P. Heathers, P. B. Corr, and L. J. Rubin, *Biochem. Biophys. Res. Commun.* **156,** 485 (1988).
3. S. Palmer and M. J. O. Wakelam, *Biochim. Biophys. Acta* **1014,** 239 (1989).
4. R. F. Irvine (ed.) "Methods in Inositide Research." Raven, New York, 1990.
5. N. M. Dean and M. A. Beaven, *Anal. Biochem.* **183,** 199 (1989).
6. W. R. Sherman, K. E. Ackerman, R. G. Berger, B. G. Gish, and M. Zinbo, *Biomed. Environ. Mass Spectrom.* **13,** 333 (1986).
7. F.-F. Hsu, H. D. Goldman, and W. R. Sherman, *Biomed. Environ. Mass Spectrom.* **19,** 597 (1990).
8. H. D. Goldman, F.-F. Hsu, and W. R. Sherman, *Biomed. Environ. Mass Spectrom.* **19,** 771 (1990).
9. S. D. DaTorre, P. B. Corr, and M. H. Creer, *J. Lipid Res.* **31,** 1925 (1990).
10. W. R. Sherman, P. M. Packman, M. H. Laird, and R. L. Boshans, *Anal. Biochem.* **78,** 119 (1977).
11. C. P. Downes and R. H. Michell, *Biochem. J.* **198,** 133 (1981).
12. S. E. Rittenhouse and W. G. King, "Methods in Inositide Research" (R. F. Irvine, ed.), p. 109. Raven, New York, 1990.
13. B. A. Wittenberg, R. L. White, R. D. Ginzberg, and D. C. Spray, *Circ. Res.* **59,** 143 (1986).
14. L. Stehno-Bittel, M. H. Laughlin, and M. Sturek, *Am. J. Physiol.* **259,** H643 (1990).

[20] Characterization of Inositol Phosphates by High-Performance Liquid Chromatography

Nobuyuki Sasakawa, Toshio Nakaki, and Ryuichi Kato

Introduction

It is well established that inositol polyphosphates play important roles in regulating the functions of a variety of cells. Inositol 1,4,5-trisphosphate [Ins(1,4,5)P$_3$] is the primary factor in an agonist-induced mobilization of intracellular Ca^{2+} (1, 2). Inositol 1,3,4,5-tetrakisphosphate [Ins(1,3,4,5)P$_4$] also exerts effects on Ca^{2+} influx (3, 4), Ca^{2+} sequestration (5), and membrane current (6, 7). The number of inositol phosphates known to exist in mammalian cell types has increased and now stands at over 20, including cyclic inositol polyphosphates, inositol pentakisphosphate (InsP$_5$), and inositol hexakisphosphate (InsP$_6$).

It has been reported that exogenously added InsP$_5$ and InsP$_6$ play some role in neuronal cells which have specific binding sites for InsP$_6$ (8–10). We have shown that several kinds of stimulants cause a rapid accumulation of Ins(1,3,4,5,6)P$_5$ in adrenal chromaffin cells (11, 12) and of Ins(1,3,4,6)P$_4$, Ins(1,3,4,5,6)P$_5$, and InsP$_6$ in N1E-115 neuroblastoma cells (13). These results suggest that the inositol lipid signaling pathways may generate both intracellular and extracellular signals in neuronal cells (14). In this chapter, we describe the experimental procedures used in our laboratory for the measurement of inositol polyphosphate accumulation in cultured adrenal chromaffin cells and N1E-115 neuroblastoma cells by high-performance liquid chromatography (HPLC).

Principles

[^{3}H]Inositol taken up into cells is incorporated into phosphatidylinositol, which is eventually phosphorylated to phosphatidylinositol 4,5-bisphosphate. This compound is the major precursor of most [^{3}H]inositol polyphosphates. Use of cultured cells has facilitated the incorporation of radiolabeled [^{3}H]inositol to full isotopic equilibrium. High-performance liquid chromatography offers high-resolution separations of inositol polyphosphates, including isomers of InsP$_3$, InsP$_4$, and InsP$_5$, by a strong anion-exchange column using a gradient of ammonium phosphate. Radioactivity in HPLC effluents is quantitated by liquid scintillation counting in an on-line radioactivity flow detector equipped with a computer-aided analytical program, which offers a rapid method of quantitatively detecting [^{3}H]inositol polyphosphates.

Experimental Procedure

Primary Culture of Bovine Adrenal Chromaffin Cells

Chromaffin cells are isolated from fresh bovine adrenal medulla by retrograde perfusion with 0.025% (w/v) collagenase (15), then purified by differential plating (16) and plated on plastic 35-mm diameter dishes (2.8×10^6 cells/ dish) in 3 ml minimum essential medium (GIBCO, Grand Island, NY), supplemented with 10% fetal calf serum (17, 18). The purity of the chromaffin cells is over 95%. They are cultured at 37°C in an atmosphere of 95% (v/v) air/ 5% (v/v) CO_2 and used for experiments 5 days after plating. Most cells have attached to the dishes by this time. The culture medium contains the following antibiotics: penicillin G (100 units/ml), streptomycin sulfate (100 μg/ml), gentamicin sulfate (40 μg/ml), and mycostatin (25 units/ml). The medium also contains fluorodeoxyuridine (10 μM), cytosine arabinoside (10 μM), and uridine (10 μM) to prevent the proliferation of nonneuronal cells.

Protocol

1. Ten fresh bovine adrenal glands are obtained within 30 min of the death of the animal. The glands are placed in ice-cold phosphate-buffered saline containing 200 units/ml of penicillin G, 200 μg/ml streptomycin sulfate, and 80 μg/ml of gentamicin sulfate and transported to the laboratory.
2. External fat is removed, and ice-cold phosphate-buffered saline (20 ml) is injected through the adrenal vein.
3. The cortexes are removed with a pair of scissors as thoroughly as possible, taking care to leave some tissue surrounding the adrenal vein. The blood vessels should be kept intact.
4. The adrenal vein is cannulated and the cannula is connected to a peristaltic pump.
5. The medulla is flushed with 10 ml of the phosphate-buffered saline.
6. The cannula is connected to a peristaltic pump. The medulla is perfused in a recirculating system using a multichannel peristaltic pump at a rate of 20 ml/min for 30 min with 300 ml of Hanks' solution containing 0.025% collagenase and antibiotics, as above. The medulla is placed in the Hanks' solution.
7. The solution is discarded.

8. The Hanks' solutions are changed for fresh ones. The medulla is perfused again for 60 min. At the end of the second perfusion, the medulla becomes fluffy.

9. Remove the cannula and the surrounding cortex. Dissect the medulla with a pair of forceps and dissociate the tissue completely. It is important to carry out this step rapidly.

10. The cell suspension is filtered once through gauze.

11. The filtrate is filtered through 80-μm nylon mesh.

12. The filtrate is centrifuged at 150 g for 10 min at room temperature.

13. The pellet is resuspended in 150 ml of Hanks' solution containing 1% (w/v) bovine serum albumin (BSA) and the antibiotics.

14. Centrifuge the cell suspension at 100 g for 8 min.

15. The pellet is resuspended in 150 ml of culture medium containing 10% fetal calf serum and the antibiotics.

16. Centrifuge the cell suspension at 30 g for 4 min.

17. The pellet is resuspended in culture medium 4×10^5 cells/ml.

18. The cells are transferred to a plastic tissue culture flask at a density of 10×10^6 cells/25 ml/75 cm^2 surface area.

19. After 4–5 hr at 37°C in a 95% air/5% CO_2 atmosphere, the nonattached cells (chromaffin cells) are collected.

20. The purified chromaffin cells are plated on 35-mm diameter dishes (2.8×10^6 cells/dish) in a volume of 3 ml of minimal essential medium (GIBCO).

Culture of N1E-115 Cells

Mouse neuroblastoma clone N1E-115 cells (passage 9–13) are grown in 75-cm^2 tissue culture flasks and seeded onto plastic collagen-coated 35-mm diameter dishes (1.2×10^6 cells/35-mm dish at seeding, 3×10^6 cells/35-mm dish at the time of experiments) in a volume of 3 ml of Dulbecco's modified Eagle's medium (DMEM) with high glucose (GIBCO), containing streptomycin (25 μg/ml) and penicillin G (50 units/ml), and supplemented with 10% fetal calf serum.

Labeling Cells

The cells are labeled with [^{3}H]inositol (50 μCi/ml) in 35-mm diameter dishes with 1 ml of culture medium for 48 hr (11–13, 17–20). To achieve a high level of [^{3}H]inositol in the medium, the original [^{3}H]inositol solution is concentrated. For this purpose, 50 μl of the solvent-containing original [^{3}H]inositol solution (17 Ci/mmol) provided by the supplier (see below) is evaporated and reconstituted with 1 ml of the culture medium to obtain a final isotopic concentration of [^{3}H]inositol of 50 μCi/ml. However, the addition of up to 5% (v/v) [^{3}H]inositol solution to the incubation medium does not affect the labeling efficiency and subsequent response to stimulants. Thus, the same results are obtained by direct addition of 50 μl (50 μCi) of the original [^{3}H]inositol solution to 1 ml of the culture medium. In some experiments, cells are doubly labeled with H$_3$^{32}PO$_4$ (50 μCi/ml) and [^{3}H]inositol (50 μCi/ml) (11). For this purpose, inorganic phosphate is added directly to the medium in addition to [^{3}H]inositol.

Changes in the radioactivity of [^{3}H]inositol phosphates reflect changes in the amount thereof only when cells are radiolabeled to isotopic equilibrium. The basal accumulations of [^{3}H]Ins(1,4,5)P$_3$, [^{3}H]Ins(1,3,4,6)P$_4$, and [^{3}H]InsP$_5$ attain equilibrium with [^{3}H]inositol within 48 hr. [^{3}H]InsP$_6$ reaches equilibrium within 72 hr. As in the case of cells labeled for 48 hr, carbachol (100 μM) also induces accumulations of [^{3}H]inositol polyphosphates in cells labeled for 96 hr, and to a similar extent. Therefore, if the cells are labeled for 48 hr or longer, stimulant-induced increases in the radioactivty of [^{3}H]inositol polyphosphates reflect an increase in the amount of inositol polyphosphate, but not an increase in the isotopic specific activity.

Measurement of Inositol Polyphosphate Accumulation in Intact Cells

The culture medium is aspirated and replaced with Locke's solution (for adrenal chromaffin cells) or Hanks' solution (for N1E-115 cells) containing 10 mM HEPES and 0.1% (w/v) BSA (pH 7.4). The cell layers are washed twice with the solution. They are then preincubated at 37°C for 25 min in a 10 mM LiCl-containing solution. Omission of the preincubation step causes larger variation among samples. Stimulants are added to the incubation mixture in a small volume (e.g., 5–10 μl), and the cells are incubated for various times. It is important that the small added volumes be mixed well with gentle pipetting (Gilson, Middleton, WI, P-1000). Because N1E-115 cells are only loosely adherent to the dishes, care should be taken not to detach the cells. At the end of the incubation period, the incubation mixture is removed by aspiration, and 1.5 ml of 10% (w/v) trichloroacetic acid is added to the culture dishes. We use trichloroacetic acid to extract inositol phosphates from the cells. It should be kept in mind, however, that the use of acid for extraction destroys cyclic inositol polyphosphates. For the extraction of cyclic inositol phosphates, another solvent such as chloroform/methanol should be employed (21). The attached cells are homogenized by sonication (20 sec), and the homogenate is transferred to 1.5-ml plastic tubes (Eppendorf) followed by centrifugation at 8000 g for 5 min. The supernatant is transferred to

10-ml glass tubes, and the trichloroacetic acid is extracted four times with 4 ml of water-saturated diethyl ether. The aqueous phase is dried with a concentrator (Speed Vac, Savant, Farmingdale, NY). Dried residue is reconstituted with 240 μl of distilled water.

Protocol

1. Culture cells under the following conditions: chromaffin cells, 2.8×10^6 cells/35-mm dish with 3 ml of culture medium; N1E-115 cells, 1.2×10^6 cells/35-mm dish.
2. Three days after the cell preparation (chromaffin cells) or two days after seeding (N1E-115 cells), 2ml of culture medium is discarded from the dishes.
3. Add 50 μl of [^{3}H]inositol (17 Ci/mmol) solution to the 1 ml of culture medium and incubate cells for 2 days under a 5% CO_2 atmosphere.
4. Wash the cell layer with 0.1% BSA-containing Locke's solution (2 ml); repeat.
5. Preincubate cells with 1 ml of 0.1% BSA- and 10 mM LiCl-containing Locke's solution for 20 min (chromaffin cells) or 25 min (N1E-115 cells) on a hot plate adjusted to 37°C.
6. Add 10 μl of stimulant solution (100 $\times$ concentration) and incubate cells for the desired time periods.
7. Aspirate the medium and add 10% trichloracetic acid (1.4 ml).
8. Homogenize cells still attached to the dishes by sonication for 20 sec.
9. Transfer the homogenate to a 1.5-ml plastic tube (Eppendorf).
10. Centrifuge the tube at 8000 g for 5 min at room temperature.
11. Transfer the supernatant to a 10-ml glass tube.
12. Add 4 ml of water-saturated diethyl ether, mix well, and centrifuge the tube at 1500 g for 5 min at room temperature. Remove the upper phase. Repeat this procedure four times.
13. Lyophilize with a Speed Vac concentrator.
14. Reconstitute the sample with 240 μl of water.
15. Subject 200 μl of the sample to HPLC.

Separation of Inositol Polyphosphates by High-Performance Liquid Chromatography

Isomers of inositol polyphosphates are separated by anion-exchange HPLC (8–10, 15, 16, 19). The reconstitutted sample (200 μl) is subjected to HPLC with an Adsorbosphere SAX 5 μm column (Alltech Applicd Science Labs, Deerfield, IL), as originally used by Balla *et al.* (22) with minor modifications.

For the samples from adrenal chromaffin cells, a linear gradient (1% increase/min) of ammonium phosphate (pH 3.35 with phosphoric acid) at a flow rate of 1 ml/min is used. For the samples from N1E-115 cells, we use a gradient delivered from two independent pumps drawing on reservoirs containing water (pump A) and 1 M ammonium phosphate (pH 3.35 with phosphoric acid; pump B) at a flow rate of 1 ml/min as follows: 0 min, 0% B; 5 min, 0% B; 25 min, 25% B; 45 min, 30% B; 65 min, 65% B; 70 min, 100% B; 75 min, 100% B; 80 min, 0% B. The latter gradient conditions are better than the former for separation of the isomers of $InsP_3$ and $InsP_4$. The effluent radioactivity is monitored by an on-line flow detector with an efficiency of 30% (Flow-1 beta, Packard Japan, Co., Ltd., Tokyo, Japan). Peaks are quantified by integration, and the background is set at 50 counts/min (cpm).

Accumulation of Inositol Polyphosphates in Cultured Adrenal Chromaffin Cells

The typical elution profiles of the extracts obtained from [3H]inositol-prelabeled chromaffin cells are shown in Fig. 1. Each standard of $[^3H]Ins(1,3,4)P_3$, $[^3H]Ins(1,4,5)P_3$, $[^3H]Ins(1,3,4,6)P_4$, $[^3H]Ins(1,3,4,5)P_4$, $[^3H]Ins(3,4,5,6)P_4$, $[^3H]Ins(1,3,4,5,6)P_5$, and $[^3H]InsP_6$ is eluted from the column as one major peak at the position indicated by the arrows. Inositol trisphosphate isomers, $[^3H]Ins(1,3,4)P_3$ and $[^3H]Ins(1,4,5)P_3$, inositol tetrakisphosphate isomers, $[^3H]Ins(1,3,4,6)P_4$, $[^3H]Ins(1,3,4,5)P_4$, and $[^3H]Ins(3,4,5,6)P_4$, $[^3H]Ins(1,3,4,5,6)P_5$ and $[^3H]InsP_6$ are eluted at about 0.3, 0.5, 0.6, and 0.7 M ammonium phosphate, respectively. When the cells are doubly labeled with [^3H]inositol and inorganic ^{32}P, $[^3H]Ins(1,3,4,5)P_4$, $[^3H]Ins(1,3,4,5,6)P_5$, and $[^3H]InsP_6$ peaks coincide with those of ^{32}P radioactivity (Fig. 2). Under these conditions, ^{32}P counts with retention times corresponding to $[^3H]Ins(1,4,5)P_3$ and $[^3H]Ins(1,3,4)P_3$ contain numerous peaks and cannot be assigned to each $[^3H]InsP_3$ species.

Nicotine and angiotensin II induce significant increases in $[^3H]Ins(1,4,5)P_3$ formation at 15 sec after stimulation, whereas high K^+ induces a slight increase in $[^3H]Ins(1,4,5)P_3$ formation (Fig. 1). Stimulation with high K^+ (56 mM), nicotine (10 μM), and angiotensin II (10 μM) increased $[^3H]InsP_5$ formation in cultured adrenal chromaffin cells. Small rises in $[^3H]Ins(1,3,4,5)P_4$ and $[^3H]InsP_6$ accumulations are observed at 15 sec after stimulation with all agents. Although the basal and stimulated levels are slightly reduced in the absence of lithium, Li^+ does not modify carbachol-induced inositol polyphosphate accumulation, suggesting that the accumulation of inositol polyphosphates is induced through lithium-insensitive pathways.

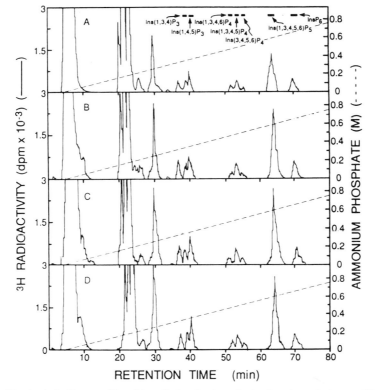

Fig. 1   Typical elution profile of inositol polyphosphates in adrenal chromaffin cells separated by HPLC. The cells were stimulated as follows for 15 sec. (A) Basal levels; (B) high K$^+$ (56 mM); (C) nicotine (10 μM); (D) angiotensin II (10 μM). The standard of each [^{3}H]inositol polyphosphate was eluted from the column as a single peak at the position indicated by the arrow. [From N. Sasakawa, T. Nakaki, and R. Kato, *J. Biol. Chem.* **265,** 17700 (1990).]

Accumulation of Inositol Polyphosphates in N1E-115 Neuroblastoma Cells

Figure 3 shows a typical elution profile of extracts prepared from [^{3}H]inositol-prelabeled N1E-115 cells. [^{3}H]Ins(1,3,4)P$_3$ and [^{3}H]Ins(1,4,5)P$_3$ are eluted at 0.3 M ammonium phosphate. Inositol tetrakisphosphate isomers, [^{3}H]Ins-(1,3,4,6)P$_4$, [^{3}H]Ins(1,3,4,5)P$_4$, and [^{3}H]Ins(3,4,5,6)P$_4$, are eluted at about 0.5 M. [^{3}H]Ins(1,3,4,5,6)P$_5$ and [^{3}H]InsP$_6$ are eluted at about 0.6 and 0.7 M, respectively. These results are consistent with the data obtained from the cultured chromaffin cells.

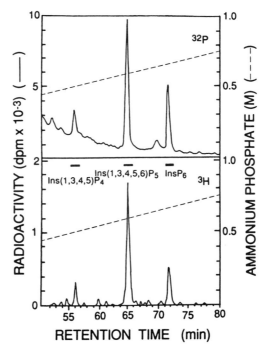

FIG. 2   Elution profile of inositol polyphosphates doubly labeled with [³H]inositol and ³²P produced in adrenal chromaffin cells. The cells were doubly labeled with [³H]inositol (50 μCi/ml) and H₃³²PO₄ (50 μCi/ml) for 2 days. Data from unstimulated cells are shown. (*Top*) ³²P radioactivity; (*bottom*) ³H radioactivity. [From N. Sasakawa, T. Nakaki, and R. Kato, *FEBS Lett.* **261**, 378 (1990).]

When [³H]inositol-prelabeled N1E-115 cells are stimulated with carbachol and high K⁺ for 15 sec, increases in [³H]Ins(1,4,5)P₃, [³H]Ins(1,3,4,6)P₄, [³H]InsP₅, and [³H]InsP₆ accumulation are observed. Although prostaglandin E₁ (PGE₁) (10 μM) also induces these accumulations, the effects are smaller than with carbachol and high K⁺. Other inositol polyphosphates, such as [³H]Ins(1,3,4)P₃, [³H]Ins(1,3,4,5)P₄, and [³H]Ins(3,4,5,6)P₄, have not changed noticeably at 15 sec after stimulation. It should be noted that [³H]Ins(1,3,4,6)P₄ and [³H]InsP₆ increase rapidly in N1E-115 cells, which does not occur in chromaffin cells.

It has been reported that inositol pentakisphosphate isomers, Ins-(1,3,4,5,6)P₅, Ins(1,2,3,4,6)P₅, and Ins(1,2,4,5,6)P₅, exist in the slime mold *Dictyostelium* (23). It is possible, therefore, that the InsP₅ peak eluted from N1E-115 cell extracts contains isomers other than Ins(1,3,4,5,6)P₅.

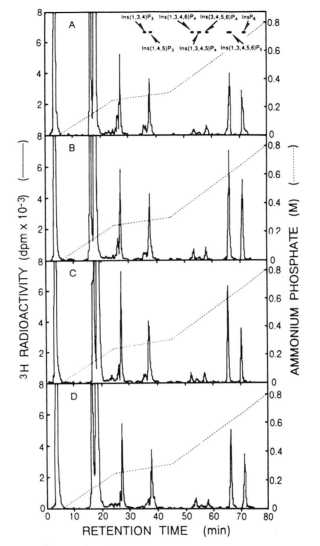

FIG. 3   Typical elution profile of inositol polyphosphates in N1E-115 cells separated by HPLC. The cells were stimulated as follows for 15 sec (A) Basal levels; (B) carbachol (100 μM); (C) high K^+ (60 mM); (D) prostaglandin (PGE$_1$) (10 μM). The standard of each [^{3}H]inositol polyphosphate was eluted from the column as a single peak at the position indicated by the arrow. [Reproduced with permission from N. Sasakawa, T. Nakaki, R. Kashima, S. Kanba, and R. Kato, *J. Neurochem.* **58,** 2116 (1992).]

Chemicals

The following chemicals are obtained from the companies indicated. *myo*-[2-^{3}H]Inositol (17 Ci/mmol) and $H_3{}^{32}PO_4$ are from Amersham International Inc. (Bucks, UK); *myo*-[1-^{3}H]Ins(1,4,5)P$_3$ (17 Ci/mmol), *myo*-[1-^{3}H]inositol 1,3,4-trisphosphate [Ins(1,3,4)P$_3$] (17 Ci/mmol), *myo*-[1-^{3}H]Ins(1,3,4,5)P$_4$ (17 Ci/mmol), and *myo*-[2-^{3}H]InsP$_6$ (12 Ci/mmol) are from New England Nuclear (Boston, MA). The standard mixture of [^{3}H]Ins(1,3,4,5)P$_4$, [^{3}H]inositol 1,3,4,6-tetrakisphosphate [Ins(1,3,4,6)P$_4$], [^{3}H]inositol 3,4,5,6-tetrakisphosphate [Ins(3,4,5,6)P$_4$], and [^{3}H]inositol pentakisphosphate (InsP$_5$) was generously provided by Dr. K. J. Catt (Endocrinology and Reproduction Research Branch National Institute of Child Health and Human Development, National Institutes of Health, Bethesda, MD). The standard of [^{3}H]Ins(1,3,4,5,6)P$_5$ was generously provided by Dr. P. T. Hawkins (Department of Cellular Pharmacology, Smith Kline and French Research Ltd., The Frythe, Welwyn, Herts, UK).

Summary

Stimulus-induced formation of [^{3}H]inositol phosphates including [^{3}H]Ins-(1,4,5)P$_3$, [^{3}H]Ins(1,3,4,6)P$_4$, [^{3}H]InsP$_5$, and [^{3}H]InsP$_6$ can be detected in cultured neuronal cells. High-performance liquid chromatography combined with an on-line radioactivity flow detector offers a powerful tool for simultaneously separating and radiochemically quantitating many [^{3}H]inositol phosphates from intact cells.

Acknowledgments

This work was supported in part by a Grant-in-Aid for Encouragement of Young Scientists, a Grant-in-Aid for Scientific Research on Priority Areas, and a Grant-in-Aid for Developmental Scientific Research from the Ministry of Education, Science, and Culture, Japan.

References

1. M. J. Berridge and R. F. Irvine, *Nature (London)* **312,** 315 (1984).
2. M. J. Berridge and R. F. Irvine, *Nature (London)* **341,** 197 (1989).
3. J. P. Heslop, D. M. Blakeley, K. D. Brown, R. F. Irvine, and M. J. Berridge, *Cell (Cambridge, Mass.)* **47,** 703 (1986).

4. R. F. Irvine and R. M. Moor, *Biochem. Biophys. Res. Commun.* **146,** 284 (1987).
5. T. D. Hill, N. M. Dean, and A. L. Boynton, *Science* **242,** 1176 (1988).
6. H. Higashida and D. A. Brown, *FEBS Lett.* **208,** 283 (1986).
7. L. Changya, D. V. Gallacher, R. F. Irvine, B. V. L. Potter, and O.H. Petersen, *J. Membr. Biol.* **109,** 85 (1989).
8. F. Nicoletti, V. Bruno, L. Fiore, S. Cavallaro, and P. L. Canonico, *J. Neurochem.* **53,** 1026 (1989).
9. F. Nicoletti, V. Bruno, S. Cavallaro, A. Copani, M. A. Sortino, and P. L. Canonico, *Mol. Pharmacol.* **37,** 689 (1990).
10. M. A. Sortino, F. Nicoletti, and P. L. Canonico, *Eur. J. Pharmacol.* **189,** 115 (1990).
11. N. Sasakawa, T. Nakaki, and R. Kato, *FEBS Lett.* **261,** 378 (1990).
12. N. Sasakawa, T. Nakaki, and R. Kato, *J. Biol. Chem.* **265,** 17700 (1990).
13. N. Sasakawa, T. Nakaki, R. Kashima, S. Kanba, and R. Kato, *J. Neurochem.* **58,** 2116 (1992).
14. M. R. Hanley, T. R. Jackson, M. Vallejo, S. I. Patterson, O. Thastrup, S. Lightman, J. Rogers, G. Henderson, and A. Pini, *Philos. Trans. R. Soc. London B* **320,** 381 (1988).
15. K. Kumakura, A. Guidotti, and E. Costa, *Mol. Pharmacol.* **16,** 865 (1979).
16. J. C. Waymire, W. F. Bennet, R. Boehme, L. Hankins, K. G. Waymire, and J. W. Haycock, *J. Neurosci. Methods* **7,** 329 (1983).
17. N. Sasakawa, T. Nakaki, S. Yamamoto, and R. Kato, *Cell. Signaling* **1,** 75 (1989).
18. N. Sasakawa, T. Nakaki, S. Yamamoto, and R. Kato, *J. Neurochem.* **52,** 441 (1989).
19. N. Sasakawa, T. Nakaki, S. Yamamoto, and R. Kato, *FEBS Lett.* **223,** 413 (1987).
20. T. Nakaki, N. Sasakawa, S. Yamamoto, and R. Kato, *Biochem. J.* **251,** 397 (1988).
21. J. F. Dixon and L. E. Hokin, *J. Biol. Chem.* **260,** 16068 (1985).
22. T. Balla, G. Guillemette, A. J. Baukall, and K. J. Catt, *J. Biol. Chem.* **262,** 9952 (1987).
23. L. R. Stephens and R. F. Irvine, *Nature (London)* **346,** 580 (1990).

[21] Measurement of Inositol 1,4,5-Trisphosphate, Inositol 1,3,4,5-Tetrakisphosphate, and Phosphatidylinositol 4,5-Bisphosphate in Brain

R. A. John Challiss and Stefan R. Nahorski

Introduction

Intensive research has resulted in the establishment of the phosphoinositide cycle as a major pathway by which a plethora of hormones, neurotransmitters, and other extracellular signaling molecules can generate intracellular second messengers in many cells including those of the central nervous system (CNS) (1–3). Agonist-stimulated hydrolysis of phosphatidylinositol 4,5-bisphosphate (PtdInsP$_2$) proceeds via phosphodiesteratic cleavage by phosphoinositide-specific phospholipase C (PI–PLC) with the consequent generation of sn-1,2-diacylglycerol and inositol 1,4,5-trisphosphate [Ins(1,4,5)P$_3$]. Elucidation of the pathways by which the second messenger molecules are metabolized has been achieved almost exclusively by employing methodologies that involve the incorporation of radioisotopic labels into phosphoinositide cycle intermediates (4, 5). Such studies have given rise to the concept that the complexity of the phosphoinositide cycle may be necessary to allow the production of further biologically active molecules, as well as to allow efficient resynthesis of inositol phospholipids.

Although many of the original observations implicating inositol phospholipid involvement in transmembrane signaling events were obtained using ortho[^{32}P]phosphate, by far the most popular strategy for selective radiolabeling has been to use myo-[^{3}H]inositol to achieve head group labeling of the inositol phospholipids. The discovery that the enzyme responsible for inositol monophosphate dephosphorylation is uncompetitively inhibited by low millimolar concentrations of lithium (6) allowed the development of a simple assay for agonist-stimulated phosphoinositide hydrolysis (7) and firmly established the [^{3}H]inositol labeling method as a mainstay of research in this area. It should be noted that quantitative interpretation of data requires labeling of preparations to isotopic equilibrium. This is often impractical, as extended preincubation periods are usually required for isotopic equilibrium labeling to be achieved, and is therefore rarely attempted [or experimentally verified (8, 9)], particularly in slice or acutely dissociated tissue preparations. How-

Methods in Neurosciences, Volume 18

ever, radioisotopic labeling methods have provided valuable qualitative information on the formation and fate of $Ins(1,4,5)P_3$.

In spite of the above proviso and the corollary that changes in the incorporation of radiolabel cannot necessarily be extended to imply a change in pathway intermediate concentration, *myo*-[^{3}H]inositol labeling of cells has continued to provide valuable new knowledge of the cellular pathways of phosphoinositide metabolism. Thus, the discovery of the 3-kinase route of $Ins(1,4,5)P_3$ metabolism, by which the putative second messenger inositol 1,3,4,5-tetrakisphosphate [$Ins(1,3,4,5)P_4$] is formed (10, 11), was made using acutely [^{3}H]inositol-labeled cerebral cortex slices. Similarly, the elegant work of Stephens and Irvine (12) toward the elucidation of pathways by which higher inositol polyphosphates might be synthesized and their cellular levels regulated has depended on radiolabeling pathway intermediates.

In general, high throughput assays, which allow simultaneous processing and quantitation of multiple samples, have been acheived using the method of Berridge *et al.* (7). Batch recovery of the total [^{3}H]inositol phosphate fraction from cell or tissue preparations prelabeled with [^{3}H]inositol and incubated in the presence of a sufficient concentration of LiCl (routinely 5–10 mM) to prevent completely inositol monophosphate dephosphorylation provides a simple and sensitive method for assessing agonist-stimulated PI–PLC activity. However, this method has a number of limitations: such measurements rarely reflect the time course or magnitude of changes in inositol polyphosphate second messenger levels, do not allow definition of the inositol phospholipid species acted on by PI–PLC, and do not take into account the disruption of the phosphoinositide cycle which might occur in the presence of lithium (13, 14). Resolution of cell extracts into fractions dependent on the extent of phosphorylation of the inositol moiety is also possible (4); however, each fraction is likely to contain multiple inositol phosphate isomers [e.g., the inositol trisphosphate fraction resolved by ion-exchange chromatography on Dowex 1 (formate form) minicolumns will routinely contain both $Ins(1,4,5)P_3$ and $Ins(1,3,4)P_3$, in addition to other possible trisphosphate isomers]. Although a method has been reported which allows the selective dephosphorylation of $Ins(1,3,4)P_3$, and thus the resolution of the major inositol trisphosphate isomers using minicolumn technology (15), most workers employ high-performance liquid chromatography (HPLC) methods to achieve separation of inositol (poly)phosphate metabolites.

An impressive range of HPLC methods are now available (4, 16–19), but all rely on extended gradient elution programs (typically 80–150 min) to achieve isomer resolution and are therefore time-consuming and unsuitable for routine analysis of multiple samples. Furthermore, as with all methods that rely on incorporation of radiolabels into pathway intermediates, it is generally not possible to extrapolate from changes in radioactivity to changes in actual tissue concentrations as the specific activities may change significantly during the time course of the experiment. Therefore, as our knowledge of the structure and physiological regulation of the phosphoinositide pathway has developed, there has become an increasingly urgent need for suitable methods for accurate quantitation of the cellular concentrations of important pathway intermediates such as $Ins(1,4,5)P_3$ and $Ins(1,3,4,5)P_4$.

Mass Assay of Inositol Phosphates

Methods for assessing mass changes in phosphoinositide cycle intermediates are not a recent technological innovation. For example, the first evidence linking the antimanic actions of lithium salts to *in vivo* changes in the concentrations of inositol phosphates in the brain were made by Allison, Sherman, and colleagues in the late 1970s (20, 21). In an elegant series of experiments these workers demonstrated that administration of LiCl to rats caused a 20-fold increase in inositol 1-monophosphate (20), which was primarily due to an increase in the concentration of the D-isomer (21). These seminal findings were achieved by derivatization of inositol phosphates in lyophilized brain regions and subsequent separation by gas chromatography and detection by flame photometry.

More recent developments to allow mass determination of a broader range of phosphoinositide cycle intermediates have also relied on multistage separation and detection procedures (22). Most of the reported methods require (1) extraction of the cell/tissue preparation, (2) chromatographic separation of inositol (poly)phosphates, (3) postcolumn desalting, (4) dephosphorylation of inositol phosphate fractions, and (5) quantitation of the *myo*-inositol liberated by step (4). The quality of information yielded by such procedures is dependent on the chromatographic step [e.g., simple ion-exchange chromatography on Dowex (formate form) will provide information only on mixtures of inositol trisphosphate isomers unless some further step is introduced to selectively remove or quantify one or more of the isomeric species (23, 24)], the precautions taken to monitor recovery through such a multistep protocol (note that inositol phosphate isomers differ considerably in their susceptibility to dephosphorylation by alkaline phosphatase, with vicinal phosphate substitutions being particularly resistant to enzyme attack), and the sensitivity of the *myo*-inositol quantitation step (22, 24–27).

Other methods have attempted to combine chromatographic separation with on-line derivatization/detection. Methods of this type include on-line dephosphorylation and quantitation of inorganic phosphate release (28), metal–dye detection (29), and a novel HPLC separation employing stepwise isocratic elutions in NaOH with postcolumn ion conductivity detection (30).

All of the above methods can provide quantitative measurements of a wide range of inositol (poly)phosphate species, but they have a common major disadvantage in that they are time-consuming, laborious, and require specialized (and often costly) instrumentation. Therefore, the possibility of specifically measuring concentrations of physiologically important products of phosphoinositide metabolism [such as Ins(1,4,5)P$_3$ and Ins(1,3,4,5)P$_4$] without the need for extensive isomer resolution prior to assay or the need for major financial investment in specialist instrumentation is particularly attractive. The remainder of this chapter concentrates on a description and critical assessment of such methods.

Radioreceptor Assays for Inositol 1,4,5-Trisphosphate

The original proposal that stimulation of phosphinositide turnover was intimately linked to cellular Ca^{2+} homeostasis (31) was substantiated by the observation that Ins(1,4,5)P$_3$, generated by hydrolysis of PtdInsP$_2$, could mobilize organellar-sequestered Ca^{2+} (32, 33). The concept that Ins(1,4,5)P$_3$ exerted this second messenger action by interaction with the endoplasmic reticulum was demonstrated by the use of [^{32}P]Ins(1,4,5)P$_3$ to characterize saturable binding sites in permeabilized cells (34), and quickly led to a competitive binding assay being reported which allowed estimation of Ins(1,4,5)P$_3$ mass in cell extracts using saponin-permeabilized neutrophils as a source of cellular Ins(1,4,5)P$_3$ recognition sites (35).

Using this mass assay, Bradford and Rubin (35) were able to demonstrate a transient increase in Ins(1,4,5)P$_3$ accumulation evoked by fMet-Leu-Phe in neutrophils (6 to 8-fold increase over basal within 10 sec, returning to basal values by 120 sec). Despite this early promise the assay required the synthesis of a radioligand not commercially available at the time, produced a poor dynamic range for Ins(1,4,5)P$_3$ displaceable binding [specific binding ~250 disintegrations/min (dpm)], and was open to the criticisms that the specificity of the binding site population for D-Ins(1,4,5)P$_3$ was largely uncharacterized and the preparation retained endogenous complements of Ins(1,4,5)P$_3$ generating and metabolizing activities which might interfere with accurate quantitation. Unfortunately, as a consequence, the assay seems to have been universally ignored.

Further characterization of cellular Ins(1,4,5)P$_3$ binding sites defined the pharmacology of ligand–receptor interaction and demonstrated the impressive stereospecificity and positional specificity of the Ins(1,4,5)P$_3$ receptor for Ins(1,4,5)P$_3$ (36, 37). Comparative studies of Ins(1,4,5)P$_3$ binding site densities in a range of tissues revealed that the densities of Ins(1,4,5)P$_3$ binding sites varied considerably, with particularly high densities of sites being found in cerebellum (37, 38). The latter finding allowed the cerebellar Ins(1,4,5)P_3-binding protein to be purified (39) and characterized as an Ins(1,4,5)P_3-gated Ca^{2+} channel present in the endoplasmic reticulum (40, 41).

A common finding of the initial attempts to characterize Ins(1,4,5)P_3 binding sites was that lower equilibrium dissociation constants were reported for peripheral compared to neuronal preparations. For example, typical K_D values for the cerebellar Ins(1,4,5)P_3 receptor were 20–50 nM (37, 38, 42) compared to 2–5 nM for peripheral tissues (43–45). Although with hindsight it is possible that these early observations may have arisen, at least in part, because of differences in assay conditions employed, such observations suggested that use of a peripheral source of the Ins(1,4,5)P_3-binding protein might allow the development of a more sensitive radioligand binding assay for the determination of cellular Ins(1,4,5)P_3 mass. Indeed, the first descriptions of a mass assay for Ins(1,4,5)P_3 employed a crude microsomal fraction of bovine adrenal cortex (46–48). The preparation of the adrenal binding protein, the sample extraction procedure, and a description of the Ins(1,4,5)P_3 mass assay are given in the Appendix (Procedures 1–3).

The affinity of the adrenal cortex receptor for Ins(1,4,5)P_3 (Fig. 1) allows accurate quantitation of solutions containing as little as 0.5 nM Ins(1,4,5)P_3. Such sensitivity is adequate for most studies [e.g., agonist-stimulated Ins(1,4,5)P_3 mass accumulations in cerebral cortex slices (Fig. 2)]; however, if this proves insufficient [e.g., for primary cultures of cerebellar granule cells (50)], a high volume modification of the Ins(1,4,5)P_3 mass assay has been described (51).

The mass assay is dependent on the assumption that only Ins(1,4,5)P_3 interacts with the Ins(1,4,5)P_3 receptor, while other inositol (poly)phosphate isomers present in cell/tissue extracts are much poorer displacers of [^{3}H]Ins(1,4,5)P_3 binding and are therefore not present at sufficient concentrations to affect accurate Ins(1,4,5)P_3 mass determination. A wide range of inositol (poly)phosphates have now been tested for their ability to displace Ins(1,4,5)P_3 binding (37, 44–48, 51–53), and these studies have generally provided supporting evidence for the selectivity of the mass assay. Although a large number of inositol (poly)phosphates which might occur in biological systems have yet to be investigated, it should be noted that displacing activity in the mass assay can be eliminated by treating samples with preparations of Ins(1,4,5)P_3 5-phosphatase or 3-kinase (51). The specificity of these enzymes for Ins(1,4,5)P_3 (53) makes a persuasive argument for the fidelity of the assay: thus, the initial criticism that other inositol polyphosphates may artifactually contribute to the cell/tissue Ins(1,4,5)P_3 concentration determined by this method has become increasingly muted as the assay has gained wide acceptance.

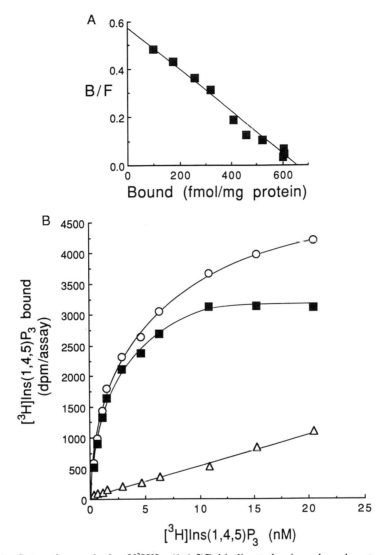

FIG. 1   Saturation analysis of [^{3}H]Ins(1,4,5)P$_3$ binding to bovine adrenal cortex membranes. A P$_2$ fraction was prepared from bovine adrenal cortex (BAC) as described in Procedure 1 (Appendix). Under the assay conditions given in Procedure 3 (Appendix), increasing concentrations of [^{3}H]Ins(1,4,5)P$_3$ (17 Ci/mmol) were incubated with BAC (137 μg protein/assay) in the absence ($\bigcirc$) or presence ($\triangle$) of 10 μM Ins(1,4,5)P$_3$. Bound and free ligand were resolved by vacuum filtration. Specific binding ($\blacksquare$) was calculated as the difference between total and nonspecific binding and was transformed to produce the Scatchard plot shown in (A). For the data shown here, a K_D of 1.3 nM and a B_{max} of 647 fmol/mg of protein were obtained by linear regression analysis of Scatchard transformation.

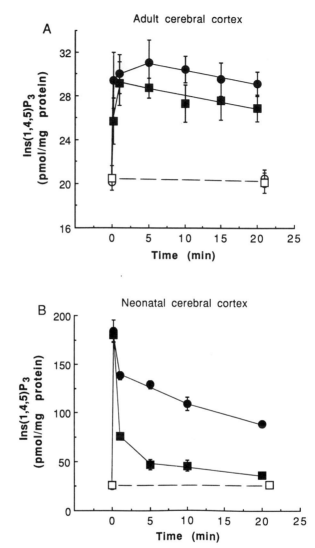

FIG. 2   Assessment of agonist-stimulated Ins(1,4,5)P$_3$ mass accumulations in preparations of adult and neonatal rat cerebral cortex slices. Cerebral cortex slices (350
× 350 μg) were prepared from either (A) adult (70–80 days of age) or (B) neonatal
(7–8 days of age) rats. Incubations were performed as described previously (15) and
were terminated and processed for mass assay as described in Procedure 2 (Appendix). Time courses for Ins(1,4,5)P$_3$ mass accumulations are shown for stimulations
with either carbachol (1 mM; ●) or quisqualate (10 μM; ■). Values are means ±
S.E.M. for three experiments performed in triplicate. The large difference in ordinate
values between the two graphs should be noted.

Therefore, the Ins(1,4,5)P$_3$ mass assay provides a simple, sensitive method for processing multiple cell/tissue extracts with a high degree of interassay reproducibility (47); it is also noteworthy that the assay does not require specialist instrumentation (beyond a suitable centrifuge or vacuum filtration facility) and is relatively inexpensive (5 μCi of [^{3}H]Ins(1,4,5)P$_3$ provides sufficient radioligand for at least 1500 assays). Furthermore, provided suitable precautions are taken (e.g., ensuring that the filtration wash buffer is maintained at 0–4°C), the assay can be performed using a semiautomated vacuum filtration protocol (e.g., a Brandel cell harvester, Gaithersburg, Maryland).

Subsequent to the publication of the assay described here, Bredt and co-workers (54) reported a similar assay based on the use of a crude microsomal fraction from rat cerebellum. To overcome the higher apparent K_D reported for the Ins(1,4,5)P$_3$ receptor in this tissue, a high assay pH was used. This modification was reported to increase the Ins(1,4,5)P$_3$ affinity of the preparation to a value approaching that obtained in peripheral receptor preparations (54). Our own experiments using a P$_2$ fraction (see Procedure 1 in Appendix) of pig cerebellum (Fig. 3) support the finding that alkalinization of the assay buffer decreases the K_D value (obtained by Scatchard transformation of isotope dilution data), albeit modestly [K_D at pH 7.6, 15.9 ± 1.8 nM; at 8.4, 10.0 ± 2.3 nM ($n = 3$)]. However, use of this preparation for Ins(1,4,5)P$_3$ mass assay, with resolution of bound and free ligand by vacuum filtration, is not recommended. The reason for this caution is illustrated in Fig. 4, which shows the rates of dissociation of [^{3}H]Ins(1,4,5)P$_3$ from adrenal cortex and cerebellar preparations following sample dilution in 20 volumes of assay wash buffer (see Appendix, Procedure 3). It is clear that the initial rate of dissociation is more rapid in the cerebellar membrane preparation, with about 20% of specific binding being lost over the first 10 sec following sample dilution. This potential problem can be obviated by employing centrifugation to separate bound and free assay components; however, this precludes semiautomation of the assay for high-throughput screening (see above).

Use of Inositol 1,4,5-Trisphosphate Mass Assay for Phosphatidylinositol 4,5-Bisphosphate Determination

A number of methods are available for isolation of membrane phospholipids and efficient hydrolysis of the polar head group (see Ref. 4). In the case of PtdIns(4,5)P$_2$, such methods can release Ins(1,4,5)P$_3$ as a major product, and this can then be quantified using the Ins(1,4,5)P$_3$ mass assay described above. A suitable method for processing cell/tissue preparations for subsequent Ins(1,4,5)P$_3$ mass assay has been presented by Chilvers et al. (55) and is described in the Appendix, Procedure 4. Application of this method affords

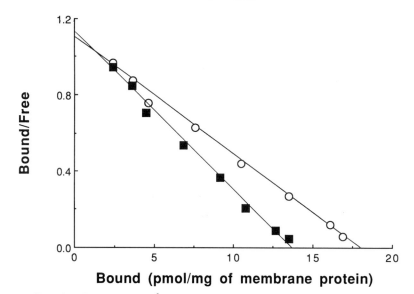

Bound (pmol/mg of membrane protein)

FIG. 3   Scatchard analysis of [³H]Ins(1,4,5)P₃ binding to pig cerebellar membranes at different assay pH. A P₂ fraction was prepared from pig cerebellum exactly as descirbed in Procedure 1 (Appendix). Assays were initiated by addition of 38 μg cerebellar protein to [³H]Ins(1,4,5)P₃ (~7500 dpm; 1.67 nM) and increasing concentrations of Ins(1,4,5)P₃ (1–100 nM) in Tris-HCl/EDTA buffer at pH 7.6 (○) or 8.4 (■). Nonspecific binding was defined in the presence of 10 μM Ins(1,4,5)P₃. Assays were performed as described in Procedure 3 (Appendix), with bound and free ligand being separated by centrifugation (12,000 g, 3 min, 4°C). Mean K_D and B_{max} values obtained from this and two other experiments are given in the text.

the opportunity to study mass changes in both PtdIns(4,5)P₂ and Ins(1,4,5)P₃ in the same preparation and therefore obtain information on PI–PLC sub-strate–product relationships during agonist-stimulated phosphoinositide turnover (55, 56).

Radioreceptor Assay for Inositol 1,3,4,5-Tetrakisphosphate

Since the original report that [³H]Ins(1,3,4,5)P₄ accumulates rapidly and dramatically following agonist challenge of [³H]inositol-labeled cerebral cortex slices (10), similar observations have been made in numerous cells and tissue preparations, and considerable efforts have been made to ascribe a second messenger role to this phosphorylated metabolite of Ins(1,4,5)P₃. It is considered unlikely that a pathway of Ins(1,4,5)P₃ metabolism, which proceeds via a highly regulated enzyme requiring ATP as a cosubstrate, can

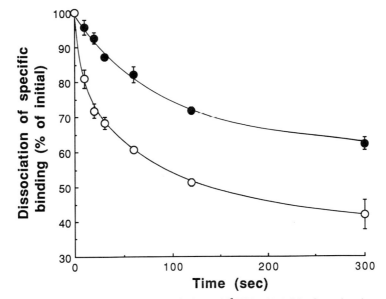

FIG. 4   Comparison of rates of dissociation of [^{3}H]Ins(1,4,5)P$_3$ from bovine adrenal cortex and pig cerebellar membranes. P$_2$ fractions prepared from (●) bovine adrenal cortex (BAC, 500 μg protein/assay) or (○) pig cerebellum (PC, 55 μg protein/assay) were incubated with [^{3}H]Ins(1,4,5)P$_3$ (8200 dpm/assay) in Tris-HCl/EDTA assay buffers at pH 8.0 and 8.4, respectively. Once at equilibrium (after 30 min, 4°C), 3.2 ml wash buffer (25 mM Tris-HCl, 1 mM EDTA, 5 mM NaHCO$_3$, pH 8.0/8.4) was added, and samples were vacuum filtered 0–300 sec after addition of wash buffer. In this case, assay tubes were rapidly rinsed once with a further 3.2 ml wash buffer, and assays were performed in triplicate. At equilibrium, specific binding was 2706 ± 23 and 4012 ± 49 dpm for BAC and PC, respectively.

have evolved simply to terminate the Ca^{2+}-mobilizing action of Ins(1,4,5)P$_3$ (57; but see Ref. 58). Such teleological reasoning is borne out by the experimental evidence implicating a number of possible roles for Ins(1,3,4,5)P$_4$ in cellular Ca^{2+} homeostasis (57, 59–64).

Another actively pursued research avenue has been the characterization of cellular proteins that exhibit high-affinity Ins(1,3,4,5)P$_4$ binding, with a view to the identification of the cellular receptor through which this inositol polyphosphate may exert its putative second messenger actions. Although early reports of Ins(1,3,4,5)P$_4$-binding proteins provided little evidence for selectivity for Ins(1,3,4,5)P$_4$ compared to other inositol (poly)phosphates (65, 66), Enyedi et al. (67) were able to distinguish Ins(1,4,5)P$_3$- and Ins(1,3,4,5)P$_4$-selective binding sites in membranes prepared from bovine parathyroid gland. In this study, the Ins(1,3,4,5)P$_4$ binding site exhibited an acidic pH optimum and a high degree of selectivity for $Ins(1,3,4,5)P_4$ over $Ins(1,4,5)P_3$, $Ins(1,3,4)P_3$, and $InsP_5$ (unspecified isomer) (67). In addition, displacement of $[^{32}P]Ins(1,3,4,5)P_4$ by $Ins(1,3,4,5)P_4$ gave rise to a curvilinear Scatchard plot, suggesting the presence of two classes of binding sites. A high-affinity $Ins(1,3,4,5)P_4$ binding site with superficially similar characteristics was subsequently reported to be present in porcine (68) and rat (69) cerebellum, with both reports presenting $Ins(1,3,4,5)P_4$ mass determinations employing the binding site as the basis of the radioligand binding assay (see Appendix, Procedure 5). The cerebellar preparation provides an excellent source of the $Ins(1,3,4,5)P_4$ binding site for mass measurements, as it exhibits remarkable selectivity for $Ins(1,3,4,5)P_4$ (53, 68–70), and the acidic assay conditions prevent possible interference from the high density of $Ins(1,4,5)P_3$ receptor sites present (70).

It should be noted that detailed analysis of the displacement of specifically bound $[^{32}P]Ins(1,3,4,5)P_4$ by D-$Ins(1,3,4,5)P_4$ [or L-$Ins(1,3,4,5)P_4$ (see Ref. 53)] produces a displacement isotherm which is best modeled by a two-site curve-fitting programme (Fig. 5). The high-affinity site present in pig cerebellar preparations displays nanomolar affinity for $Ins(1,3,4,5)P_4$ (K_H 1.8 nM) and constitutes the major component of $[^{32}P]Ins(1,3,4,5)P_4$ binding (75–85% of liganded sites). From these data it can be calculated that the high-affinity $Ins(1,3,4,5)P_4$ binding site is present in this preparation at a modest density (B_{max} 220–250 fmol/mg of protein).

Unlike the binding protein used for the $Ins(1,4,5)P_3$ mass assay, which is clearly the $Ins(1,4,5)P_3$ receptor, the cerebellar $Ins(1,3,4,5)P_4$ binding site(s) has an unknown physiological significance at present. However, considerable progress has been made toward its purification and characterization (71, 72). In addition, a complex array of inositol polyphosphate-binding proteins have been identified in neuronal membrane preparations (73, 74), raising the possibility that $Ins(1,3,4,5)P_4$ may exert its proposed cellular actions through multiple receptor proteins.

Use of the $Ins(1,3,4,5)P_4$ mass assay described here has allowed estimates of basal and agonist-stimulated concentrations to be made in neuronal preparations such as cerebral cortex slices (69, 75). Compared to $Ins(1,4,5)P_3$, basal levels of $Ins(1,3,4,5)P_4$ are about 10-fold lower in cerebral cortex (2–4 pmol/mg protein); however, levels can increase dramatically on agonist stimulation [e.g., a maximally effective concentration of muscarinic cholinoceptor agonist causes a rapid and sustained 15- to 25-fold increase in $Ins(1,3,4,5)P_4$ (69)], consistent with previous results obtained in [^3H]inositol-labeled preparations. Furthermore, agonist stimulation of cerebral cortex slices in the presence of a depolarizing stimulus (high K^+) synergistically increases both $Ins(1,4,5)P_3$ and $Ins(1,3,4,5)P_4$ mass accumulations (Table I) to such an extent that the specificity of the respective mass assays might be called into question. When this issue is addressed, it can be estimated that

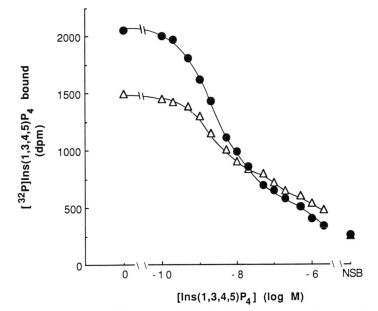

FiG. 5   Displacement of [^{32}P]Ins(1,3,4,5)P$_4$ binding from cerebellar membranes by Ins(1,3,4,5)P$_4$. A P$_2$ microsomal fraction of rat ($\triangle$) or pig ($\bullet$) cerebellum was prepared as described in Procedure 1 (Appendix). Assays were performed as described in Procedure 5 (Appendix), except that the final assay volume was 160 μl. Each assay contained 9700 dpm [^{32}P]Ins(1,3,4,5)P$_4$ ($\sim$0.17 nM) and 245 or 250 μg cerebellar membrane protein for rat and pig preparations, respectively. Nonspecific binding (NSB) was defined by inclusion of 3 mM 2,3-bisphosphoglycerate [identical estimates of NSB were also obtained using 1 mM InsP$_6$ or 100 μg/ml heparin (M_r 4000–6000)]. Displacement data were best fitted by a two site model: for rat and pig cerebellar preparations K_H values were 2.5 and 1.8 nM (56 and 79% of sites), respectively.

the crossover between assays is such that detection of Ins(1,4,5)P$_3$ by the Ins(1,3,4,5)P$_4$ mass assay [EC$_{50}$ for displacement of ^{32}P-labeled Ins(1,3,4,5)P$_4$ by Ins(1,4,5)P$_3$ is about 20 μM (69)] is essentially zero, whereas Ins(1,3,4,5)P$_4$ may account for less than 7% of Ins(1,4,5)P$_3$ detected by the Ins(1,4,5)P$_3$ assay [assuming only a 50-fold selectivity for the adrenal cortical Ins(1,4,5)P$_3$ receptor (51)]. This extreme case of cellular inositol polyphosphate accumulations is given to illustrate the impressive specificity of both mass assays.

Concluding Remarks

The development of simple methods for the routine assay of cellular concentrations of key phosphoinositide cycle intermediates represents a highly significant advance in the experimental tools available for interrogation of

TABLE I   Muscarinic Cholinoceptor- and Depolarization-Stimulated Inositol Polyphosphate Mass Accumulations in Rat Cerebral Cortex Slices[a]

Stimulus addition	Inositol polyphosphate accumulation (pmol/mg protein)			
	$Ins(1,4,5)P_3$	Increase over basal	$Ins(1,3,4,5)P_4$	Increase over basal
Control	21.2 ± 0.8	—	3.8 ± 0.3	—
+CCH	28.1 ± 1.0	6.9	50.1 ± 6.6	46.3
+KCl	34.9 ± 1.1	13.7	14.8 ± 1.2	11.0
+CCH, +KCl	73.7 ± 2.9	52.5	364.3 ± 20.5	360.5
+Atropine, +CCH, +KCl	30.8 ± 4.6	9.6	10.4 ± 3.0	6.6

[a] Cerebral cortex slices were prepared from adult rats and incubated as described in Ref. 75. All incubations (except control) were for 5 min in the presence of 1 mM carbachol (CCH) and/or 25 mM (29.7 mM final concentration) KCl. Where indicated atropine (10 μM) was added 10 min prior to CCH/KCl addition. Incubations were terminated as described in Procedure 2 (Appendix), and mass assays were performed as described in Procedures 3 and 5 (Appendix). Values are means $\pm$ S.E.M. for at least three experiments performed in triplicate. The increase over basal columns are included to indicate the synergistic effects on both $Ins(1,4,5)P_3$ and $Ins(1,3,4,5)P_4$ mass accumulations of costimulation with CCH plus KCl.

this important cellular signaling pathway. Direct assay of endogenous second messenger levels should supercede the use of the lithium block, total [^{3}H]inositol phosphate assay employed at present, particularly in experimental paradigms designed to address complex cellular cross talk between signaling pathways. Furthermore, application of these methods will prove invaluable in the future in many aspects of phosphoinositide research, including, for example, investigation of the precise, quantitative relationship between inositol polyphosphate generation and calcium mobilization from organellar stores (76) and desensitization phenomena associated with prolonged agonist–receptor occupancy (77, 78).

Appendix

Procedure 1. Preparation of Inositol 1,4,5-Trisphosphate-Binding Protein from Bovine Adrenal Glands

1. Bovine adrenal glands should be obtained as fresh as possible (if there is a gap of >45 min between slaughter and commencing dissection, glands should be trimmed of fat, wrapped in foil, and stored on ice). Once cleaned of fat, each gland is cut longitudinally and the central medulla removed. The cortex is then scraped from the outer capsule using a spatula.

2. Cortex is maintained on ice until the required number of glands have been processed. The cortex is dispensed into centrifuge tubes (5–8 g tissue per 50-ml tube) and homogenized [Polytron (Brinkmann Instruments, Westbury, NY) setting 5–6, 3 times, 15 sec each time] in ice-cold 20 mM NaHCO$_3$, 1 mM dithiothreitol, pH 8.0 (buffer A).

3. Homogenized cortex is centrifuged (5000 g, 10 min, 4°C) and the supernatants pooled and maintained on ice. The pellets are rehomogenized in buffer A and recentrifuged. The supernatant is recovered and the twice-extracted pellet discarded.

4. The supernatants from the two low-speed centrifugation steps are combined and dispensed into fresh tubes. A "P$_2$" fraction is recovered by centrifugation (40,000 g, 20 min, 4°C). The supernatant is discarded and the pellet rehomogenized in buffer A and recentrifuged. This step is repeated to wash the P$_2$ fraction 3 times following its original isolation.

5. The washed P$_2$ fraction is rehomogenized in a known volume of buffer A, and the protein concentration is determined and adjusted to 15–18 mg protein/ml. The P$_2$ fraction of known protein concentration is then dispensed as 1-ml aliquots into Eppendorf tubes and stored at −20°C until required. The binding protein can be stored for at least 6 months without significant changes in its Ins(1,4,5)P$_3$ binding properties. Furthermore, limited freeze–thawing does not cause any adverse effects.

6. For a typical preparation, 8–10 adrenal glands will yield 60–80 g of adrenal cortex, and this will produce 60–80 ml of binding protein. Note that 75 ml of binding protein is sufficient for 2500 assays using the method described in Procedure 2.

Procedure 2. Sample Preparation of Cerebral Cortex Slices for Inositol 1,4,5-Trisphosphate Mass Assay

1. For cerebral cortex slices incubated in 300 μl Krebs–Henseleit buffer (KHB), terminate by addition of 300 μl ice-cold 1 M trichloroacetic acid (TCA). Transfer the sample to an ice bath and extract for 20 min with intermittent vortex mixing.

2. Centrifuge (3000 g, 15 min, 4°C) and remove 500 μl supernatant [the slice pellet can be washed in 0.9% NaCl and digested in 1 M NaOH for determination of protein concentration, or processed for PtdInsP$_2$ mass measurement (see Procedure 3)]. Wash the acid supernatant 4 times with 3 volumes each time of water-saturated diethyl ether [alternatively, samples can be neutralized using Freon/tri-n-octylamine (49)].

3. Following acid extraction by diethyl ether, samples are allowed to stand for 30–60 min at 4°C. A known volume of sample (200 μl) is transferred

to an Eppendorf tube, and 50 μl of 60 mM NaHCO$_3$ and 50 μl of 30 mM EDTA (pH adjusted to 7) are added. Under these conditions samples may be stored at 4°C for up to 14 days prior to assay of Ins(1,4,5)P$_3$.

4. A buffer blank is also prepared to provide a suitable diluent for construction of the Ins(1,4,5)P$_3$ mass assay standard curve. This is achieved by mixing equal volumes of KHB and 1 M TCA, extracting 4 times with 3 volumes of diethyl ether, and adding appropriate volumes of NaHCO$_3$ and EDTA (see above).

Procedure 3. Mass Determination of Inositol 1,4,5-Trisphosphate

1. Recommended materials are as follows: D-Ins(1,4,5)P$_3$ from Research Biochemicals Inc. (Natick, MA) or Rhode Island University (Kingston, RI) and [^{3}H]Ins(1,4,5)P$_3$ from NEN–Du Pont (Boston, MA; NET-911, 17–20 Ci/mmol) or Amersham International (Bucks, UK; TRK.999, 30–50 Ci/mmol).

2. D-Ins(1,4,5)P$_3$ can be stored in aqueous solution at 1 mM at −20°C. For short periods (<3 months) aliquots of 40 μM Ins(1,4,5)P$_3$ can also be stored for daily preparation of standard curves. Standard curves are constructed by dilution of 40 μM stocks to give final concentrations of 1, 3, 10, 30, and 100 nM (for definition of nonspecific binding the 40 μM stock is used) in the prepared buffer blank. The final assay volume is 120 μl, and therefore these concentrations correspond to 0.12–12 pmol Ins(1,4,5)P$_3$ per assay.

3. To 30 μl of standard Ins(1,4,5)P$_3$ or unknown is added 30 μl of 100 mM Tris-HCl, 4 mM EDTA, pH 8.0, and 30 μl [^{3}H]Ins(1,4,5)P$_3$ (appropriately diluted to give 6000–8000 dpm/assay). Care should be taken to maintain assay tubes at 0–4°C at all times by performing the procedure in an ice bath.

4. The assay is initiated by addition of 30 μl of the bovine adrenal cortical preparation (it may be necessary to rehomogenize the preparation on thawing). Samples are incubated for 30 min on ice with intermittent vortex mixing.

5. Separation of bound and free radioligand can be achieved by either centrifugation or rapid vacuum filtration. In our experience the high protein concentration in the assay (routinely 450–600 μg) can result in loose pellets following centrifugation, and this causes problems with supernatant removal and may affect the quality of data obtained. Although this problem can be overcome (e.g., by introduction of a sucrose cushion to aid separation of pellet and supernatant, or by increasing the salt concentration in the assay buffer), we routinely resolve bound and free ligand by filtration and recommend its use.

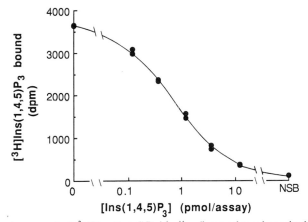

FIG. A.1   Displacement of [³H]Ins(1,4,5)P₃ binding from adrenal cortical preparation.

6. For filtration, it is crucial that the wash buffer (25 mM Tris-HCl, 1 mM EDTA, 5 mM NaHCO₃, pH 8.0) is ice-cold. Millipore (Bedford, MA) vacuum manifolds are loaded with GF/B filters and wetted with wash buffer. Assay samples are diluted with 3 ml wash buffer and immediately filtered, and the sample tube is then rapidly washed 2 times with 3 ml wash buffer; this procedure should be completed within 5–10 sec.

7. Following filtration, GF/B filter disks are transferred to vials, and 4 ml of a suitable scintillant is added. Samples should be allowed to extract for at least 6 hr prior to scintillation counting.

8. A typical standard curve is shown in Fig. A.1. In this case, each assay tube contained 7523 dpm [³H]Ins(1,4,5)P₃ and 504 μg bovine adrenal–cortical preparation. In the absence of unlabeled Ins(1,4,5)P₃ about 50% binding was obtained, with the nonspecific binding being less than 4%. Addition of 0.12 pmol unlabeled Ins(1,4,5)P₃ resulted in 17.5% displacement of specific binding, whereas 50% displacement of binding occurred at 0.87 pmol/assay [i.e., EC₅₀ for Ins(1,4,5)P₃ binding was 7.25 nM].

Procedure 4. Extraction/Hydrolysis of Phosphatidylinositol 4,5-Bisphosphate for Mass Determination

1. Pellets from TCA-terminated incubations (see Procedure 2) are sequentially washed with 2 ml of 5% (w/v) TCA/1 mM EDTA and 2 ml water. Following thorough aspiration of the supernatant, 0.94 ml chloroform/methanol/concentrated HCl (40:80:1, by volume) is added to the pellet

and intermittently vortex mixed for 20 min. Phases are resolved by addition of 0.31 ml chloroform and 0.56 ml of 0.1 M HCl and centrifugation (1000 g, 15 min, at room temperature).

2. A known volume of lower phase is dried under N_2. The lipid extract is deacylated by addition of 0.25 ml of 1 M KOH; the tubes are then tightly capped and heated in a boiling water bath for 15 min. Samples are transferred to an ice bath, neutralized by addition to columns [prepared by adding 0.5 ml of a 50% slurry of Dowex 50 (200–400 mesh; H^+ form)], and then eluted with 2.25 ml water.

3. The total eluate (2.5 ml) is washed 2 times with 2 ml 1-butanol/light petroleum ether (5 : 1, v/v); if necessary, tubes are centrifuged (1000 g, 15 min, at room temperature) to resolve the phases. A 1-ml aliquot of the lower phase is taken and lyophilized.

4. The lyophilizate is redissolved in the required volume of water and aliquots taken for Ins(1,4,5)P_3 mass measurement as detailed in Procedure 3.

5. It should be noted that the efficiency of alkaline hydrolysis of PtdIns(4,5)P_2 must be determined using [^{3}H]PtdIns(4,5)P_2 (55). Hydrolysis yields Ins(2,4,5)P_3 and Ins(4,5)P_2 as well as Ins(1,4,5)P_3, and the molar ratio of these products must also be established; Chilvers *et al.* (55) obtained a ratio of 20 : 14 : 66. Note that Ins(2,4,5)P_3 and Ins(4,5)P_2 are 100–400 times weaker in their displacing activity in the Ins(1,4,5)P_3 mass assay and therefore do not interfere with the mass determination. There may also be a small loss of Ins(1,4,5)P_3 during the neutralization step; thus, it is imperative that the recovery of Ins(1,4,5)P_3 through this procedure be determined for each cell/tissue preparation to which it is applied.

Procedure 5. Mass Determination of Inositol 1,3,4,5-Tetrakisphosphate

1. Recommended materials are as follows: D-Ins(1,3,4,5)P_4 is from Rhode Island University; an alternative is Boehringer Mannheim (Mannheim, Germany), but in our experience D-Ins(1,3,4,5)P_4 from this source often contains significant Ins(1,4,5)P_3 contamination. We are unaware of a commercial source of [^{32}P]Ins(1,3,4,5)P_4 at present; therefore, preparation requires phosphorylation of [^{32}P]Ins(1,4,5)P_4 (NEN–Du Pont, NEG-066, 200–250 Ci/mmol) (65). Alternatively, [^{3}H]Ins(1,3,4,5)P_4 (NEN–Du Pont, NET-941, 15–30 Ci/mmol; or Amersham International, TRK 998, 20–60 Ci/mmol) can be used, although in our hands this radioligand yields inferior data compared to the ^{32}P-labeled ligand.

2. Stocks of D-Ins(1,3,4,5)P_4 can be stored at millimolar concentrations at −20°C. Standard curves are constructed to give 0.3–1000 nM final concen-

trations [i.e., 0.036–12 pmol Ins(1,3,4,5)P$_4$ per assay for a 120 μl final assay volume]. A P$_2$ fraction of porcine cerebellum is prepared exactly as described in Procedure 1. The binding protein can be stored at 6–8 mg of protein/ml for at least 4 months at $-20°$C without significant loss of binding activity.

3. To 30 μl of standard Ins(1,3,4,5)P$_4$ or unknown is added 30 μl of 50 mM sodium acetate, 50 mM KH$_2$PO$_4$, 2 mM EDTA, 0.25% bovine serum albumin, pH 5.0 (buffer B), and 30 μl radiolabeled Ins(1,3,4,5)P$_4$ in buffer B. If [^{32}P]Ins(1,3,4,5)P$_4$ is used, 10,000–12,000 dpm/assay is recommended. Care should be taken to maintain assay tubes at 0–4°C at all times.

4. The assay is initiated by the addition of 30 μl of the cerebellar preparation (it is important to rehomogenize the preparation prior to dispensing). Samples are incubated for 30 min on ice with intermittent vortex mixing.

5. Separation of bound and free radioligand is best achieved by rapid vacuum filtration over GF/B filter disks [separation by centrifugation following introduction of a sucrose cushion has also been used (67)]: it is crucial that the wash buffer (25 mM sodium acetate, 25 mM KH$_2$PO$_4$, 5 mM NaHCO$_3$, 1 mM EDTA, pH 5.0) be ice-cold. The sample is diluted with 3 ml wash buffer and immediately filtered, and the sample tube is then rapidly washed 2 times with 3 ml wash buffer; this procedure should be completed within 5–10 sec.

6. Filter disks are transferred to vials and 4 ml of a suitable scintillant added. Samples should be allowed to extract for 6 hr prior to scintillation counting.

7. Examples of Ins(1,3,4,5)P$_4$ displacement curves are given in Fig. 5. The biphasic displacement of [^{32}P]Ins(1,3,4,5)P$_4$ from preparations of rat and pig cerebellar membranes does not compromise the mass assay, as displacement between 0.036 and 12 pmol Ins(1,3,4,5)P$_4$ per assay can be adequately modeled using simple curve-fitting programs. The pig cerebellar preparation offers the advantage of a greater dynamic range for mass determination, owing to the high affinity and greater proportion of high-affinity binding sites. The assay can reproducibly detect 0.1 pmol Ins(1,3,4,5)P$_4$ in a 30-μl sample.

Acknowledgments

We thank the Wellcome Trust and the Science and Engineering Research Council for financial support. We also gratefully acknowledge NEN Du Pont (Boston, MA) for providing as gifts much of the [^{3}H]Ins(1,4,5)P$_3$ and [^{32}P]Ins(1,3,4,5)P$_4$ used in our work toward the development of the methods described here.

References

1. M. J. Berridge, *Biochem. J.* **220,** 345 (1984).
2. C. J. Fowler and G. Tiger, *Neurochem. Int.* **19,** 171 (1991).
3. S. K. Fisher, A. M. Heacock, and B. W. Agranoff, *J. Neurochem.* **58,** 18 (1992).
4. C. M. F. Simpson, I. H. Batty, and J. N. Hawthorne, *in* "Neurochemistry: A Practical Approach" (A. J. Turner and H. S. Bachelard, eds.), p. 193. IRL Press, Oxford, 1987.
5. S. B. Shears, *Pharmacol. Ther.* **49,** 79 (1991).
6. L. M. Hallcher and W. R. Sherman, *J. Biol. Chem.* **255,** 10896 (1980).
7. M. J. Berridge, C. P. Downes, and M. R. Hanley, *Biochem. J.* **206,** 587 (1982).
8. D. A. Horstman, H. Takemura, and J. W. Putney, *J. Biol. Chem.* **263,** 15297 (1988).
9. G. St.J. Bird, K. G. Oliver, D. A. Horstman, J. Obie, and J. W. Putney, *Biochem. J.* **273,** 541 (1991).
10. I. H. Batty, S. R. Nahorski, and R. F. Irvine, *Biochem. J.* **232,** 211 (1985).
11. R. F. Irvine, A. J. Letcher, J. P. Heslop, and M. J. Berridge, *Nature (London)* **320,** 631 (1986).
12. L. R. Stephens and R. F. Irvine, *Nature (London)* **346,** 580 (1990).
13. M. J. Berridge, C. P. Downes, and M. R. Hanley, *Cell (Cambridge, Mass.)* **59,** 411 (1989).
14. S. R. Nahorski, C. I. Ragan, and R. A. J. Challiss, *Trends Pharmacol. Sci.* **12,** 297 (1991).
15. E. D. Kennedy, I. H. Batty, E. R. Chilvers, and S. R. Nahorski, *Biochem. J.* **260,** 283 (1989).
16. N. M. Dean and J. D. Moyer, *Biochem. J.* **242,** 361 (1987).
17. I. H. Batty, A. J. Letcher, and S. R. Nahorski, *Biochem. J.* **258,** 23 (1989).
18. L. R. Stephens, P. T. Hawkins, A. F. Stanley, T. Moore, D. R. Poyner, P. J. Morris, M. R. Hanley, R. R. Kay, and R. F. Irvine, *Biochem. J.* **275,** 485 (1991).
19. J.-C. Sulpice, C. Bachelot, P. Gascard, and F. Giraud, *in* "Methods in Inositide Research" (R. F. Irvine, ed.), p. 45. Raven, New York, 1990.
20. J. H. Allison, M. E. Blisner, W. H. Holland, P. P. Hipps, and W. R. Sherman, *Biochem. Biophys. Res. Commun.* **71,** 664 (1976).
21. W. R. Sherman, A. L. Leavitt, M. P. Honchar, L. M. Hallcher, and B. E. Phillips, *J. Neurochem.* **36,** 1947 (1981).
22. J. A. Maslanski and W. B. Busa, *in* "Methods in Inositide Research" (R. F. Irvine, ed.), p. 113. Raven, New York, 1990.
23. S. E. Rittenhouse and J. P. Sasson, *J. Biol. Chem.* **260,** 8657 (1985).
24. A. P. Tarver, W. G. King, and S. E. Rittenhouse, *J. Biol. Chem.* **262,** 17268 (1987).
25. J. A. Shayman, A. R. Morrison, and O. H. Lowry, *Anal. Biochem.* **162,** 562 (1987).
26. G. P. Heathers, T. Juehne, L. J. Rubin, P. B. Corr, and A. S. Evers, *Anal. Biochem.* **176,** 109 (1989).
27. S. A. Prestwich and T. B. Bolton, *Biochem. J.* **274,** 663 (1991).
28. J. L. Meek, *Proc. Natl. Acad. Sci. U.S.A.* **83,** 4162 (1986).
29. G. W. Mayr, *Biochem. J.* **254,** 585 (1988).

30. G. Y. Sun, T.-N. Lin, N. Premkumar, S. Carter, and R. A. MacQuarrie, *in* "Methods in Inositide Research" (R. F. Irvine, ed.), p. 135. Raven, New York, 1990.

31. R. H. Michell, *Biochim. Biophys. Acta* **415**, 81 (1975).

32. H. Streb, R. F. Irvine, M. J. Berridge, and I. Schulz, *Nature (London)* **306**, 67 (1983).

33. M. Prentki, T. J. Biden, D. Janjic, R. F. Irvine, M. J. Berridge, and C. B. Wollheim, *Nature (London)* **309**, 562 (1984).

34. A. Spät, P. G. Bradford, J. S. McKinney, R. P. Rubin, and J. W. Putney, *Nature (London)* **319**, 514 (1986).

35. P. G. Bradford and R. P. Rubin, *J. Biol. Chem.* **261**, 15644 (1986).

36. S. R. Nahorski and B. V. L. Potter, *Trends Pharmacol. Sci.* **10**, 139 (1989).

37. A. L. Willcocks, A. M. Cooke, B. V. L. Potter, and S. R. Nahorski, *Biochem. Biophys. Res. Commun.* **146**, 1071 (1987).

38. P. F. Worley, J. M. Baraban, S. Supattapone, V. S. Wilson, and S. H. Snyder, *J. Biol. Chem.* **262**, 12132 (1987).

39. S. Supattapone, P. F. Worley, J. M. Baraban, and S. H. Snyder, *J. Biol. Chem.* **263**, 1530 (1988).

40. C. A. Ross, J. Meldolesi, T. A. Milner, T. Satoh, S. Supattapone, and S. H. Snyder, *Nature (London)* **339**, 468 (1989).

41. C. D. Ferris, R. L. Huganir, S. Supattapone, and S. H. Snyder, *Nature (London)* **342**, 87 (1989).

42. S. K. Joseph and H. L. Rice, *Mol. Pharmacol.* **35**, 355 (1989).

43. A. Spät, G. L. Lukacs, I. Eberhardt, L. Kiesel, and B. Runnebaum, *Biochem. J.* **244**, 493 (1987).

44. G. Guillemette, T. Balla, A. J. Baukal, and K. J. Catt, *J. Biol. Chem.* **263**, 4541 (1988).

45. A. L. Willcocks, R. A. J. Challiss, and S. R. Nahorski, *Eur. J. Pharmacol.* **189**, 185 (1990).

46. S. Palmer, K. T. Hughes, D. Y. Lee, and M. J. O. Wakelam, *Biochem. Soc. Trans.* **16**, 991 (1988).

47. R. A. J. Challiss, I. H. Batty, and S. R. Nahorski, *Biochem. Biophys. Res. Commun.* **157**, 684 (1988).

48. S. Palmer, K. T. Hughes, D. Y. Lee, and M. J. O. Wakelam, *Cell. Signalling* **1**, 147 (1989).

49. E. S. Sharps and R. L. McCarl, *Anal. Biochem.* **124**, 421 (1982).

50. E. M. Whitham, R. A. J. Challiss, and S. R. Nahorski, *Eur. J. Pharmacol.* **206**, 181 (1991).

51. R. A. J. Challiss, E. R. Chilvers, A. L. Willcocks, and S. R. Nahorski, *Biochem. J.* **265**, 421 (1990).

52. P. J. M. Van Haastert, *Anal. Biochem.* **177**, 115 (1989).

53. R. A. J. Challiss, S. T. Safrany, B. V. L. Potter, and S. R. Nahorski, *Biochem. Soc. Trans.* **19**, 888 (1991).

54. D. S. Bredt, R. J. Mourey, and S. H. Snyder, *Biochem. Biophys. Res. Commun.* **159**, 976 (1989).

55. E. R. Chilvers, I. H. Batty, R. A. J. Challiss, P. J. Barnes, and S. R. Nahorski, *Biochem. J.* **275,** 373 (1991).
56. R. Plevin and M. J. O. Wakelam, *Biochem. J.* **285,** 759 (1992).
57. R. F. Irvine, *BioEssays* **13,** 419 (1991).
58. T. Balla, S. S. Soo, T. Iida, K. Y. Choi, K. J. Catt, and S. G. Rhee, *J. Biol. Chem.* **266,** 24719 (1991).
59. T. D. Hill, N. M. Dean, and A. L. Boynton, *Science* **242,** 1176 (1988).
60. L. Changya, D. V. Gallacher, R. F. Irvine, and O. H. Petersen, *J. Membr. Biol.* **109,** 85 (1989).
61. P. J. Cullen, R. F. Irvine, and A. P. Dawson, *Biochem. J.* **271,** 549 (1990).
62. D. J. Gawler, B. V. L. Potter, and S. R. Nahorski, *Biochem. J.* **272,** 519 (1990).
63. A. Lückhoff and D. E. Clapham, *Nature (London)* **355,** 356 (1992).
64. S. DeLisle, D. Pittet, B. V. L. Potter, P. D. Lew, and M. J. Welsh, *Am. J. Physiol.* **262,** C1456 (1992).
65. A. B. Theibert, S. Supattapone, P. F. Worley, J. M. Baraban, J. L. Meek, and S. H. Snyder, *Biochem. Biophys. Res. Commun.* **148,** 1283 (1987).
66. P. Enyedi and G. H. Williams, *J. Biol. Chem.* **263,** 7940 (1988).
67. P. Enyedi, E. Brown, and G. H. Williams, *Biochem. Biophys. Res. Commun.* **159,** 200 (1989).
68. F. Donié and G. Reiser, *FEBS Lett.* **254,** 155 (1989).
69. R. A. J. Challiss and S. R. Nahorski, *J. Neurochem.* **54,** 2138 (1990).
70. R. A. J. Challiss, A. L. Willcocks, B. Mulloy, B. V. L. Potter, and S. R. Nahorski, *Biochem. J.* **274,** 861 (1991).
71. F. Donié and G. Reiser, *Biochem. J.* **275,** 453 (1991).
72. G. Reiser, R. Schaefer, F. Donie, E. Huelser, M. Nehls-Sahabandu, and G. W. Mayr, *Biochem. J.* **280,** 533 (1991).
73. C. C. Chadwick, A. P. Timerman, A. Saito, M. Mayrleitner, H. Schindler, and S. Fleischer, *J. Biol. Chem.* **267,** 3473 (1992).
74. A. B. Theibert, V. A. Estevez, R. J. Mourey, J. F. Marecek, R. K. Barrow, G. D. Prestwich, and S. H. Snyder, *J. Biol. Chem.* **267,** 9071 (1992).
75. R. A. J. Challiss and S. R. Nahorski, *J. Neurochem.* **57,** 1042 (1991).
76. R. J. H. Wojcikiewicz, S. T. Safrany, R. A. J. Challiss, J. Strupish, and S. R. Nahorski, *Biochem. J.* **272,** 269 (1990).
77. R. J. H. Wojcikiewicz and S. R. Nahorski, *J. Biol. Chem.* **266,** 22234 (1991).
78. F. Donié and G. Reiser, *Biochem. Biophys. Res. Commun.* **181,** 997 (1991).

Section V

Inositol Phosphate Receptors and Their Regulation

[22] Molecular Analysis of Inositol 1,4,5-Trisphosphate Receptors

Gregory A. Mignery and Thomas C. Südhof

Introduction

Stimulation of eukaryotic cell surface receptors results in the activation of several intracellular signaling pathways, many of which are mediated by intracellular second messengers. Inositol 1,4,5-trisphosphate (IP$_3$) is one of the most important second messengers. Production of IP$_3$ is caused by activation of receptors for hundreds of biologically active substances. Studies have shown that IP$_3$ has a function in a multitude of physiological processes, ranging from muscle contraction to lymphocyte activation, and from cell division to neuronal excitation (reviewed in Ref. 1).

Initial clues to the presence of the phosphatidylinositol signaling pathway were obtained in experiments on the cholinergic stimulation of the pancreas (2). In the classic experiments, Hokin and Hokin demonstrated that cholinergic agonists caused a rapid turnover of phosphatidylinositol in pancreatic cells. Nearly 20 years elapsed until Michell proposed that the receptor-activated breakdown of phosphatidylinositol might release a soluble mediator which causes mobilization of intracellular calcium (3). This hypothesis was confirmed in experiments using permeabilized pancreatic cells in which IP$_3$, a product of phosphatidylinositol hydrolysis, caused release of Ca^{2+} from intracellular stores (4). Innumerable studies have extended these observations to demonstrate that a multitude of extracellular messengers stimulate intracellular IP$_3$ production and Ca^{2+} release from intracellular stores. As discussed below, these stores correspond to the endoplasmic reticulum, on which IP$_3$ acts by binding to specific, saturable receptors.

Receptor-activated hydrolysis of phosphatidylinositol 4,5-bisphosphate in cells leads to the generation of at least two messengers: diacylglycerol (DAG), an activator of protein kinase C, and IP$_3$, which releases Ca^{2+} from intracellular stores. The two messenger pathways are interconnected because the Ca^{2+} released by IP$_3$ activates protein kinase C, and protein kinase C phosphorylation may modulate aspects of the IP$_3$ pathway. After production, IP$_3$ is quickly metabolized to a large number of derivatives, some of which may be intracellular messengers in their own right (such as inositol 1,3,4,5-tetrakisphosphate) (5). The metabolic pathway of IP$_3$ in cells is very complex. It eventually leads to the generation of inositol monophosphate, which has to be hydrolyzed to inositol in order to be recycled to phosphatidylinositol for reentry into the signaling pathway (6).

Hydrolysis of inositol monophosphate to inositol is catalyzed by an inositol-phosphatase that is inhibited by Li^+ in an uncompetitive manner. As an uncompetitive inhibitor of inositol-phosphatases, Li^+ prevents the recycling of inositol phosphates to phosphatidylinositol. As a consequence, membrane inositol lipids used to generate the second messengers IP_3 and DAG are depleted after chronic lithium treatment (7). Li^+ is used successfully to treat manic-depressive psychosis, suggesting that the phosphatidylinositol signaling pathway may be affected in this disease.

The inositol phosphate signaling pathway may also be involved in early development in vertebrate embryos (8). Mesoderm induction in *Xenopus* embryos is accompanied by a doubling of IP_3 concentrations. Injection of Li^+ at this stage into a ventral vegetal cell redirects the developmental fates of the progeny cells toward dorsal mesodermal derivatives and dorsal organizer tissue. When embryos were treated with a teratogenic dose of Li^+, IP_3 levels significantly declined. The teratogenic effects of lithium can be inhibited if coinjected with *myo*-inositol, suggesting that they arose from phosphatidylinositol depletion.

Purification of Inositol 1,4,5-Trisphosphate Receptors

Intracellular IP_3 causes Ca^{2+} release by binding to specific receptors on the endoplasmic reticulum. For unknown reasons, cerebellar Purkinje cells have more IP_3 receptors than any other tissue, making the cerebellum the most common starting material for receptor preparations. The IP_3 receptor was initially solubilized with Triton X-100 from rat cerebellar microsomes and purified in multiple chromatography steps using DEAE-cellulose, heparin-agarose, and concanavalin A (Con A)-Sepharose (9). This purification procedure was modified and improved by Hingorani and Agnew (10) who utilized wheat germ agglutinin affinity columns instead of Con A-Sepharose. The purified receptor in these studies was shown to contain a single subunit of approximately 300 kDa and to bind IP_3 with affinities similar to those observed in cerebellar microsomes.

For our studies, we have developed an alternative purification procedure (11) based on the high apparent molecular weight of native IP_3 receptors. Membrane proteins are solubilized from cerebellar microsomes in 1% CHAPS and subjected to sucrose gradient centrifugation (Fig. 1). On the gradients, the IP_3 receptor exhibits a high apparent molecular weight of slightly more than 1 million daltons. The receptor is separated from most other proteins on the gradient except for the ryanodine receptor. Similar to

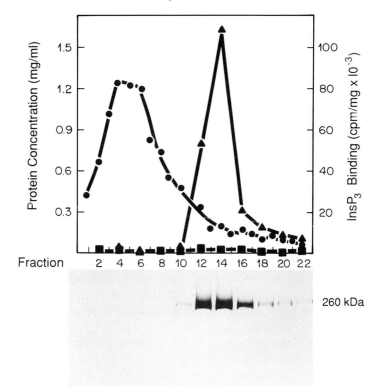

FIG. 1 Purification of cerebellar IP₃ receptors by sucrose gradient centrifugation. The graph demonstrates the distribution of total protein (circles), specific IP₃ binding (triangles), and nonspecific binding (squares) in a 5 to 20% sucrose gradient. The immunoblot shows the distribution of IP₃ receptors in the gradient using an antipeptide antibody against the carboxyl terminus of the type I IP₃ receptor. IP₃ binding and immunoreactivity for IP₃ receptors peak at the same position at an apparent molecular mass of slightly more than 1 million daltons. At this position in the sucrose gradient, few other cellular proteins are found, making sucrose gradients an effective means of purification. [Reprinted with permission from *Nature* (11). Copyright 1989 Macmillan Magazines Limited.]

the ryanodine receptor, IP₃ receptors are composed of multiple subunits that self-associate, producing apparent sizes in excess of 1 million daltons, whereas most other proteins are much smaller. After sedimentation on sucrose gradients, the receptor can be further purified by anion-exchange or heparin-agarose chromatography.

Biochemically, the purified IP_3 receptor is composed of multiple identical subunits with an apparent molecular weight on sodium dodecyl sulfate–polyacrylamide gel electrophoresis (SDS-PAGE) of approximately 300,000. The size of the IP_3 receptor on the sucrose gradients suggests that it is composed of four identical subunits. This suggestion is also supported by Chadwick et al. (12), who purified the receptor by a similar procedure and showed by electron microscopy that the receptor is a tetramer. Binding studies demonstrated binding specifities of the purified receptor for different inositol phosphates that were similar to the specificity of Ca^{2+} release from permeabilized cells for the different inositol phosphates. These studies strongly suggest that the purified receptor corresponds to the protein responsible for IP_3-triggered Ca^{2+} release from the endoplasmic reticulum.

IP_3 receptors have many similarities with ryanodine receptors, the Ca^{2+}-triggered Ca^{2+} release channels of muscle and brain. Both the IP_3 and the ryanodine receptors constitute Ca^{2+} channels found in elements of the endoplasmic reticulum (see below). Structurally, the two classes of receptors share sequence similarity in their carboxyl-terminal regions. Biochemically, both form tetrameric structures, as judged by sucrose gradient sedimentation, negative staining, and chemical cross-linking (11–13). Transmission electron microscopy shows that both receptors form large structures with similar size and 4-fold symmetry. The purified IP_3 receptor has surface geometries of 0.025 μm^2 and resembles a pinwheel with apparently mobile arms (12). The ryanodine receptor, on the other hand, resembles a clover leaf whose individual leaves are fixed and immobile (14).

Ferris et al. (15) have demonstrated that the purified IP_3 receptor contains an intrinsic calcium channel. In these experiments, the purified receptor is reconstituted into liposomes, and the ability to sequester $^{45}Ca^{2+}$ in an IP_3-dependent fashion is monitored. The IP_3-triggered flux into liposomes is discontinuous or graded, suggesting that the graded-release phenomenon (also referred to as quantal release) is a function of the receptor (16). These experiments establish the functionality and autonomy of purified IP_3 receptors.

Molecular cloning has revealed that the IP_3 receptor belongs to a multigene family of related proteins (17). At least three different receptor genes exist that are ubiquitously expressed. The different receptors are referred to as type I, type II, and type III IP_3 receptors, with the cerebellar receptor corresponding to the type I receptor. Although all of the biochemical work described was carried out on IP_3 receptors purified from cerebellum, the high degree of sequence similarity between the different receptors suggests that they will be biochemically very similar (see below).

Localization of Inositol 1,4,5-Trisphosphate Receptors

Specific antibodies have been raised against IP$_3$ receptors using either purified receptor, synthetic peptides from different regions of the receptor, or different recombinant protein fragments. In our hands, the best immunogen for the IP$_3$ receptor is a synthetic peptide corresponding to the carboxyl terminus of the cerebellar (type I) receptor (11). Some of the antibodies generated in this manner, in particular those generated against larger protein fragments, react with multiple receptors. The peptide antibodies, on the other hand, are often specific for one receptor type because the sequences of the peptides usually contain one or several nonconserved residues that appear to be crucial for antibody reactivity.

The IP$_3$ receptor antibodies have been used to investigate the tissue distribution of the type I IP$_3$ receptor (18). In general, most tissues are found to contain very low levels of type I receptor with the exception of cerebellum, which exhibits signals corresponding to levels more than a 1000 times higher than those observed in peripheral tissues. In addition, comparatively high levels are observed in other brain regions and in PC12 cells. Considerable variation in the levels of IP$_3$ receptors is also observed between peripheral tissues.

RNA blotting experiments constitute an independent method to assess the tissue distribution of IP$_3$ receptors (17). They allow a more specific assessment of the relative tissue distributions of different receptor types. RNA blotting experiments demonstrate that the type I receptor is the most abundant of the receptor types and is completely responsible for the enrichment of IP$_3$ receptors in cerebellum. These studies also show that all of the currently known three types of receptors are ubiquitous, with each showing a different profile of expression in different tissues (T. C. Südhof, Y. A. Ushkaryov, C. L. Newton, and G. A. Mignery, unpublished observation, 1991).

Antibodies against IP$_3$ receptors are used to perform immunocytochemical studies on their localization. In most tissues, the levels of receptors are below detection levels. In those tissues in which a signal is observed, a uniform distribution of IP$_3$ receptors in smooth intracellular membranes corresponding to the endoplasmic reticulum is found. In cerebellum, the receptor is found to be highly concentrated in Purkinje cells.

The high levels of IP$_3$ receptors in cerebellar Purkinje cells allow localization of the receptor by immunoelectron microscopy. The results of several groups using this technique are generally in agreement and demonstrate an exclusive localization of the receptor to the endoplasmic reticulum of Purkinje cells (11, 19, 22). The most striking finding is that the receptor is present in all elements of the endoplasmic reticulum in Purkinje cells. Our own studies (primarily carried out in collaboration with Dr. Pietro de Camilli at

Yale University, New Haven, CT) indicate that the receptor is present on endoplasmic reticulum that extends into all arborizations of both axons and dendrites (11, 23). It is possible to demonstrate clearly the presence of IP_3 receptors in presynaptic nerve terminals, suggesting that IP_3-mediated intracellular Ca^{2+} release may have a modulatory function in neurotransmitter release. The receptor is also found in all sections of the dendrites, including the dendritic spines. In these the receptor is localized to the spine apparatus, suggesting that the spine apparatus represents a Ca^{2+} compartment (11).

In addition to the localization studies, the distribution of IP_3 receptors in Purkinje cells has also been compared to that of ryanodine receptors (23). These studies demonstrate that the two functionally distinct Ca^{2+} release channels are colocalized in the endoplasmic reticulum with the exception of dendritic spines. Here only IP_3 receptors but not ryanodine receptors are found. These results suggest that the two receptors functionally cooperate in most compartments but have differential roles in specialized cell components.

Cloning and Polymerase Chain Reaction Analysis of Inositol 1,4,5-Trisphosphate Receptor cDNAs

The original identification of the sequence of an IP_3 receptor was achieved by our laboratory and by the laboratory of Mikoshiba using completely different approaches. However, in both laboratories the cloning of IP_3 receptor cDNAs happened more by serendipity than by strategic planning. We originally identified IP_3 receptor cDNA clones on the basis of antibodies that we made to a peptide from an unknown cDNA sequence highly expressed in cerebellum (11). Furuichi *et al.* purified a phosphoprotein of M_r 400,000 from cerebellum that on cloning was found to be identical with the IP_3 receptor (24). Together these original studies provided the baseline for all structural studies on the IP_3 receptor.

At this point, the complete primary structures of IP_3 receptors from rats, mice, and *Drosophila* as well as partial sequences from humans have been reported (11, 17, 18, 24–26). In addition to the structure of the more abundant type I IP_3 receptor, studies have also reported full-length and partial structures of further receptor types from rats and humans which are referred to as type II and III receptors (17, 26; see below for a discussion). In the following, we first discuss the conclusions derived from the cloning data on the type I receptor, which has been most extensively studied. We then discuss the presence of multiple IP_3 receptors in animal tissues produced by alternative splicing and by the expression of multiple genes.

Full-length structures for type I IP_3 receptors were reported from mice and rats (18, 24). Type I IP_3 receptors from both species contained 2749 amino acids, corresponding to 313-kDa proteins. With 99.2% identical residues, the IP$_3$ receptors were found to be highly conserved between mice and rats. In addition, the structure of an IP$_3$ receptor was recently determined from *Drosophilia* (25). The *Drosophilia* receptor is very similar to mammalian IP$_3$ receptors, although it is currently unclear to which type it corresponds (25).

Databank searches demonstrated that the type I IP$_3$ receptor is distantly related to ryanodine receptors; no other sequence similarities were found. Ryanodine receptors are large proteins of the endoplasmic and sarcoplasmic reticulum that, similarly to IP$_3$ receptors, function as Ca^{2+} release channels (27). The gating of ryanodine receptors, however, seems to be triggered either by Ca^{2+} or by a mechanical coupling with plasma membrane Ca^{2+} channels in skeletal muscle. Interestingly, the greatest degree of similarity between ryanodine and IP$_3$ receptors was observed in the carboxyl-terminal regions in the area of the putative transmembrane regions (see below), suggesting that they may have similar Ca^{2+} channel domains (11). In particular, the sequences of the last transmembrane region and flanking regions are very similar.

Hydrophobicity analysis of the amino acid sequence of the type I IP$_3$ receptor reveals clusters of hydrophobic residues at the carboxyl terminus of the protein. These hydrophobic sequences contain four clearly identifiable transmembrane regions as judged by the algorithm of Kyte and Doolittle (28). In addition, an extended hydrophobic sequence of 76 amino acids is observed that is interrupted by charged residues and contains an average hydrophobicity of 1.6. As an average hydrophobicity of 1.6 is thought to constitute an intramembraneous sequence (29), the results suggest that the 76 amino acids span the membrane several times. Judging by its length, this region most likely transverses the membrane two to three times, resulting in a total of six to seven transmembrane regions. Outside of the carboxyl-terminal hydrophobic stretch of sequence in the IP$_3$ receptor that contains the putative transmembrane regions, the receptor is generally very hydrophilic. It exhibits a high percentage of charged amino acid residues (28%) that are evenly distributed over the entire protein (18).

Biochemical and immunocytochemical experiments demonstrate that the amino and carboxyl termini of the type I IP$_3$ receptor are cytoplasmic. Therefore, the receptor must have an even number of transmembrane regions (11, 18). In addition to the six to seven putative transmembrane regions described above, a hydrophobic sequence is observed in the primary structure of the IP$_3$ receptor that does not meet the criteria of Kyte and Doolittle owing to the high content of glycine. Glycine is now recognized to be a fairly hydrophobic amino acid frequently present in transmembrane regions, and a similar sequence in the ryanodine receptor has also been postulated to constitute a transmembrane region (30). On the whole, these considerations

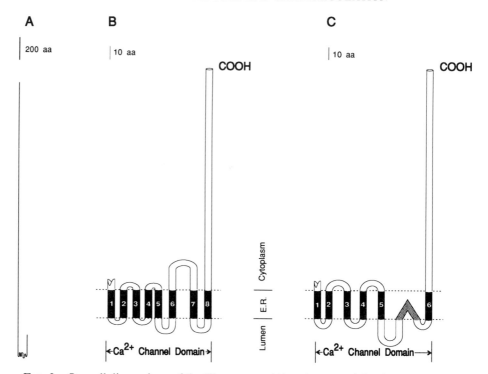

FIG. 2   Overall dimensions of the IP₃ receptor (A) and two models of transmembrane organization (B, C). In A, the IP₃ receptor is drawn to scale, illustrating the small part of the receptor occupied by the six to eight putative transmembrane regions. In B and C, two alternative models for the transmembrane organization of the IP₃ receptor are illustrated. Note the changes in scale between A and B, C as indicated above each diagram (aa, amino acids). The two models for the transmembrane orientation of the receptor differ in the number and location of the transmembrane regions. Model B proposes eight transmembrane regions, whereas model C proposes six transmembrane regions. In model C, we speculate that the relatively hydrophobic sequence that is hypothesized to constitute membrane-spanning region 7 in model B serves as a pore-forming loop analogous to the H-loops in K^+ channels (shown shaded in gray).

lead to two different models of transmembrane organization of the IP₃ receptor with either six or eight transmembrane regions (Fig. 2). In the model postulating eight transmembrane regions, the extended hydrophobic sequence would contain three membrane-spanning segments, and the glycine-rich sequence would also constitute a membrane-spanning region (Fig. 2B). In the model with six transmembrane regions, the extended hydrophobic sequence would contain only two transmembrane regions, and the glycine-rich sequence would be intraluminal in the endoplasmic reticulum (Fig. 2C).

The highest degree of sequence similarity between IP$_3$ receptors and ryanodine receptors is observed in the region of the glycine-rich hydrophobic sequence and the following transmembrane region. Above, we presented two alternative models postulating either six or eight transmembrane regions. In the model with six transmembrane regions (Fig. 2C), it is tempting to speculate that the hydrophobic glycine-rich sequence could represent a pore-forming sequence. The glycine-rich sequence would then be analogous to the H-loop in K$^+$ channels and presumably have a β-sheet structure (shown shaded in Fig. 2C). In this case the IP$_3$ receptor would be very similar to other ligand-gated ion channels, containing subunits with six transmembrane regions in a tetrameric configuration.

In most membrane proteins, positive charges flank the membrane-spanning sequences on the cytoplasmic side (31). This may relate to the presence of negatively charged phospholipids in the membranes and to the function of positively charged residues on the cytoplasmic side of membrane-spanning regions as stop–transfer sequences. Most of the putative transmembrane regions in the IP$_3$ receptor also contain cytoplasmic positively charged flanking residues. However, some of the putative transmembrane regions are flanked by negative charged instead of positively charged residues in a pattern that is also found in the ryanodine receptors (18). Negatively charged residues would be expected to line a calcium channel, suggesting that transmembrane regions containing negatively charged flanking residues may be part of the Ca^{2+} channel.

Multiple IP$_3$ receptors are expressed in many tissues, with the multiple receptor types being generated both by alternative splicing and by the expression of multiple genes. The type I IP$_3$ receptor is extensively alternatively spliced (18, 32). In addition, at least three different IP$_3$ receptor genes exist that are ubiquitously expressed (17). The presence of multiple receptors implies that intracellular calcium signaling may be complex and involve multiple pathways with different regulatory properties.

Two regions of alternative splicing of the type I receptor have been described. The initial cloning of the rat receptor demonstrated that there were two classes of cDNA clones that differed by the presence and absence of a 45-base pair (bp) sequence, suggesting that this sequence is differentially spliced (18). This was later confirmed by polymerase chain reaction (PCR) analysis of the mouse receptor (32). In addition, cloning and PCR experiments demonstrated that a sequence in the middle of the receptor exists in at least four forms in mouse and two forms in rat (Fig. 3). Although the significance of these alternative splicing events is currently unknown, their conservation between rat and mouse suggests that they may be functional.

A

```
                      311                                    350
                       ↓                                      ↓
Rat 1 SIa     GHYLAAEVDPDFEEECLEFQPSVDPDQDASRSRL RNAQEK
Mouse 1 SIa   GHYLAAEVDPDFEEECLEFQPSVDPDQDASRSRL RNAQEK
Rat 1 SIb     GHYLAAE[          ]VDPDQDASRSR LRNAQEK
Mouse 1 SIb   GHYLAAE[          ]VDPDQDASRSRLR NAQEK
Rat 2         GNYLAAELN PDYRDAQNEGKT VRDGEL PTSK–KKHQAGEK
Drosophila    GHYLAAEAE I DVSAGAKSA TSASGHD LHLGDCSKDSG LSC
```

B

```
                P                                                          P
                |                                                          |
              1586  1692                                        1733     1752
               ↓     ↓                                           ↓         ↓
Rat 1 SIIa    GYGEKQISIDELENAELPQPPEAENSTEQELEPSPPLRQLEDHKRGEALR
Mouse 1 SIIa  GYGEKQISIDESENAELPQAPEAENSTEQELEPSPPLRQLEDHKRGEALR
Rat 1 SIIb    GYGEKQISIDELENAELPQPPEAENSTE□ELEPSPPLRQLEDHKRGEALR
Mouse 1 SIIb  GYGEKQISIDESENAELPQAPEAENSTE□ELEPSPPLRQLEDHKRGEALR
Mouse 1 SIIc  GYGEKQISIDESENAELPQAPEAENSTE□[          ]GEALR
Mouse 1 SIId  GYGEK[          ]□□[          ]GEALR
Rat 1 SIId    GYGEK[          ]□□[          ]GEALR
Rat 2         SFMEE[                                 ]SSTLR
Drosophila    NYCEK[                                 ]GDALR
```

FIG. 3   Alternatively spliced sequences of the type I IP$_3$ receptor. The type I IP$_3$ receptor contains two known alternatively spliced sequences, one at an amino-terminal site (18) called S1 (shown in A) and a second in the middle of the protein called S2 (13) (shown in B). The differentially spliced sequences and their flanking regions are shown in single-letter code for the mouse and rat type I receptors, the rat type II receptor, and the *Drosophila* receptor. The different variants are referred to by lowercase letters following the splice site designation (e.g., SIb for the second variant of the first splice site). The spliced out sequences are indicated by open boxes. Residues that are identical in the majority of the sequences are shown on a shaded background, and the residue numbers corresponding to the rat type I receptor are indicated above the sequences. In B, the localization of the second alternatively spliced sequence between the two cAMP-dependent protein kinase phosphorylation sites is illustrated by indicating the positions of the phosphorylation sites.

At least three IP$_3$ receptor genes are expressed in multiple tissues, as determined by cDNA cloning and PCR experiments. We have determined the full-length structure of the rat type II IP$_3$ receptor from multiple overlapping cDNA clones from rat brain and a partial structure of the human type III receptor from human kidney (17). In addition, Ross *et al.* (26) reported partial structures for type II and type III receptors from human placenta. These investigators also described a partial clone encoding a receptor which they labeled type IV but which shares sequence identity with the type III receptor. The putative type IV receptor likely represents a splice variant of the type III receptor or a cloning artifact.

The sequences of the rat type I and type II receptors are 69% identical. Alignment of the sequences demonstrates that the sequence similarity extends over the entire length but shows a patchy distribution, with regions of identity separated by dissimilar sequence stretches. This is particularly evident in the hydrophobic amino acid sequence regions. The hydrophobicity plots for the two receptors are virtually identical. Some of the putative transmembrane regions are also highly conserved in sequence and not only in hydrophobicity. Conversely, other transmembrane regions show very little sequence similarity. In addition, many of the loops connecting transmembrane regions are poorly conserved. Similar patches of identical or divergent sequences are distributed across the entire sequence, indicating that the divergent sequences are either functionally irrelevant or specify properties which differ between the two types of receptors.

Northern blotting and PCR experiments have been performed to determine which tissues express which receptors. Surprisingly, all receptors were found to be expressed in all tissues (17; and T. C. Südhof, Y. A. Ushkaryov, C. L. Newton, and G. A. Mignery, unpublished observation, 1991). A distinct pattern of expression levels was observed, with the type I receptor, for example, being more than 1000 times higher in expression in cerebellar Purkinje cells than in the periphery, and the type III receptor showing higher levels in intestine and kidney than in any other tissues. On the whole, however, the expression data suggest that the receptor types are not simply isoforms with distinct, mutually exclusive tissue distributions, but rather that they also serve distinct functions.

Structure–Function Relationships of Inositol 1,4,5-Trisphosphate Receptors

The IP₃ receptors and the ryanodine receptors are surprisingly large proteins. They are larger than any other current described ligand-gated ion channel. The ryanodine receptor is regulated in a complex manner and also serves as a mechanical link between the sarcoplasmic reticulum and the plasma membrane in muscle, providing a potential explanation for its large size. However, the IP₃ receptor is known only to gate Ca^{2+} ions as a function of IP₃. There is no reason *a priori* why the IP₃ receptor has to be larger than other gated and modulated ion channels. This poses the challenge to delineate the

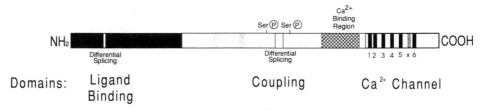

FIG. 4 Domain model of the IP$_3$ receptor illustrating the relative positions of the amino-terminal ligand-binding domain, the carboxyl-terminal Ca^{2+} channel domain, and the middle coupling domain in the receptor. The receptor is tetramerized via interactions in the Ca^{2+} channel domain, allowing the ligand-binding and the coupling domains to move freely (the "arms" of the receptor). The relative positions of the two differentially spliced sequences are indicated, as well as the region of Ca^{2+} binding. The coupling domain of the receptor constitutes the largest domain and contains potential modulatory sites for Ca^{2+} binding, phosphorylation, and possibly ATP binding. [Modified from Mignery and co-workers (17).]

sizes of the active domains of the IP$_3$ receptors and raises the question if the receptors might have additional, presently unanticipated functions.

The IP$_3$ receptor has four currently known functional properties that can be partially investigated using mutagenesis and protein expression: (1) ligand (IP$_3$) binding; (2) tetramerization; (3) IP$_3$-dependent Ca^{2+} channel gating; and (4) modulation of IP$_3$-dependent Ca^{2+} channel gating. Of the four properties, the first two are readily testable and are discussed below. Functional expression of IP$_3$ receptors whose Ca^{2+} gating could be investigated has not yet been possible, making it currently unfeasible to investigate the last two properties of IP$_3$ receptors. The reason for the inability to investigate Ca^{2+} gating at the present time is that all cells already contain a very efficient InsP$_3$-gated Ca^{2+} release pathway. This makes it impossible to use simple Ca^{2+} flux measurements in transfected cells. Future approaches to investigate these questions will have to utilize expressed receptor that must be studied as single molecules using sensitive electrophysiological techniques.

To investigate the domains of the IP$_3$ receptor responsible for ligand binding and receptor tetramerization, we have expressed receptor constructs by transfection in COS cells. Expressed receptors were then assayed for IP$_3$ binding and tetramerization, the former using radioligand binding assays and the latter using sucrose gradient centrifugation. The combined results of these studies led to a domain model of the IP$_3$ receptor (summarized in Fig. 4).

Our initial mutagenesis of expressed IP$_3$ receptors was guided by the cluster of hydrophobic sequences that is found close to the carboxyl terminus of the IP$_3$ receptors. Because the IP$_3$ receptor is an intrinsic membrane protein, these hydrophobic residues presumably represent transmembrane regions.

In addition, Furuichi *et al.* (28) had reported that deletion of the carboxyl terminus from the receptor abolished ligand binding, suggesting that transmembrane regions and ligand-binding domains for the receptor were colocalized in the carboxyl terminus of the receptor.

Our initial mutants were therefore designed to test the role of the putative transmembrane regions in IP$_3$ receptor function. For this purpose, the putative transmembrane regions were deleted. The membrane association, tetramerization, and ligand binding of the mutant protein were then investigated (33). As expected, a significant portion of the mutant-expressed protein lacking transmembrane regions was soluble, whereas none of several mutant proteins containing transmembrane regions was. Sucrose gradient centrifugations of the mutant soluble protein without the transmembrane regions demonstrated that it was a monomer. This suggested that the transmembrane regions not only insert the IP$_3$ receptor into the membrane but are also necessary for tetramerization (33).

This result agrees well with the hypothesis that the transmembrane regions of the IP$_3$ receptor form its intrinsic Ca^{2+} channel. The channel domain is multimeric in all currently known ligand-gated receptor channels. It would make most sense if the point at which the subunits are attached to each other is in the vicinity of the pore. Therefore, these results suggest that the hydrophobic regions of the IP$_3$ receptor form its channel and tetramerization domain.

IP$_3$ binding measurements on the mutant receptor demonstrate that it bound IP$_3$ with high affinity. This result proved that tetramerization is not required for ligand binding. Therefore, each subunit of the native IP$_3$ receptor tetramer must contain an independent ligand binding site. Needless to say, the ligand-binding and transmembrane regions must also be well separated.

To localize the IP$_3$ binding site within the receptor, further deletion mutants have been constructed. Successive carboxyl-terminal deletions demonstrated that only the amino-terminal 25% of the IP$_3$ receptor sequence is required for IP$_3$ binding (11). This result demonstrates that the ligand binding site of the IP$_3$ receptor is localized to its amino-terminal tip. Because the transmembrane regions are located in the carboxyl-terminal one-fourth of the protein, the putative Ca^{2+} channel domain of the receptor is separated from its ligand binding domain by more than 1500 amino acids. Although most of the studies have been carried out with type I IP$_3$ receptors, limited studies with the type II receptor reach similar results. This suggests that the different receptors have similar domain structures, as would be expected from the high degree of sequence identity.

Based on these results, we postulated the domain model of the IP$_3$ receptor shown in Fig. 4. In this model, three basic domains are present, an amino-terminal ligand-binding domain, a carboxyl-terminal Ca^{2+} channel domain,

InsP$_3$ cooperativity model (Meyer & Stryer)

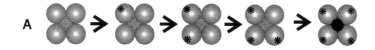

InsP$_3$ redundancy/subunit cooperativity model: single conductance state model

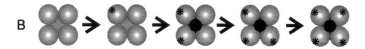

Noncooperative models with multiple conductance states

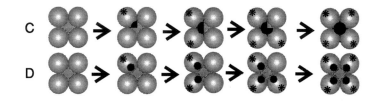

InsP$_3$ redundancy/subunit cooperativity model: multiple conductance states model

(Watras, Brezprozvanny & Ehrlich)

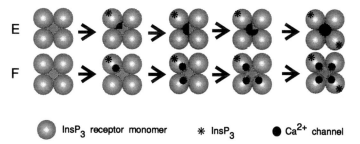

FIG. 5   Models of IP$_3$ receptor gating. In model A, the Ca^{2+} channels in the IP$_3$ receptor tetramers are thought to open only if all four independent ligand binding sites are occupied. This model predicts cooperatively of Ca^{2+} channel gating with respect to IP$_3$ and would allow only a single Ca^{2+} conductance state. In model B, occupation of a single binding site in the IP$_3$ receptor with IP$_3$ is thought to open the receptor, suggesting a noncooperative relationship between IP$_3$ binding and Ca^{2+} channel gating and a single conductance state for the receptor. We term this the IP$_3$ redundancy model because three of the four binding sites for IP$_3$ would be redundant in the receptor. Models C to F are models incorporating different Ca^{2+} conductance states that differ in the cooperativity properties and the manner in which different

and a connecting domain. The sequence connecting the ligand-binding and Ca^{2+} channel domains was called the coupling domain because it presumably serves to couple ligand binding to channel gating.

We initially posed the question of why IP$_3$ receptors are so large. Part of the answer is that the ligand-binding domain of the receptor, with more than 600 amino acids, is larger than most ligand-binding domains. The largest domain of the IP$_3$ receptors, however, is the coupling domain. This domain would be in an ideal position to serve as the target for modulatory signals on the IP$_3$ receptor that change the relation between ligand binding and channel gating. Several such signals have been described (see below). It is conceivable that this modulatory activity together with the transduction of the ligand-binding signal to the channel opening requires a very large protein domain. However, in view of the fact that other ligand-gated channels achieve the same result with much smaller sizes makes this highly unlikely and suggests, rather, that the coupling domain may have additional, currently unknown functions.

Another question that arises is why there should be multiple IP$_3$ receptor types. IP$_3$ binding measurements using the ligand-binding domains of the type I and type II receptors indicate that the type II receptor has a much higher affinity than the type I receptor (17). This suggests that different receptor types may respond to different IP$_3$ levels in the cell. However, this is probably only a partial answer because, of all domains, the ligand-binding domain is the most conserved between the receptors. The greater divergence in other domains between the receptors suggests that there may be additional functional differences, for example, in the channel gating and in the modulation of the signal.

Molecular Basis of Inositol 1,4,5-Trisphosphate Receptor Regulation

It is likely that the gating of Ca^{2+} release by IP$_3$ via the receptor is subject to multiple regulatory events. The most convincing type of regulation was

---

conductance states are generated. In the noncooperative models C and D, occupancy of each of the four binding sites in the receptor tetramer would open the Ca^{2+} channel incrementally, whereas in the subunit cooperativity models E and F occupation of a single binding site would already impart a certain probability on the receptor tetramer to open the receptor to multiple conductance states. Models C and E postulate that the multiple conductance states of the receptor are due to a single pore in the receptor that can assume different sizes, whereas models D and F suggest that each receptor subunit contains a separate pore (a rather unlikely but not impossible event in view of the limited number of transmembrane regions per receptor subunit).

shown to occur by Ca^{2+}. At low concentrations, Ca^{2+} is a necessary coagonist for Ca^{2+} release by IP_3, whereas at high concentrations Ca^{2+} blocks IP_3-triggered Ca^{2+} release (34). These results suggest that Ca^{2+} acts directly or indirectly on the receptor to modulate its response to IP_3.

One way in which Ca^{2+} could act is by regulating IP_3 binding to the receptor. Indeed, the initial studies on purification of the receptor demonstrated that Ca^{2+} inhibited IP_3 binding to the receptor in membranes. However, Ca^{2+} had no effect on the properties of the purified receptor (9, 35). These results led to the model that Ca^{2+} could act via a second protein named calmedin to selectively modulate IP_3 binding to the receptor (36). Although this idea is attractive, more recent experiments from our laboratory suggest that cerebellar membranes contain a very potent Ca^{2+}-activated phospholipase C (37). Apparently most if not all inhibition of the binding of radiolabeled ligand to IP_3 receptors in crude fractions that was previously observed is due to activation of phospholipase C. This activation produces unlabeled IP_3 which competes with the labeled ligand for binding, thereby creating the impression of inhibition. On the other hand, it is clear that Ca^{2+} has an effect on IP_3 receptor function. This effect most likely appears to be due to a direct effect. Indeed, Ca^{2+} binding measurements suggested that purified receptor binds Ca^{2+} (36), and the receptor seems to have at least one Ca^{2+} binding site in the coupling domain that is conserved between the type I and type II receptors (37).

In addition to being affected by Ca^{2+}, the receptor is functionally modulated by ATP (38). Micromolar concentrations of ATP enhance Ca^{2+} fluxes of reconstituted IP_3 receptors, and purified IP_3 receptors bind ATP specifically with a K_d of 17 μM (13). These studies demonstrate that ATP binds to the receptor and modulates it, although they do not clarify if this modulation has a functional role *in vivo*.

Finally, the IP_3 receptor is a prominent substrate for multiple protein kinases. The receptor was actually originally identified primarily as a prominent cerebellar substrate for cAMP-dependent protein kinase (39, 40). Later, *in vitro* studies using purified components demonstrated it to be a substrate for multiple protein kinases (41). The initial cloning of the rat receptor suggested that there are only two possible phosphorylation sites for cAMP-dependent protein kinases in the receptor structure (18), which were later shown to be utilized *in vitro* (41). Interestingly, these phosphorylation sites have been localized to the middle of the coupling domain and would therefore be in an ideal position to regulate Ca^{2+} gating as a function of IP_3. However, no effect of phosphorylation on receptor function has yet been demonstrated, making it currently impossible to determine if phosphorylation has a true regulatory role.

How Do Inositol 1,4,5-Trisphosphate Receptors Work?

The studies discussed above reveal that the IP$_3$ receptor is composed of a tetramer of four identical subunits, each of which contains an independent IP$_3$ binding site. How does IP$_3$ binding trigger Ca^{2+} channel opening? Several hypotheses have been proposed and are illustrated in Fig. 5. One model is that the release of Ca^{2+} by the receptor is cooperative, suggesting that occupancy of all four binding sites is required for channel gating. This hypothesis is supported by the cooperativity for gating observed in permeabilized rat basophilic leukemia cells (42). Another model postulates that each binding event opens the receptor incrementally, either in a cooperative manner or in a noncooperative manner. This model is supported by the measurements of IP$_3$-gated channel activity in planar lipid bilayers at different IP$_3$ concentrations and the observation of multiple subconductance states (43). The different models currently proposed appear to be mutually exclusive.

The structural studies allow some conclusions with regard to different models of IP$_3$ receptor function. First, the fact that the receptor is a tetramer with independent ligand binding sites but multimerized IP$_3$ channel domains suggests that any cooperativity between the subunits occurs at the level of the Ca^{2+} channel. Second, the presence of multiple receptors with different ligand affinities and probably also different regulatory properties indicates that the cell can respond to different levels of IP$_3$ in a different manner. This differential sensitivity to IP$_3$ could provide one explanation for the observed "quantel release" phenomenon described by Muallem *et al.* (44). Third, it is hard to envision four different conductance states in a transmembrane structure consisting at most of four times eight transmembrane regions, and more likely four times six transmembrane regions. Such a number of transmembrane regions resembles more closely those observed in voltage- and ligand-gated channels that exhibit only a single conductance state, suggesting that the multiple levels of conductance states observed could potentially have been due to interactions between receptors.

Acknowledgments

The work described in this chapter was supported by the National Institutes of Health (Grant RO1-MH47510). We thank our colleagues Christopher L. Newton and Ilya Bezprozvanny for valuable comments on the manuscript.

References

1. M. J. Berridge, *Annu. Rev. Biochem.* **56,** 159 (1987).
2. M. R. Hokin and L. E. Hokin, *J. Biol. Chem.* **203,** 967 (1953).

3. R. H. Michell, *Biochim. Biophys. Acta* **415,** 81 (1975).
4. H. Streb, R. F. Irvine, M. J. Berridge, and I. Schulz, *Nature (London)* **306,** 67 (1983).
5. P. W. Majerus, T. S. Ross, T. W. Cunningham, T. K. Caldwell, A. B. Jefferson, and V. S. Bansal, *Cell (Cambridge, Mass.)* **63,** 459 (1990).
6. M. J. Berridge, *JAMA, J. Am. Med. Assoc.* **262,** 1834 (1989).
7. M. J. Berridge, C. P. Downes, and M. R. Hanley, *Biochem J.* **206,** 587 (1982).
8. J. A. Maslanski, L. Leshko, and W. B. Busa, *Science* **256,** 243 (1992).
9. S. Suppattapone, P. F. Worley, J. M. Baraban, and S. H. Snyder, *J. Biol. Chem.* **263,** 1530 (1988).
10. S. R. Hingorani and W. S. Agnew, *in* ''Methods in Enzymology'' (B. Rudy and L. E. Iverson, eds.), Vol. 207, p. 573. Academic Press, San Diego, 1992.
11. G. A. Mignery, T. C. Südhof, K. Takei, and P. DeCamilli, *Nature (London)* **342,** 192 (1989).
12. C. C. Chadwick, A. Saito, and S. Fleischer, *Proc. Natl. Acad. Sci. U.S.A.* **87,** 2132 (1990).
13. N. Maeda, T. Kawasaki, S. Nakade, N. Yokota, and T. Taguchi, *J. Biol. Chem.* **266,** 1109 (1991).
14. T. Wagenknecht, R. Grassucci, J. Frank, A. Saito, M. Inui, and S. Fleischer, *Nature (London)* **338,** 167 (1989).
15. C. D. Ferris, R. Huganir, S. Supattapone, and S. H. Snyder, *Nature (London)* **342,** 87 (1989).
16. C. D. Ferris, A. M. Cameron, R. L. Huganir, and S. H. Snyder, *Nature (London)* **356,** 350 (1992).
17. T. C. Südhof, C. L. Newton, B. T. Archer III, Y. A. Ushkaryov, and G. A. Mignery, *EMBO J.* **10,** 3199 (1991).
18. G. A. Mignery, C. L. Newton, B. T. Archer, and T. C. Südhof, *J. Biol. Chem.* **265,** 12679 (1990).
19. H. Otsu, A. Yamamoto, N. Maeda, K. Mikoshiba, and Y. Tashiro, *Cell Struct. Funct.* **15,** 163 (1990).
20. C. A. Ross, J. Meldolesi, T. A. Milner, T. Satoh, and S. Supattapone, *Nature (London)* **339,** 468 (1989).
21. T. Satoh, C. A. Ross, A. Villa, S. Supattapone, and T. Pozzan, *J. Cell Biol.* **111,** 615 (1990).
22. P. D. Walton, J. A. Airey, J. L. Sutko, C. F. Beck, G. A. Mignery, T. C. Südhof, T. J. Deerinck, and M. H. Ellisman, *J. Cell Biol.* **113,** 1145 (1991).
23. K. Takei, H. Stukenbrok, A. Metcalk, G. A. Mignery, T. C. Südhof, P. Volpe, and P. De Cemilli, *J. Neurosci.* **12,** 489 (1992).
24. T. Furuichi, S. Yoshikawa, A. Miyawaki, K. Wada, N. Maeda, and K. Mikoshiba, *Nature (London)* **342,** 32 (1989).
25. S. Yoshikawa, T. Tanimura, A. Miyawaki, M. Nakamura, M. Yuzaki, T. Furuichi, and K. Mikoshiba, *J. Biol. Chem.* **257,** 16613 (1992).
26. C. A. Ross, S. K. Danoff, M. J. Schell, S. H. Snyder, and A. Ullrich, *Proc. Natl. Acad. Sci. U.S.A.* **89,** 4625 (1992).
27. S. Fleischer and M. Inui, *Annu. Rev. Biophys. Biophys. Chem.* **18,** 333 (1989).

28. J. Kyte and R. F. Doolittle, *J. Mol. Biol.* **157,** 105 (1992).
29. P. Klein, M. Kanehisa, and C. DeLisi, *Biochim. Biophys. Acta* **815,** 468 (1985).
30. F. Zorzato, J. Fujii, K. Otsu, M. Phillips, N. M. Green, F. A. Lai, G. Meissner, and D. H. MacLennan, *J. Biol. Chem.* **265,** 2244 (1990).
31. G. von Heijne and Y. Gavel, *Eur. J. Biochem.* **174,** 671 (1988).
32. T. Nakagawa, T. H. Okano, T. Furuichi, J. Aruga, and K. Mikoshiba, *Proc. Natl. Acad. Sci. U.S.A.* **88,** 6244 (1991).
33. G. A. Mignery and T. C. Südhof, *EMBO J.* **9,** 3893 (1990).
34. I. Bezprozvanny, J. Watras, and B. E. Ehrlich, *Nature (London)* **351,** 751 (1991).
35. P. F. Worley, J. M. Baraban, S. Supattapone, V. S. Wilson, and S. H. Snyder, *J. Biol. Chem.* **262,** 12132 (1987).
36. S. K. Danoff, S. Supattapone, and S. H. Snyder, *Biochem. J.* **245,** 701 (1988).
37. G. A. Mignery, P. A. Johnston, and T. C. Südhof, *J. Biol. Chem.* **267,** 7450 (1992).
38. C. D. Ferris, R. L. Huganir, and S. H. Snyder, *Proc. Natl. Acad. Sci. U.S.A.* **87,** 2147 (1990).
39. G. Weeks, M. Picciotto, A. C. Nairn, S. I. Walaas, and P. Greengard, *Synapse* **2,** 89 (1988).
40. H. Yamamoto, N. Maeda, M. Niinobe, E. Miyamoto, and K. Mikoshiba, *J. Neurochem.* **53,** 917 (1989).
41. C. D. Ferris, R. L. Huganir, D. S. Bredt, A. M. Cameron, and S. H. Snyder, *Proc. Natl. Acad. Sci. U.S.A.* **88,** 2232 (1991).
42. T. Meyer, T. Wensel, and L. Stryer, *Biochemistry* **29,** 32 (1990).
43. J. Watras, I. Bezprozvanny, and B. E. Ehrlich, *J. Neurosci.* **11,** 3239 (1991).
44. S. Muallem, S. J. Pandol, and T. G. Beeker, *J. Biol. Chem.* **164,** 205 (1989).

[23] Inositol 1,4,5-Trisphosphate Receptor Down-Regulation

Richard J. H. Wojcikiewicz and Stefan R. Nahorski

Introduction

Inositol 1,4,5-trisphosphate (IP$_3$) is formed during phosphoinositidase C-catalyzed phosphatidylinositol 4,5-bisphosphate hydrolysis in response to activation of certain cell surface receptors (1). The primary role of IP$_3$ appears to be to mobilize Ca^{2+} from intracellular stores (2). The precise nature of these stores, however, is presently unknown, although the sequestered Ca^{2+} is clearly intravesicular and nonmitochondrial and may be contained within an endoplasmic reticulum-like compartment (2–4). The cloning and sequencing of a gene encoding an IP$_3$ receptor in 1989 (5) confirmed previous indications that IP$_3$-induced Ca^{2+} mobilization was mediated by a specific receptor (2, 4). The existence of several IP$_3$ receptor subtypes has also been recognized (6) (see [22] in this volume), and studies are currently underway to define their location and roles in intracellular signaling.

In addition, we have begun to examine whether the IP$_3$ receptor concentration is regulated during cell stimulation. As a model system we have utilized a human neuroblastoma cell line (SH-SY5Y). These cells express muscarinic receptors (predominantly the M3 subtype) (7) that when activated stimulate phosphoinositide hydrolysis, and they also possess substantial IP$_3$-sensitive Ca^{2+} stores (8). Here we summarize the methods that we have used to study muscarinic agonist-induced IP$_3$ receptor regulation in this and other cell lines.

Quantification of Inositol 1,4,5-Trisphosphate-Induced Calcium Ion Mobilization in Control and Agonist-Pretreated Cells

Release of Intracellular Stores Labeled with ^{45}Ca^{2+}

The essential features of the procedure are permeabilizing the cell plasma membrane, loading of intracellular stores with ^{45}Ca^{2+}, and, following experimental incubations and ^{45}Ca^{2+} mobilization, effectively separating released ^{45}Ca^{2+} from that remaining in intracellular stores.

Methods in Neurosciences, Volume 18

Permeabilization

Permeabilization is required both to allow $^{45}Ca^{2+}$ unhindered access to the intracellular sites that mediate its sequestration and to allow IP_3, which is normally membrane-impermeant, into the cell. The method that we have used most frequently to permeabilize cells is electroporation. This is performed as follows, the volumes of buffer quoted being that per flask of cells. Medium from control or agonist-pretreated SH-SY5Y cells, cultured as monolayers in a 175-cm² flask (9), is removed and 20 ml of ice-cold 155 mM NaCl, 10 mM HEPES, pH 7.4 (HEPES-buffered saline, HBS) plus 0.02% EDTA is added. This causes cells to detach after several minutes. Cells are then centrifuged (500 g for 2 min at 4°C), resuspended in 20 ml ice-cold HBS, recentrifuged, resuspended in 5 ml ice-cold buffer A (120 mM KCl, 6 mM MgCl$_2$, 5 mM sodium succinate, 20 mM HEPES, 2 mM KH$_2$PO$_4$, 5 mM Na$_2$ATP, 5–10 μM EGTA, pH 7.0, pCa 7.3–7.0), centrifuged again, and finally resuspended in 0.8 ml ice-cold buffer A. Cells are then permeabilized with three discharges of a 3-μF capacitor with a field strength of 3.75 kV/cm and a time constant of approximately 0.1 msec (Gene Pulser, Bio-Rad, Richmond, CA), diluted to 4 ml with ice-cold buffer A, and centrifuged (500 g for 2 min at 4°C). At this point the cells are deemed to be permeable by a number of criteria, for example, the inability to exclude trypan blue or to retain [³H]inositol phosphates (9). We have employed other means to permeabilize cells that yield preparations with $^{45}Ca^{2+}$ release characteristics no different from those obtained with electrically permeabilized cells (see below). These include incubation with the detergents saponin, digitonin, and β-escin at approximately 0.1 mg/ml for 1 min. The remainder of this section, however, deals with experiments performed with electrically permeabilized cells.

Loading with $^{45}Ca^{2+}$

Pellets of permeabilized cells are resuspended in 0.8–1.2 ml buffer A (2.0–3.5 mg cell protein/ml) supplemented with 1.3–1.6 μCi $^{45}Ca^{2+}$/ml. This supplement is achieved using $^{45}CaCl_2$ (1000 Ci/mmol) and shifts the pCa to 6.4–6.2. Cells are then incubated for 15 min at 20°C to allow uptake of $^{45}Ca^{2+}$, which occurs via Ca^{2+}-ATPase(s) (3, 4) and is, therefore, dependent on the presence of ATP and Mg^{2+} in buffer A. For SH-SY5Y cells incubated under these conditions, uptake reaches equilibrium at approximately 10 min with a half-time of about 1 min and amounts to 1–2 nmol Ca^{2+}/mg protein.

Experimental Incubations and Assessment of $^{45}Ca^{2+}$ Release

Experimental incubations are conducted in two ways: at 20°C so as to monitor $^{45}Ca^{2+}$ mobilization under steady-state conditions and at 1–2°C in order to obtain a measure of unidirectional Ca^{2+} efflux. At 1–2°C, IP_3 is still fully capable of releasing Ca^{2+} stores but Ca^{2+}-ATPase is inactive.

$^{45}Ca^{2+}$ mobilization under steady-state conditions is initiated by addition of 50 μl of labeled cell suspension to 10 μl of buffer A plus stimuli (IP_3 or ionomycin) in 1.5-ml microcentrifuge tubes. Experimental incubations are for 2 min at 20°C, at which point $^{45}Ca^{2+}$ release is maximal and no significant reuptake, which parallels IP_3 metabolism, has occurred (10). Indeed, the initial reason for performing experiments at 20°C rather than at 37°C was to slow down IP_3 metabolism, which begins as soon as it is added to the cells (10). Incubations are terminated by addition of 0.25 ml silicone oil (Dow Corning, Midland, MI, 550/556, 9:11, v/v) and centrifugation (16,000 g for 3 min) to separate cells from buffer before assay of the radioactivity in the pellet. Release of $^{45}Ca^{2+}$ in the presence of stimuli is calculated from the amount remaining in the cell pellet, expressed as a percentage of that remaining after control incubations [80,000–150,000 disintegrations/min (dpm)/tube].

Data obtained using this protocol from control and carbachol-pretreated SH-SY5Y cells are shown in Fig. 1. In control cells, IP_3 releases maximally 65 ± 2% of $^{45}Ca^{2+}$ with EC_{50} = 0.32 ± 0.05 μM (mean ± SEM, n = 12). Pretreatment with carbachol for 3, 6, or 24 hr reduces significantly ($p \leq$ 0.01) maximal release to 49 ± 2, 36 ± 2, and 34 ± 3%, respectively ($n \geq 5$), and increases significantly ($p \leq 0.01$) EC_{50} values to 0.78 ± 0.18 , 1.17 ± 0.29, and 0.92 ± 0.13 μM, respectively ($n \geq 5$). In contrast, release caused by 10 μM ionomycin (84 ± 1% in control cells, n = 10) is unaltered by carbachol pretreatment (8). It is also important to note that neither the amount of protein per flask nor the characteristics of $^{45}Ca^{2+}$ uptake (in terms of rate and extent) are altered by pretreatment with carbachol (8). Thus, the effect of carbachol appears to be specific to the action of IP_3.

Data obtained using this procedure in another series of experiments on Chinese hamster ovary (CHO) cells transfected with human muscarinic M1, M2, and M3 receptor cDNA (11) and rat pituitary GH_3 cells that express thyrotropin-releasing hormone (TRH) receptors (12) are shown in Table I. Clearly, the efficacy and potency of IP_3 vary considerably in the different cell lines, and for muscarinic receptors, only persistent activation of those subtypes linked directly to activation of phosphoinositidase C (i.e., M1 and M3) (11) suppresses IP_3 action. The reason why TRH, which also stimulates phosphoinositidase C (12), is unable to suppress IP_3 action may be related to the fact that in control GH_3 cells IP_3 is only a relatively weak stimulus of $^{45}Ca^{2+}$ mobilization.

For measurement of unidirectional $^{45}Ca^{2+}$ efflux, incubations are initiated by addition of 50 μl labeled cell suspension to 350 μl ice-cold buffer A plus stimuli (the labeled permeabilized cells are cooled rapidly to 1–2°C by the excess of ice-cold buffer A). After 0.5–5 min on ice, incubations are termi-

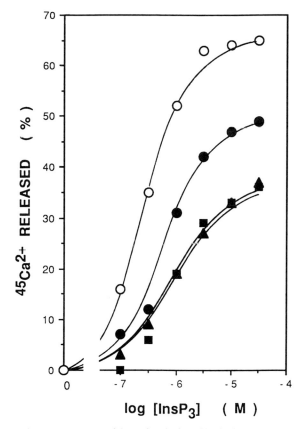

FIG. 1 Effects of pretreatment with carbachol on IP_3-induced mobilization of $^{45}Ca^{2+}$ in permeabilized SH-SY5Y cells incubated under steady-state conditions. Cells in culture were not pretreated (○) or were exposed to 2 mM carbachol for 3 hr (●), 6 hr (■), or 24 hr (▲). Cells were then permeabilized, incubated with $^{45}Ca^{2+}$ for 15 min at 20°C, and added to tubes containing IP_3, giving the final concentrations indicated. $^{45}Ca^{2+}$ released was then assessed after incubation for 2 min at 20°C. Data shown (means; $n \geq 5$; error bars omitted for clarity) are adapted with permission from Ref. 8.

nated by addition of 4.4 ml ice-cold buffer A without ATP, followed by immediate filtration through Whatman (Clifton, NJ) GF/B filters. The $^{45}Ca^{2+}$ content is calculated as a percentage of that retained after filtration of unincubated samples. Data obtained using this method are shown in Fig. 2. Incubation of control permeabilized cells at 1–2°C results in a gradual fall in $^{45}Ca^{2+}$ content (20 ± 3% in 5 min), reflecting gradual leakage from Ca^{2+} stores in a manner described by a single exponential function (4). In control cells, a maximal dose of IP_3 (10 μM) causes a rapid burst of $^{45}Ca^{2+}$ efflux, accounting for 71 ± 1% of that sequestered, which is complete by 0.5 min and which

TABLE I   Effects of Pretreatment with Agonist on Inositol
1,4,5-Trisphosphate-Induced $^{45}Ca^{2+}$ Mobilization[a]

	Released $^{45}Ca^{2+}$			
	Control		Agonist pretreated	
Cell line	Maximum release (%)	EC_{50} (μM)	Maximum release (%)	EC_{50} (μM)
SH-SY5Y ($n = 5$)	61 ± 1	0.25 ± 0.2	27 ± 3^b	1.21 ± 0.15^b
CHO-M1 ($n = 3$)	73 ± 3	0.10 ± 0.01	61 ± 1^b	0.27 ± 0.01^b
CHO-M2 ($n = 3$)	69 ± 2	0.11 ± 0.01	68 ± 2	0.11 ± 0.02
CHO-M3 ($n = 5$)	70 ± 2	0.14 ± 0.02	49 ± 5^b	0.28 ± 0.05^b
GH_3 ($n = 3$)	24 ± 1	1.01 ± 0.33	24 ± 3	1.09 ± 0.17

[a] Cells in culture either were not pretreated or were exposed for 20 hr to 1 mM carbachol or, in the case of
GH_3 cells, to 2 μM TRH. Cells were then permeabilized, and $^{45}Ca^{2+}$ mobilization was assessed as in Fig.
1. Data shown are means ± SEM.
[b] $p < 0.05$ as compared to control.

is followed by a return to gradual leakage (Fig. 2). In carbachol-pretreated
cells the rate of leakage is unchanged, but the extent to which IP_3 lowers
$^{45}Ca^{2+}$ content in the initial burst is reduced to $24 \pm 6\%$ (Fig. 2).

Calcium Ion Mobilization from Unlabeled Stores Measured with Ca²⁺-Sensitive Electrodes

As an alternative means of measuring modulation of IP_3-induced Ca^{2+}
release, the free Ca^{2+} concentration, $[Ca^{2+}_{free}]$, in permeabilized cell suspensions can be monitored directly with a Ca^{2+}-sensitive electrode. Cells are
pretreated and prepared for experiments exactly as for $^{45}Ca^{2+}$ mobilization
studies except that, in an attempt to reduce clumping of cells, buffer A
is supplemented with 0.1% (w/v) bovine serum albumin (buffer B) and
cells are permeabilized with 10 electrical discharges and are finally resuspended in buffer B without $^{45}Ca^{2+}$ (0.6 ml/flask of cells). The cells (4.0–4.8
mg cell protein/ml) are then stirred continuously at 20°C in a polypropylene
vial with the Ca^{2+}-sensitive membrane and reference electrode immersed
in the suspension. The principles of construction of the Ca^{2+}-sensitive
electrode have been described elsewhere (13) and are summarized in Fig.
3. The system is calibrated by adding small amounts of Ca^{2+} or EGTA
to buffer B and comparing changes in the absolute value of $[Ca^{2+}_{free}]$,
measured from the fluorescence of added quin 2 or Fura-2 (14), with
voltage changes between the Ca^{2+}-sensitive and reference electrodes. As

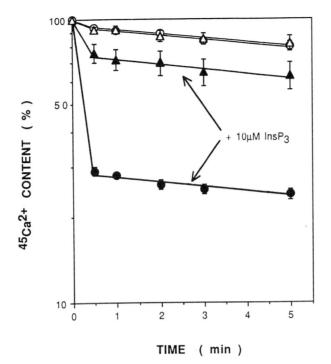

FIG. 2 IP$_3$-induced ^{45}Ca^{2+} efflux from permeabilized control or carbachol-pretreated SH-SY5Y cells. Cells in culture either were not pretreated (circles) or were exposed to 1 mM carbachol for 24 hr (triangles). Cells were then harvested, permeabilized, and incubated at 20°C with ^{45}Ca^{2+} for 15 min. Aliquots of cells were then added to tubes on ice containing an excess of buffer without ($\circ$, $\triangle$) or with ($\bullet$, $\blacktriangle$) IP$_3$ (10 μM, final concentration). The ^{45}Ca^{2+} content was then assessed at the times stated. Data shown (means $\pm$ SEM; $n = 3$) are adapted with permission from Ref. 8.

voltage is directly proportional to pCa ($-\log[Ca^{2+}_{free}]$) (13), this enables the changes in voltage seen during experiments with cell suspensions to be equated to changes in [Ca$^{2+}_{free}$]. [Ca$^{2+}_{free}$] reaches a steady-state level of 50–100 mM, 10–20 min after resuspension of cells (15). At this stage small volumes of IP$_3$ are added to obtain the final concentration stated.

Data obtained using this procedure with control and pretreated cells are shown in Fig. 4. In these experiments, responses to IP$_3$ are transient because of IP$_3$ metabolism and rapid Ca^{2+} resequestration (10, 15). Consistent with the data in Figs. 1 and 2, responses to IP$_3$ are reduced by pretreatment with carbachol, although as the dose of IP$_3$ used (1 μM) was submaximal (see

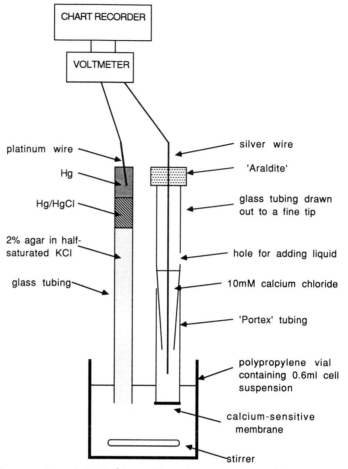

FIG. 3   Construction of the Ca^{2+}-sensitive electrode. The Ca^{2+}-sensitive membrane was made using reagents from Fluka (Ronkonkoma, NY) as follows. One milligram sodium tetraphenylborate (dissolved in ~5 μl tetrahydrofuran), 89 mg 2-nitrophenyl octyl ether, and 10 mg Ca^{2+} ionophore I (ETH 1001) were mixed together and added to 0.6 ml of a solution of 10% high molecular weight polyvinyl chloride in tetrahydrofuran. Five-centimeter lengths of Portex tubing (internal diameter 2 mm) were then dipped into the mixture such that approximately 15 μl is drawn into the tube (suction applied to the other end of the tube helped this process). After drying overnight, the tubing was filled with 10 mM $CaCl_2$ and was pushed onto a drawn-out glass pipette containing a silver wire. The reference electrode consists of a glass tube with a platinum wire sealed in one end, into which was packed sequentially Hg, Hg|HgCl, and 2% agar made up in half-saturated KCl. Screened cables were used to connect the electrode terminals to a voltmeter and chart recorder. The apparatus was set up in a Faraday cage, to which the screened cables, pH meter, and chart recorder were grounded. The reference electrode is stable for up to 3 months, whereas the Ca^{2+}-sensitive membrane is discarded every 2 weeks.

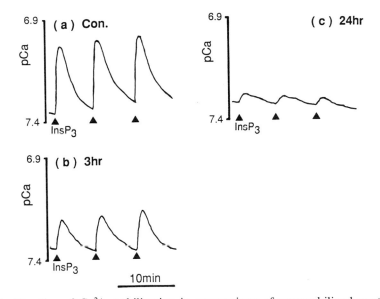

FIG. 4   Kinetics of Ca^{2+} mobilization in suspensions of permeabilized control or carbachol-pretreated SH-SY5Y cells. Cells in culture were not pretreated (a) or were exposed to 2 mM carbachol for 3 hr (b) or 24 hr (c). Cells were then harvested, permeabilized, and assayed for Ca^{2+} release at 20°C with a Ca^{2+}-sensitive electrode. Additions of IP_3 (final concentration of 1 μM) were made at the points indicated by arrowheads. Data shown are representative of at least 3 independent experiments with similar results and are adapted with permission from Ref. 8.

Fig. 1), the responses to IP_3 in Fig. 4 are suppressed more strongly by a combination of decreased potency and maximal effect.

Comments on Quantification of Calcium Ion Mobilization

During measurement of IP_3-induced Ca^{2+} mobilization it is very important to monitor and control $[Ca^{2+}_{free}]$ in buffers A and B used to prepare and incubate the permeabilized cells, as both the potency and efficacy of IP_3 are influenced by changes in $[Ca^{2+}_{free}]$ (4). $[Ca^{2+}_{free}]$ is most accurately and conveniently measured using the fluorescent Ca^{2+} indicators quin 2 or Fura-2 (14). We have found that $^{45}Ca^{2+}$ mobilization can be measured successfully when the pCa of buffer A is 7.3–7.0 and that addition of $^{45}CaCl_2$ causes a shift to pCa 6.4–6.2. We find that these concentrations can be attained by including 5–10 μM EGTA in buffer A, although depending on water quality and reagent purity more or less EGTA may be required. Indeed, in experiments with the Ca^{2+}-sensitive electrode it was often beneficial (in terms of optimizing the size of responses to IP_3) to omit EGTA from buffer B and to allow the cells to sequester the excess Ca^{2+}. It should also be noted that measurement of $^{45}Ca^{2+}$ release and changes in $[Ca^{2+}_{free}]$ with the electrode are good quantitative methods, but they do not provide an absolute measure of the rate of IP_3-induced Ca^{2+} mobilization, which stopped-flow experiments have shown to occur with a half-time of less than 1 sec (4).

Quantification of Inositol 1,4,5-Trisphosphate Receptor Concentration

Binding of Inositol 1,4,5-Trisphosphate to Membrane Preparations

The procedure is based on previously described methods (16) and relies on the use of $[^{32}P]IP_3$ to identify IP_3 binding sites in crude SH-SY5Y cell membrane preparations. In the studies described, high specific activity $[4,5-^{32}P]IP_3$ (100–155 Ci/mmol) is used to maximize the accuracy of the assay. In additional experiments, however, acceptable data are obtained using $[^3H]IP_3$ with lower specific activity (17–20 Ci/mmol).

Membrane Preparation

After removal of culture medium, control or pretreated SH-SY5Y cells are washed once with HBS, are detached with ice-cold HBS plus 0.02% EDTA, and are centrifuged (1800 g for 3 min at 4°C). Cell pellets are then resuspended in ice-cold 20 mM $NaHCO_3$, 1 mM dithiothreitol, pH 8.0 (buffer C), are disrupted (Ultra Turax homogenizer, maximum speed for 10 sec), and are centrifuged (1800 g for 10 min at 4°C). The supernatant is then collected, and the pellet is rehomogenized in ice-cold buffer C and recentrifuged (1800 g for 10 min at 4°C). The two supernatant fractions are combined and centrifuged at 38,000 g for 10 min at 4°C. The pellet is then rehomogenized in ice-cold buffer C, recentrifuged (38,000 g for 10 min at 4°C), and finally resuspended in buffer C.

Incubations

Membranes (150–360 μg/tube) are incubated in 200 μl for 45 min at 4°C with $[^{32}P]IP_3$ (~0.5 nM, 12,000 dpm/tube), a range of concentrations of nonradioactive IP_3 (1 nM–10 μM) to displace the radioligand and 5 mM $NaHCO_3$, 0.25 mM dithiothreitol, 25 mM Tris-HCl, 1 mM EDTA, pH 8.0. High-performance liquid chromatography (HPLC) of samples at the end of incubations with membranes from control or carbachol-pretreated cells revealed that less than

0.5% of IP_3 is metabolized. Bound and free ligand are separated by rapid filtration of incubation mixtures diluted with 4.3 ml of ice-cold 5 mM NaHCO$_3$, 25 mM Tris-HCl, 1 mM EDTA, pH 7.8, through Whatman GF/B filters, followed by a wash of filters with 4.3 ml of the same buffer. Using this protocol approximately 4% of [^{32}P]IP$_3$ is bound, about 20% of which is nonspecific (defined with 10 μM IP$_3$). It should be noted that filtration and washing take approximately 6 sec, during which time some [^{32}P]IP$_3$ will dissociate from its receptor (16, 17). To assess this dissociation, bound and free ligand are also separated by centrifugation (16,000 g for 5 min at 4°C) followed by rapid removal of supernatant. More binding is obtained with this method (~7%), but a much higher proportion of this is nonspecific (~55%). Specific binding after filtration is 85 $\pm$ 11% ($n = 3$) of that after centrifugation, indicating that the amount of ligand dissociation during filtration is insignificant.

[^{32}P]IP$_3$ bound to membranes from untreated SH-SY5Y cells is displaced by coincubation with nonradioactive IP$_3$, yielding K_d and B_{max} values of 64 $\pm$ 7 nM and 2.0 $\pm$ 0.1 pmol/mg protein, respectively (means $\pm$ SEM, $n = 4$). Thus, this site exhibits similar binding affinity to the well-characterized receptor in cerebellum but is present at a lower density (4, 17). Pretreatment with 1 mM carbachol for 24 hr did not alter the affinity of IP$_3$ ($K_d = 57 \pm 3$ nM) but reduced significantly ($p < 0.01$) the abundance of binding sites ($B_{max} = 1.0 \pm 0.1$ pmol/mg protein). Heterogeneity of IP$_3$ binding is not apparent, as the slopes of binding curves in both control and carbachol-pretreated cells are close to unity (1.0–1.1). Thus, as the only carbachol-induced modification to binding is a reduction in B_{max}, it appears that a simple decrease in IP$_3$ receptor concentration may have occurred. This decrease is half-maximal and maximal at approximately 3 and 6 hr, respectively, is mimicked by muscarine, and is blocked by atropine (8). Thus, muscarinic receptors mediate the inhibitory effects of carbachol, and both the extent and the time course of the decrease in IP$_3$ binding correlate well with the decrease in IP$_3$-induced Ca^{2+} mobilization seen in Fig. 1.

Inositol 1,4,5-Trisphosphate Receptor Immunoreactivity in Membrane Preparations

Although it seems likely that the reduction in B_{max} reflects a genuine decrease in IP$_3$ receptor concentration, it cannot be ignored that modification of the receptor, perhaps at the IP$_3$ binding site, could have a similar effect. This can be clarified by monitoring changes in IP$_3$ receptor concentration immunochemically, using a monoclonal antibody (MAb18A10) raised against the C terminus of mouse cerebellum IP$_3$ receptor (5).

Membrane Preparation

SH-SY5Y cells are pretreated, harvested, and centrifuged as in binding experiments. Pellets of cells or freshly excised mouse cerebella are resuspended in homogenization buffer (ice-cold 10 mM Tris, 1 mM EGTA, 0.1 mM phenylmethylsulfonyl fluoride, 1 mM dithiothreitol, 10 mM leupeptin, 10 mM pepstatin, pH 7.4), are disrupted (Ultra Turrax homogenizer, maximum speed for 12 sec), and are centrifuged (500 g for 10 min at 4°C). The supernatant is then centrifuged (38,000 g for 10 min at 4°C), and the pellet obtained is rehomogenized, centrifuged again, and finally resuspended in homogenization buffer.

Assay of Immunoreactivity

MAb18A10 was raised against a mouse IP$_3$ receptor as described (5). Its epitope is known to be within a 12-residue region very close to the C terminus (18) and should interact with human receptors, as the predicted amino acid sequence of the human (cerebellum) protein is very similar to that of the mouse (19). Western blotting is performed in the standard manner (20); samples of membrane preparations are subjected to electrophoresis in 7% (w/v) polyacrylamide gels, and proteins are transferred to nitrocellulose, which is then incubated sequentially with MAb18A10 (at a dilution of ~1 : 11 or ~1 : 2000 for crude culture medium and purified antibody, respectively), alkaline phosphatase-conjugated goat anti-rat antibody (at a dilution of ~1 : 300), and the color development reagents p-nitro blue tetrazolium chloride and 5-bromo-4-chloro-3-indolyl phosphate p-toluene salt (Bio-Rad). As the intensity of immunoreactive bands in SH-SY5Y cell preparations is relatively low and well below saturation, changes in band intensity are taken to parallel approximately changes in the concentration of immunoreactive protein (19).

As shown in Fig. 5 (lane 1) MAb18A10 recognizes a protein in 4 μg of a mouse cerebellum preparation with an apparent molecular mass of approximately 275 kDa. This is thought to correspond to the IP$_3$ receptor gene product, which has a predicted molecular mass of 313 kDa (5). Identical analysis of 40 μg of a SH-SY5Y cell preparation reveals a band of similar intensity at approximately 275 kDa that we assume corresponds to the SH-SY5Y cell IP$_3$ receptor (Fig. 5, lane 2). Weak staining of up to three additional bands at 260–220 kDa is also evident in some SH-SY5Y cell and cerebellum preparations. The origin of the minor bands is unclear, but they may reflect either limited proteolysis of the receptor during preparation or perhaps are the products of the splice variants known to occur in mouse and man (4). Of the other immunoreactivity evident in SH-SY5Y cells, only the minor band at approximately 85 kDa is recognized specifically by MAb18A10; the staining at approximately 50 kDa and at the dye front is apparent in control analyses without MAb18A10 (data not shown).

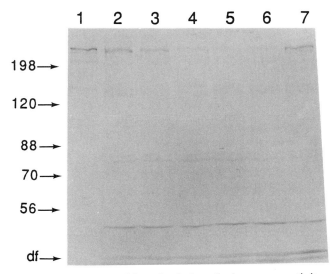

Fig. 5   Effects of pretreatment with carbachol on the immunoreactivity of SH-SY5Y cell particulate preparations. Samples of control or pretreated SH-SY5Y cells (~40 μg, lanes 2–7) or mouse cerebellum (4 μg, lane 1) were analyzed by Western blotting using MAb18A10. The positions of prestained molecular mass markers (198–56 kDa) and the dye front (df) are indicated by arrowheads. SH-SY5Y cells either were not pretreated (lane 2) or were pretreated with 0.1 mM carbachol for 1 hr (lane 3), 3 hr (lane 4), 6 hr (lane 5), or 24 hr (lane 6) or with 0.1 mM carbachol for 6 hr followed by 0.1 mM carbachol plus 10 μM atropine for a further 24 hr (lane 7).

Pretreatment of SH-SY5Y cells in culture with carbachol reduces the intensity of the band at approximately 275 kDa (Fig. 5, lanes 2–6). This reduction is maximal at 6 hr; based on visual estimates the reduction is 80–90% in all experiments and is not accompanied by a detectable change in intensity of the unknown band at approximately 85 kDa or elsewhere (Fig. 5, lanes 2–6). Recovery of immunoreactivity is evident when cells that have been incubated with carbachol for 6 hr are incubated for a further 24 hr in the presence of atropine (Fig. 5, lane 7).

Thus, chronic activation of muscarinic receptors suppresses IP_3 receptor immunoreactivity in SH-SY5Y cells, providing direct evidence that IP_3 receptor concentration can be modified by cell-surface receptor activation. These data are consistent with the findings that carbachol reduces the B_{max} of IP_3 binding sites (see above) and suppresses the Ca^{2+} mobilizing activity of IP_3 (Figs. 1, 2, and 4). As MAb18A10 recognizes an epitope within 14 residues of the C terminus of mouse IP_3 receptor (18) and the IP_3 binding site is located close to the N terminus (4), the finding that the decrease in immunoreactivity (19) concurs in terms of extent and time course with suppression of

IP$_3$ binding (8) provides strong evidence that the entire IP$_3$ receptor protein is present at a reduced concentration in carbachol-pretreated cells.

Comments on Quantification of Inositol 1,4,5-Trisphosphate Receptor Concentration

As compared to levels in cerebellum, the IP$_3$ receptor concentration in cell lines such as SH-SY5Y is relatively low (4, 8, 17). Therefore, great care must be taken, particularly during Western blotting, to follow accurately the described procedures (20). An additional point to consider is that measurement of immunoreactivity without comparison to standards is not quantitative and provides only an estimate of IP$_3$ receptor concentration. This may explain why the carbachol-induced decrease in immunoreactivity was apparently greater than the reduction in B_{max}. Alternatively, the abundance of sites with which the antibody can interact may have genuinely been reduced to a greater extent than the number of IP$_3$ binding sites. This could be due to either minor proteolytic clipping of the polypeptide at the C terminus (which is unlikely to alter IP$_3$ binding), in addition to the genuine decrease in receptor concentration, or the presence of IP$_3$ receptor subtypes in SH-SY5Y cells that are not recognized by MAb18A10.

Conclusions

The techniques described have enabled us to establish that stimulation of cell surface muscarinic receptors can down-regulate the (an?) IP$_3$ receptor in SH-SY5Y cells and, therefore, suppress the action of IP$_3$. This effect is mediated by muscarinic receptors that are linked directly to phosphoinositidase C. It will be fascinating in future studies to determine the basis of the down-regulation, by analyzing IP$_3$ receptor mRNA levels and/or the rate of IP$_3$ receptor turnover, and to establish whether different IP$_3$ receptor subtypes are regulated differently.

Acknowledgment

The work described from our laboratory was supported by the Wellcome Trust.

References

1. M. J. Berridge, *Annu. Rev. Biochem.* **56,** 159 (1987).
2. M. J. Berridge and R. F. Irvine, *Nature (London)* **341,** 197 (1989).

3. J. Meldolesi, L. Madeddu, and T. Pozzan, *Biochim. Biophys. Acta* **1055,** 130 (1990).
4. C. W. Taylor and A. Richardson, *Pharmacol. Ther.* **51,** 97 (1991).
5. T. Furuichi, S. Yoshikawa, A. Miyawaki, K. Wada, N. Maeda, and K. Mikoshiba, *Nature (London)* **342,** 32 (1989).
6. J. Meldolesi, *Curr. Biol.* **2,** 393 (1992).
7. S. J. Wall, R. P. Yasuda, M. Li, and B. B. Wolfe, *Mol. Pharmacol.* **40,** 783 (1991).
8. R. J. H. Wojcikiewicz and S. R. Nahorski, *J. Biol. Chem.* **266,** 22234 (1991).
9. R. J. H. Wojcikiewicz, D. G. Lambert, and S. R. Nahorski, *J. Neurochem.* **54,** 676 (1990).
10. S. T. Safrany, R. J. H. Wojcikiewicz, J. Strupish, J. McBain, A. M. Cooke, B. V. L. Potter, and S. R. Nahorski, *Mol. Pharmacol.* **39,** 754 (1991).
11. E. C. Hulme, N. J. M. Birdsall, and N. J. Buckley, *Annu. Rev. Pharmacol. Toxicol.* **30,** 633 (1990).
12. M. C. Gershengorn, *Annu. Rev. Physiol.* **48,** 515 (1986).
13. E. Sigel and H. Affolter, *in* "Methods in Enzymology" (P. M. Conn and A. R. Means, eds.), Vol. 141, p. 25. Academic Press, Orlando, Florida, 1987.
14. G. Grynkiewicz, M. Poenie, and R. Y. Tsien, *J. Biol. Chem.* **260,** 3440 (1985).
15. R. J. H. Wojcikiewicz, S. T. Safrany, R. A. J. Challiss, J. Strupish, and S. R. Nahorski, *Biochem. J.* **272,** 269 (1990).
16. R. A. J. Challiss, E. R. Chilvers, A. L. Willcocks, and S. R. Nahorski, *Biochem. J.* **265,** 421 (1990).
17. M. A. Varney, J. Rivera, A. Lopez Bernal, and S. P. Watson, *Biochem. J.* **269,** 211 (1990).
18. S. Nakade, N. Maeda, and K. Mikoshiba, *Biochem. J.* **277,** 125 (1991).
19. R. J. H. Wojcikiewicz, S. Nakade, K. Mikoshiba, and S. R. Nahorski, *J. Neurochem.* **59,** 383 (1992).
20. J. Sambrook, E. F. Fritsch, and T. Maniatis, "Molecular Cloning: A Laboratory Manual," 2nd Ed. Cold Spring Harbor Laboratory, Cold Spring Harbor, New York, 1989.

[24] High-Affinity Inositol 1,3,4,5-Tetrakisphosphate Receptor from Cerebellum

Georg Reiser

Introduction

Numerous neurotransmitter and growth factor receptors are coupled to phospholipase C enzymes that involve several inositol phosphates in intracellular responses (1). So far only for $Ins(1,4,5)P_3$ (D-*myo*-inositol 1,4,5-trisphosphate; IP_3) has the physiological role been clearly established by purifying (2) and functionally reconstituting the high-affinity IP_3 receptor (3). The IP_3 receptor comprises both the IP_3 binding site and an associated Ca^{2+} channel, enabling IP_3 to induce Ca^{2+} release from internal stores (4, 5).

D-*myo*-Inositol 1,3,4,5-tetrakisphosphate [$Ins(1,3,4,5)P_4$; IP_4] is formed by selective phosphorylation of IP_3 via an IP_3 3-kinase (6; see also [26] this volume). IP_4 may also take part in intracellular Ca^{2+} regulation and appears to augment IP_3-induced Ca^{2+} mobilization in mouse lacrimal acinar cells (7). Ca^{2+} release from cerebellar microsomes has been found to be triggered by IP_3 (8) and also by IP_4 (9). Physiological and biochemical experiments indicate that IP_4 might act in concert with IP_3 (7, 10). However, the actual function of IP_4 has yet to be identified. This should be possible to achieve after isolation and identification of the IP_4 receptor.

A membrane preparation from pig cerebellum contains IP_4 receptor sites that display a high selectivity for $Ins(1,3,4,5)P_4$ among several inositol phosphates tested (11). We have previously demonstrated that this binding protein preparation can be used for quantifying cellular IP_4 by a radioreceptor assay (11–13, see also [21], this volume). Subsequently we have solubilized the membrane-bound IP_4 receptor from pig cerebellum, enriched the receptor protein by heparin-agarose chromatography, and separated the IP_4 receptor from the IP_3 binding activity (14). The IP_4 receptor protein contained in the solubilized sample has been characterized biochemically (15) and identified functionally by photoaffinity labeling (16). Theibert *et al.* (17) have employed a different procedure to solubilize an IP_4-binding protein from rat cerebellum. Furthermore, they have separated the IP_4 binding activity from the IP_3 recep-

Methods in Neurosciences, Volume 18

tor and the enzymes IP_3 5-phosphatase and IP_3 3-kinase (17) and have identified several distinct proteins (18). Here methods for preparing membranes containing a high-affinity IP_4 receptor and for solubilization, purification, and functional identification of the IP_4 receptor are described.

Buffers

Test buffer (used for assaying IP_4 binding activity): Sodium acetate 100 mM, pH 5.0, KH_2PO_4/K_2HPO_4 100 mM, pH 5.0, EDTA 4 mM, and Brij 58 0.2% (w/v); the pH of both the acetate and the phosphate buffer is adjusted separately before mixing

Homogenization buffer: Tris-HCl 50 mM, pH 7.7, EDTA 1 mM, mercaptoethanol 1 mM

Solubilization buffer: Tris-HCl 50 mM, pH 7.5, EDTA 1 mM, mercaptoethanol 5 mM, NaCl 400 mM, Brij 58 1.5% (w/v)

Tris buffer: Tris-HCl 50 mM, pH 7.5, EDTA 1 mM, mercaptoethanol 1 mM, Brij 58 0.1% (w/v)

Phosphate buffer: KH_2PO_4/K_2HPO_4 25 mM, pH 7.5, EDTA 1 mM, mercaptoethanol 1 mM, Brij 58 0.1% (w/v)

Protease inhibitors: In some experiments the homogenization buffer, solubilization buffer, and Tris buffer employed for isolation of membranes and receptor have been supplemented with the following protease inhibitors: phenylmethanesulfonyl fluoride (100 μM), leupeptin (10 μM), and chymostatin (10 μM)

Assay of Inositol 1,3,4,5-Tetrakisphosphate Binding Activity

A quantitative estimate of the amount of IP_4 receptor present in the diverse fractions obtained after solubilization and chromatographic isolation of the receptor is obtained by determining the specific IP_4 binding activity. Specific IP_4 binding activity is defined as the difference between total binding (B_0) of a nanomolar concentration of [^{3}H]IP_4 and the nonspecific binding (NSB), which corresponds to the amount of [^{3}H]IP_4 bound in the presence of a micromolar concentration of nonradioactive IP_4. It should be emphasized that specific binding activity does not give the number of binding sites (B_{max}), which is calculated from Scatchard analysis.

Protocol

Step 1: Test Incubation

For the test incubation the following components are mixed in Eppendorf vials kept on ice.

> 70 μl test buffer
> 60 μl [^{3}H]IP$_4$, around 3000 disintegrations/min (dpm), as tracer
> 25 μl water (or agents whose effect on binding activity is tested)
> 50 μl of (a) water for total binding (B_0)
>   or (b) IP$_4$ (2.8 μM) for nonspecific binding (NSB)
>   or (c) IP$_4$ (4.5–280 nM) in water for Scatchard analysis

Step 2: Start of Binding Reaction

The reaction is started by adding 75 μl of protein sample. The resulting total assay volume of 280 μl contains between 1 and 400 μg protein, the tracer [^{3}H]IP$_4$ (0.5–1.0 nM) with a high specific activity (0.8–1.3 TBq/mmol, Amersham, Braunschweiger, Germany, UK, TRK 998), and the detergent Brij 58 [0.4% (w/v) in the solubilized sample and 0.08% (w/v) in all other samples]. The vials are incubated for 20 min to reach equilibrium of binding (11).

Step 3: Stop of Incubation by Spun Column Chromatography

The incubation is stopped by separating bound ligand from free ligand by gel filtration using spun column chromatography at 4°C (19).

(a) Gel columns are prepared before the test. BioGel P-4 (200–400 mesh, 65 μm, Bio-Rad, Richmond, CA) is swollen at a ratio of 1 g per 10 ml gel buffer [Tris-HCl 25 mM, pH 7.5, NaN$_3$ 0.02% (w/v)] and degassed. Columns made from 2-ml plastic syringes with nylon nets attached to the bottom are filled with 3 ml of the gel slurry.

(b) Conditioning of gel columns is carried out conveniently during test incubation (see Step 2 above). First, columns are put into 10-ml plastic tubes (inner diameter 14 mm) which fit into adaptors (Centrilab, No. 5322) of the Varifuge 3.2 (Heraeus, Osterode, Germany) and are centrifuged (2 min, 3500 g). Then the columns with a packed volume of 1 ml are equilibrated with 1 ml of test buffer, which is diluted 1:4 with water, and centrifuged (2 min, 3500 g). The flow-through is collected in the plastic tubes.

(c) For separation of bound and free ligand, the columns are transferred into centrifuge adaptors (Centrilab, No. 5322) that have been equipped with 5-ml scintillation vials, which permit one to collect the flow-through of the columns. From the total incubation volume of 280 μl (see Step 2 above), an aliquot of 250 μl is applied to the columns, which are then centrifuged immediately. The void volume containing the proteins and the tracer bound to protein is retained in the scintillation vial. The amount of bound [³H]IP₄ is determined in a scintillation counter after adding 2 ml scintillation liquid (Ultima gold, Packard, Meriden, CT).

(d) Used BioGel P-4 from several assays is collected (0.5 liter) into a column (~5 × 35 cm) and reconditioned by adding 2 liters of regeneration buffer [Tris-HCl 50 mM, pH 7.5, 0.2% (w/v) sodium dodecyl sulfate (SDS)] for washing and subsequently 1 liter of methanol (50% in water). Thus the radioactive tracer is eluted from the BioGel in the first 0.5–1 liter of the regeneration buffer. Then the BioGel is transferred into 2 liters water, reswollen overnight, washed several times with water, and finally washed with gel buffer (20).

The gel-filtration chromatography with spun columns (19, 20) allows quick and reproducible testing of a large number of samples. Alternatively, precipitation with polyethylene glycol can be used to measure binding of IP₄ in fractions with proteins solubilized by detergents (17, 21). After the binding incubation period polyethylene glycol and the carrier protein bovine γ-globulin are added, the sample is further incubated for 10 min, and the receptor–ligand complex is precipitated by centrifugation. Receptor-bound radioactivity is contained in the pellets and can thus be determined after aspirating the supernatant. However, this method might overestimate the nonspecific binding owing to radioactive tracer trapped in the pellet. Ion-exchange chromatography with Dowex AG 1-X2 resin has been used to quantify detergent-solubilized Ins(1,4,5)P₃ receptor in a spun column setup (22) similar to the one described above. This test system, which is allegedly more sensitive than a gel filtration assay, is also applicable for [³H]IP₄ binding studies.

Membrane Preparation

From a local abattoir cerebella are freshly collected, kept on ice, dissected free from meninges and white matter material, and homogenized using a Waring blendor 34BL 22 (3 times 20 sec, medium setting) in 4 volumes homogenization buffer per wet weight of tissue. This step and the following ones are carried out at 4°C.

The homogenate is centrifuged (35,000 g, 30 min, rotor A6.14) in a Centrikon H 401 centrifuge (Kontron, Eching, Germany). The pellet without the greyish bottom is resuspended in the same volume of buffer used before. For this step, however, the buffer is supplemented with 0.4 M NaCl to extract membrane-associated proteins. After homogenization (3 times 15 sec, medium setting) and centrifugation (see above) the pelleted membranes are washed two more times in homogenization buffer and again centrifuged. The membranes are resuspended in homogenization buffer (1 ml/g cerebellar tissue employed originally for the membrane preparation) at a concentration of 20–30 mg of protein/ml, then are homogenized in a glass Potter–Elvejhem homogenizer with 5 strokes and stored at −20°C in aliquots suitable for receptor binding tests (11–13) or for receptor solubilization.

Receptor Solubilization

Frozen membranes are slowly thawed at 10–15°C, mixed with an approximately equal volume of homogenization buffer, and centrifuged (10 min, 27,000 g, rotor A8.24, Centrikon H 401 centrifuge). The pellet is supplemented with 4 ml solubilization buffer per gram wet weight of membranes and gently stirred for 1 hr at 4°C. During this period the homogenate is sonicated twice (30 sec, sonifier B30 (Branson, Danbury, CT) using an emitter tip of 18 mm diameter, medium setting of 45 W, pulse mode at 50% duty cycle) and then centrifuged (60 min, 100,000 g, rotor TST 28.38) in an ultracentrifuge (Centrikon T2060, Kontron). The supernatant is collected by decanting and is dialyzed overnight in 2 × 2 liters Tris buffer without Brij 58, but with the concentration of mercaptoethanol increased to 5 mM, with one change of dialysis buffer. Owing to the low critical micellar concentration of Brij 58 (~50 μM, Ref. 23) the detergent is not dialyzed and can therefore be omitted from all dialysis buffers used.

The high-affinity IP$_4$ receptor found in pig cerebellar membranes (11) can be solubilized by treatment with the nonionic detergent Brij 58 at concentrations above 1%. The protein responsible for high-affinity IP$_4$ binding seems to be an integral membrane protein because only high concentrations of the detergent allow solubilization and the yield of the solubilized receptor is increased by addition of 0.4 M NaCl.

Purification of Inositol 1,3,4,5-Tetrakisphosphate Receptor

The chromatography employed for purifying the IP$_4$ receptor is displayed in Fig. 1. The IP$_4$ binding activities corresponding to the respective fractions are summarized in Table I. Approximately 350 ml of solubilized material after dialysis is applied to a carboxymethyl(CM)-cellulose column (35 ml, 3 cm diameter) at a flow rate of 100 ml/hr. After being washed with Tris buffer, the column is eluted by increasing the NaCl concentration as shown in Fig. 1a.

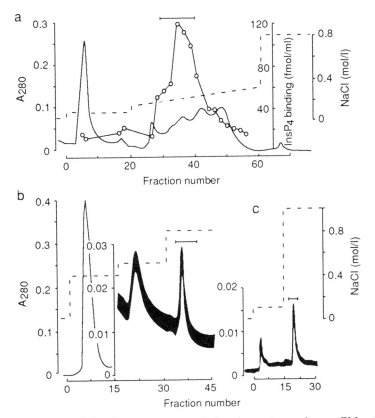

Fig. 1   Purification of the IP$_4$ receptor protein by chromatography on CM-cellulose (a), heparin-agarose (b), and hydroxylapatite (c). Graphs show the protein concentration of eluted fractions (A_{280}, continuous line), the NaCl concentration used for elution (right ordinate, dashed lines), and the IP$_4$ binding activity given as total binding of 0.1 nM [^{3}H]IP$_4$ (○). (a) Membrane extract obtained with Brij 58 applied to a CM-cellulose column was eluted with Tris buffer containing NaCl at the concentrations indicated. (b) The fractions marked by the horizontal bar in (a) were applied to heparin-agarose and eluted by Tris buffer containing NaCl as shown. The sensitivity of the photometer was increased after the first elution step by a factor of 10, resulting in a broader baseline. (c) The fractions indicated by the horizontal bar in (b) were dialyzed in phosphate buffer, applied to hydroxylapatite, and eluted with NaCl-containing phosphate buffer as indicated. The lower scale for NaCl concentrations applies to (b) and (c). Fraction sizes are 5 ml (a), 1.5 ml (b), and 0.6 ml (c). Protein concentrations and the values for specific IP$_4$ binding activity of the pooled fractions obtained in the chromatographies are included in Table I. [Reprinted with permission from Donié and Reiser (15). Copyright The Biochemical Society.]

TABLE I   Chromatographic Purification of High-Affinity Inositol 1,3,4,5-Tetrakisphosphate Receptor from Cerebellum[a]

Fraction	Protein (mg)	IP$_4$ binding activity/ml (pmol/ml)	Specific binding activity (pmol/ mg protein)	Total binding activity (pmol)	Yield (%)	Purification (-fold)
Solubilized membranes	1540	49.6	10.3	15,870	100	1
CM-cellulose						
Flow-through	1440	27.9	6.2			
Eluate 50 mM NaCl	6	0	0			
Eluate 100–300 mM NaCl	40	156	213	8580	54	21
Eluate 800 mM NaCl	3	0	0			
Heparin-agarose						
Flow-through	11	0	0			
Eluate 0.4 M NaCl	25	39.5	14			
Eluate 0.5 M NaCl	0.7	14.9	199			
Eluate 0.8 M NaCl	0.3	405	11,910	4050	25	1150
Hydroxylapatite						
Flow-through	0.02	0	0			
Eluate 1 M NaCl	0.08	860	47,780	4020	25	4625
Heparin-agarose						
Flow-through	0.04	0	0			
Eluate 0.4 M NaCl	0.017	96.6	5750			
Eluate 0.8 M NaCl	0.03	684	42,750	1370	8.6	4140

[a] Membranes from pig cerebellum (67 g) were solubilized and centrifuged, as described. The 100,000 g supernatant was subjected to CM-cellulose, heparin-agarose, and hydroxylapatite chromatography as shown in Fig. 1. The fractions of the hydroxylapatite column containing P$_4$ binding activity indicated by a horizontal bar (Fig. 1c) were dialyzed in Tris buffer and applied to a second heparin-agarose column, as described, and eluted by stepwise increases in the NaCl concentration to 0.4 and 0.8 M. IP$_4$ binding activities were determined with 0.1 nM [^{3}H]Ins(1,3,4,5)P$_4$ in the incubation mixture. Specific binding activities (i.e., total binding minus unspecific binding) of the dialyzed samples assayed in duplicate are given. For measuring unspecific binding, 0.5 μM Ins(1,3,4,5)P$_4$ was added. The overall purification factor is 20,000 when the B_{max} values obtained with membranes and with the sample from the second heparin-agarose column are compared. Reprinted with modifications from Donié and Reiser (15). Copyright The Biochemical Society.

The fraction eluted with Tris buffer containing 50 mM NaCl shows no IP$_4$ binding activity. The following gradient from 100 to 300 mM NaCl yields a complex profile of protein elution. The CM-cellulose column is washed by subsequent application of Tris buffer supplemented with 800 mM NaCl and equilibrated with Tris buffer. After several column runs the CM-cellulose is regenerated by pumping through 0.5 M NaOH and then 0.5 M HCl.

The fractions eluted in the range between 150 and 250 mM NaCl contain IP$_4$ binding activity. These are pooled and applied at a flow rate of 15 ml/hr to a heparin-agarose column (5 ml, 2 cm diameter). After washing the column with two column volumes of Tris buffer, elution is carried out at a flow rate of 30 ml/hr by increasing the NaCl concentration discontinuously to 400, 500, and 800 mM (Fig. 1b). The fraction eluted at 400 mM NaCl contains the bulk of the proteins (25 of 40 mg applied to the column). IP$_4$ binding activity, however, is detected mainly in the fraction seen at 800 mM NaCl, in which only 0.3 mg of protein is left. The heparin-agarose column is regenerated with buffer containing Tris-HCl (50 mM, pH 7.5), NaCl (1.5 M), and urea (6 M) and then equilibrated with Tris buffer.

According to the purification scheme outlined in Fig. 1 and Table I, the sample from the heparin-agarose column with binding activity (~10 ml eluted with Tris buffer containing 800 mM NaCl) is dialyzed in phosphate buffer. Then the retentate is applied at a flow rate of 0.5 ml/min to a hydroxylapatite column (0.4–0.5 ml, 1 cm diameter) filled with fresh material for each run. After washing the column with phosphate buffer, elution is carried out with phosphate buffer supplemented with 1 M NaCl. The eluate is dialyzed in Tris buffer. Omission of EDTA from the eluting buffer increases the yield of receptor slightly. After hydroxylapatite chromatography the total binding activity (Table I) of 4020 pmol is the same as after the preceding heparin-agarose chromatography step, but the amount of protein contained in the active fraction is substantially decreased from 300 to 80 μg (Table I).

To further purify the IP$_4$ receptor a second heparin-agarose step can be used. The fractions eluted from the hydroxylapatite column with phosphate buffer containing 1 M NaCl showing IP$_4$ binding activity are pooled, dialyzed in Tris buffer and applied to a small heparin-agarose column (1 $\times$ 0.3 cm) made from a 2-ml plastic syringe. The column is eluted by stepwise increases in the NaCl concentration in Tris buffer to 0.4 or 0.8 M NaCl. IP$_4$ binding activity is mainly seen in the fraction obtained with 0.8 M NaCl.

Identification of Inositol 1,3,4,5-Tetrakisphosphate Receptor

The fractions produced during purification of IP$_4$ binding activity are analyzed by SDS–polyacrylamide gel electrophoresis (SDS-PAGE). Figure 2 shows a gel after staining with Coomassie Brilliant Blue or silver. The active fraction from the CM-cellulose column (lane 3) displays a prominent band at 46 kDa and another less intensely stained band at 37 kDa, apart from a series of bands with lower molecular mass. In the fraction eluted from the first heparin-agarose column at 0.8 M NaCl, where maximal IP$_4$ binding activity is present, only three protein bands are revealed (lane 7) with approximate molecular masses of 46, 42, and 37 kDa. In the eluate from the hydroxylapatite column

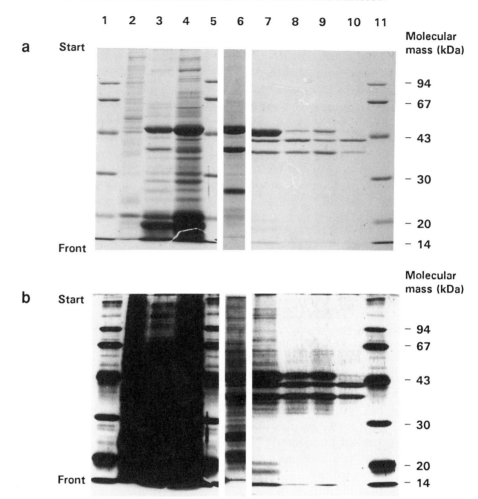

FIG. 2   SDS-PAGE analysis of fractions obtained during purification of the high-affinity IP$_4$ receptor. Fractions were analyzed by electrophoresis in a 10% polyacrylamide gel (3% polyacrylamide stacking gel), stained with Coomassie Brilliant blue R250 (a) and afterward with silver (b). Lane 2 contains the supernatant from centrifugation at 100,000 g of cerebellar membranes solubilized with Brij 58 (5 μg protein); lane 3, pooled fractions eluted between 100 and 300 mM NaCl from the CM-cellulose column showing IP$_4$ binding activity (36 μg protein); lanes 4, 6, and 7, proteins eluted by 0.4, 0.5, and 0.8 M NaCl from the first heparin-agarose column (18, 8.4, and 6.8 μg protein); lane 8, 3.6 μg eluted from the hydroxylapatite column by 1 M NaCl; lanes 9 (10), eluates from the second heparin-agarose column by 0.4 (0.8) M NaCl (0.85, 0.8 μg protein). Lanes 1, 5, and 11 contain molecular mass markers α-lactalbumin (14.4 kDa, 605 ng), trypsin inhibitor (20.1 kDa, 400 ng), carbonate dehydratase

(lane 8) the 46-kDa band is less prominent, whereas the two other bands are present at a comparable density.

A comparison of the protein bands in the two fractions obtained from the second heparin-agarose column makes the identification of the IP$_4$ receptor possible. In the 0.8 M NaCl fraction, even with intense silver staining (Fig. 2b, lane 10), only two bands (37 and 42 kDa) are visible. The relative amount of the 37-kDa band in the 0.8 M NaCl fraction (Fig. 2a, lane 10) is largely reduced in comparison with the 0.4 M NaCl fraction (Fig. 2a, lane 9). Because specific binding activity is 8-fold higher in the sample obtained at 0.8 M NaCl (Table I), the protein with approximate molecular mass of 42 kDa most likely represents the high-affinity IP$_4$ receptor from cerebellum.

Addition of protease inhibitors to the buffers used for preparation of membranes, solubilization, and receptor purification did not affect the results. Under these conditions the final eluate from the hydroxylapatite column also contains the 42-kDa protein as the most prominent protein band.

For a 42-kDa protein the maximum specific binding is 24 nmol/mg protein, assuming a stoichiometry of one ligand (IP$_4$) binding site per receptor molecule. The value obtained here (4.6 nmol/mg protein) is one-fifth of the theoretical maximum. The stoichiometry of 1 : 5 may be partly due to the artificial detergent environment or to nonaccessible binding sites.

Properties of High-Affinity Inositol 1,3,4,5-Tetrakisphosphate Receptor

The IP$_4$ receptor from the cerebellum membranes is successfully solubilized by detergent treatment since Scatchard analysis of the IP$_4$ binding both in membranes and in the solubilized preparation reveals an IP$_4$ receptor with the same affinity (K_D of 1–2 nM). The maximal binding capacity (B_{max}) is 0.22 pmol binding sites/mg protein in the membranes and 1.5 pmol/mg protein in the solubilized material. In the eluate from the hydroxylapatite column or in the final fraction from the second heparin-agarose column, the dissociation constant (K_D) for IP$_4$ varies between 2 and 9 nM (5.6 ± 3.5 nM, $n = 4$). The

---

30 kDa, 415 ng), ovalbumin (43 kDa, 735 ng), bovine serum albumin (67 kDa, 415 ng), and phosphorylase b (94 kDa, 320 ng). For electrophoresis, proteins were precipitated by incubating samples with 4-fold volume of methanol/acetone (1 : 1, v/v) for 10 min at 37°C, centrifuged at 10,000 g, and incubated at 4°C overnight in sample buffer (final concentrations: Tris 125 mM, pH 6.8, urea 4 M, mercaptoethanol 5%, SDS 2%, and bromphenol blue 0.002%). [Reprinted with modifications from Donié and Reiser (15). Copyright The Biochemical Society.]

maximal binding capacity (B_{max}) is 1500 pmol/mg protein for the fraction eluted from the hydroxylapatite column and 4600 pmol/mg protein for the active fraction (0.8 M NaCl) from the second heparin-agarose column. Thus, in comparison with the original membrane preparation, a final overall purification factor of 20,000 is obtained.

The fact that the IP_3 receptor (2) and the high-affinity IP_4 receptor represent different proteins has already been clearly demonstrated in experiments in which partial purification of the IP_4 receptor has been achieved (14). In those experiments the solubilized material was applied to heparin-agarose and eluted by increasing the NaCl concentration stepwise to 0.25, 0.4, 0.5, and 0.8 M NaCl. The latter fraction showed maximal IP_4 binding, whereas maximal IP_3 binding was found in the fraction obtained with 0.4 M NaCl (14). Thus, IP_3 and IP_4 binding activities could be separated.

The specificity of binding to the purified IP_4 receptor is comparable to that of the membrane-bound receptor. Binding of [^{3}H]IP_4 to the purified receptor can be displaced by $Ins(1,3,4,5)P_4$ and $Ins(1,3,4,5,6)P_5$ with a similar affinity and to the same extent, whereas IP_6 displaces [^{3}H]IP_4 binding with a half-maximal inhibitory concentration (IC_{50}) about 80 times higher. In the membrane preparation the affinity for $Ins(1,3,4,5,6)P_5$ is 100 times lower than for $Ins(1,3,4,5)P_4$. After purification, however, $Ins(1,3,4,5,6)P_5$ inhibits [^{3}H]$Ins(1,3,4,5)P_4$ binding with an IC_{50} close to that for nonradioactive $Ins(1,3,4,5)P_4$. Thus, the selectivity of the receptor appears to be regulated by an accessory protein. This is an intriguing possibility because (i) in many cells IP_5 is present at high concentrations (24) and (ii) IP_5 can mimic some of the cellular effects of $Ins(1,3,4,5)P_4$ (25). The following inositol oligophosphates displace binding of [^{3}H]$Ins(1,3,4,5)P_4$ from the purified receptor half-maximally in a narrow concentration range between 600 nM and 2 μM (15, 16): $Ins(1,3,4,5)P_4$, $Ins(1,2,5,6)P_4$, $Ins(1,2,3,4,5)P_5$, $Ins(1,3,4,5,6)P_5$, $Ins(1,3,4,6)P_4$, $Ins(3,4,5,6)P_4$, $Ins(1,4,5,6)P_4$, $Ins(1,2,3,4,6)P_5$, $Ins(1,2,4,5,6)P_5$. $Ins(1,4,5)P_3$, however, cannot displace IP_4 binding at concentration up to 10 μM.

Heparin suppresses high-affinity IP_3 binding and blocks IP_3-induced Ca^{2+} release (see citations in Ref. 15). Therefore the disappearance of a cellular effect after injection of heparin has frequently been taken as evidence for the involvement of $Ins(1,4,5)P_3$. However, IP_4 binding to the high-affinity receptor is also inhibited by heparin (IC_{50} 15 ng/ml) and related polyglycans with high potency (14). Therefore suppression by heparin does not allow a clear-cut conclusion since $Ins(1,4,5)P_3$ or $Ins(1,3,4,5)P_4$ might be involved in the activation process.

The influence of pH indicates a further possibly important regulatory property of the $Ins(1,3,4,5)P_4$ receptor. Changing the pH from 5 to 7 alters the K_D of the purified protein for IP_4 from 2 to 14 nM and enhances the amount of unspecific (low-affinity) binding from 13 to 45%. At neutral pH the IP_4

receptor has reduced affinity for Ins(1,3,4,5)P$_4$ and increased unspecific binding (apparently reflecting a binding site with very low affinity), whereas at acidic pH the affinity increases. Therefore, cellular pH changes occurring during Ca^{2+} regulation might modify the binding properties of the IP$_4$ receptor.

The IP$_4$ receptor is retained by CM-cellulose at pH 7.5. Therefore, the receptor is expected to be a basic protein, whereas the IP$_3$ receptor is an acidic protein (2). These opposite overall electrical charges could favor a mutual binding of the two receptors. This is compatible with the notion of a direct interaction of the IP$_4$ receptor with the IP$_3$ receptor, predicted by the model of IP$_4$ action proposed by Irvine (25).

The high affinity IP$_4$ receptor described here is most likely not the Inositol 1,3,4,5-tetrakisphosphate-3-phosphatase, which is mostly soluble, or a kinase as there is no evidence that under physiological conditions Ins(1,3,4,5)P$_4$ is phosphorylated (26). In the membrane preparation variation of the Ca^{2+} concentration from 10 nM to 10 mM did not alter binding of IP$_4$ by more than 20%. This shows a further difference between the IP$_4$ receptor and the IP$_3$ receptor; IP$_4$ binding is not regulated by Ca^{2+}, in contrast to the binding of IP$_3$ to its receptor which is inhibited by Ca^{2+} (27) through a Ca^{2+}-binding protein of 15 kDa molecular mass (28).

Photoaffinity Labeling of Inositol 1,3,4,5-Tetrakisphosphate Receptor

A photoactivatable ligand for the IP$_4$ receptor, AsaIP$_4$ [AsaIns(1,3,4,5)P$_4$: N-(4-azidosalicyl)aminoethanol(1)-1-phospho-D-myo-inositol 3,4,5-trisphosphate], has been synthesized by Dr. G. Mayr (Ruhr-Universität, Bochum, Germany) [described by Reiser et al. (16)]. AsaIP$_4$ inhibits [^{3}H]Ins(1,3,4,5)P$_4$ binding to the purified receptor with an apparent affinity only about 3 times lower than that of Ins(1,3,4,5)P$_4$ (16). A competitive interaction of AsaIP$_4$ and IP$_4$ at the IP$_4$ binding site is further demonstrated by experiments testing the binding of [^{125}I]AsaIP$_4$ performed with samples in the dark without subsequent irradiation. Binding of the iodinated photoaffinity analog [^{125}I]AsaIP$_4$ to the purified receptor is suppressed by 0.5 μM IP$_4$ by 80% but is not affected by 2 μM Ins(1,4,5)P$_3$ (16). Thus, AsaIP$_4$ specifically interacts with the high-affinity IP$_4$ receptor.

Protocol

Samples of column eluates are incubated in phosphate buffer supplemented with [^{125}I]AsaIP$_4$ (20 nM) in a 48-well culture plate (Costar, Cambridge, MA) kept on ice for 20 min and shielded from light. Photolysis is achieved

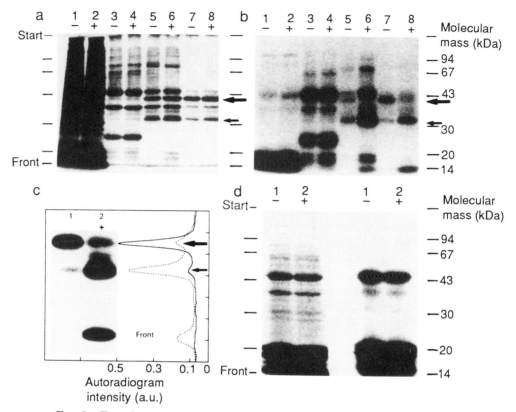

FIG. 3   Functional identification of a high-affinity IP_4 receptor by photoaffinity labeling with $[^{125}I]AsaIP_4$ demonstrating that only the 42-kDa protein band specifically
binds $[^{125}I]AsaIP_4$. Binding reaction mixtures used for lanes marked "−" contained
$[^{125}I]AsaIP_4$ without unlabeled IP_4, and those marked "+" contained in addition 5
μM IP_4. (a) SDS-PAGE analysis (10% polyacrylamide running gel, 3% stacking gel)
as in Fig. 2, gel stained with Coomassie Brilliant Blue R250 and silver. Lanes 1–6
contain samples from the heparin-agarose column: lanes 1 and 2, eluted by 0.4 M
NaCl (84 μg of protein); lanes 3 and 4, eluted by 0.5 M NaCl (35 μg of protein);
lanes 5 and 6, eluted by 0.8 M NaCl (6.7 μg of protein). Lanes 7 and 8 contain
samples from the hydroxylapatite column eluted by 1 M NaCl (8.2 μg of protein).
(b) Autoradiogram of the gel shown in (a). The position of the protein band stained
specifically by $[^{125}I]AsaIP_4$ in lanes 7 and 8 is marked by a large arrow. In the presence
of 5 μM nonradioactive IP_4 the radioactive label is mainly bound to a protein marked
by a small arrow (lane 8). Note that lanes 5 and 6 correspond to replica incubations
carried out with identical samples eluted by 0.8 M NaCl from the heparin-agarose
column; however, the amount of radioactive $[^{125}I]AsaIP_4$ during the incubation of
the mixture used for lane 5 was incidentally lower than that employed in lane 6 (see
Ref. 16). In the samples used for lanes 1, 2, 3, 4, 6, 7, and 8 the amount of radioactivity

by a subsequent 20-min irradiation at 4°C of the continuously stirred samples, using ultraviolet light from an HPK lamp (Philips, Eindhaven, the Netherlands) (125 W, distance 15 cm) directed through a filter of a saturated copper sulfate solution (10 mm light path). After irradiation the proteins are precipitated by adding a 4-fold volume of methanol/acetone (1 : 1, v/v) and incubated for 10 min at 37°C. The mixture is centrifuged at 10,000 g and washed. For electrophoresis the samples are treated as described in legend to Fig. 2. The SDS-PAGE gel is stained by Coomassie Brilliant Blue R250 or silver, dried, and placed on Hyperfilm MP (Amersham). Films are exposed at −70°C for 2–20 hr.

Results of Photoaffinity Labeling

Analysis by SDS-PAGE (Fig. 3a) and autoradiography (Fig. 3b) demonstrates that among the proteins obtained after the hydroxylapatite chromatography one single protein band specifically binds [^{125}I]AsaIP$_4$. In the absence of nonradioactive IP$_4$ only one protein band with an apparent molecular mass of 42 kDa is strongly labeled, and a comparatively negligible amount of binding is associated with a protein band of 32 kDa molecular mass (Fig. 3a,b, lane 7). In the presence of a high concentration (5 μM) of nonradioactive IP$_4$, binding of [^{125}I]AsaIP$_4$ is mostly displaced from the 42-kDa protein band and associated with the small molecular mass band. The optical density scan of an autoradiogram (Fig. 3c) allows a quantitative estimate: In the absence of nonradioactive IP$_4$ 84% of the bound label is attached to the 42-kDa protein band (Fig. 3c, continuous trace), whereas in the presence of 5 μM IP$_4$ 60% of the label is bound to the 32-kDa band and only 20% to the 42-kDa protein band (Fig. 3c, dotted trace).

---

used was identical. (c) Densitometric scan of autoradiogram obtained with partially purified receptor eluted from the hydroxylapatite column. Samples with 9 μg of protein from the hydroxylapatite column were incubated with [^{125}I]AsaIP$_4$ in the absence (−) or presence (+) of 5 μM IP$_4$ and subjected to SDS-PAGE; the autoradiogram (left-hand side of the diagram) was scanned with a laser densitometer (Pharmacia, Freiburg, Germany, gel scanner). The continuous and dotted curves correspond to lanes 1 ("−") and 2 ("+"), respectively. The position of the 42-kDa protein is marked by the large arrow, that of the 32-kDa protein by the small arrow. (d) Sample (45 μg of protein) eluted by 0.2 M NaCl from CM-cellulose analyzed by SDS-PAGE (left-hand side) and autoradiography (right-hand side). Further details are as in (a) and (b). [Reprinted with permission from Reiser et al. (16). Copyright The Biochemical Society.]

The 32-kDa protein band binds $AsaIP_4$ with low affinity. This unspecific binding is very small in lane 7 (Fig. 3a,b), because the binding reaction is carried out with a concentration of receptor binding sites exceeding by approximately 20-fold the concentration of $[^{125}]AsaIP_4$. Thus, the concentration of the free ligand is reduced to such an extent that the binding to the low-affinity sites becomes negligible. Only at the high concentration of nonradioactive IP_4 (lane 8, Fig. 3a,b) is sufficient $[^{125}I]AsaIP_4$ displaced from the 42-kDa protein and thus available for the low-affinity binding sites of the 32-kDa protein and of the low molecular mass proteins running with the front in the gel electrophoresis. The identity of this protein still has to be clarified.

In the eluate obtained after the first purification step (CM-cellulose), which contains many different proteins (Fig. 3d), a whole range of proteins binds $[^{125}I]AsaIP_4$ (note that the gel shown in Fig. 3d has been stained with Coomassie blue only, because with these samples after silver staining individual protein bands can no longer be resolved). However, bound $[^{125}I]AsaIP_4$ cannot be displaced by IP_4, suggesting only low-affinity binding. In the fractions obtained both from the CM-cellulose (Fig. 3d) and from the heparin-agarose column (Fig. 3a,b, lanes 1–6), low-affinity binding of $[^{125}I]AsaIP_4$ is mainly associated with the 46-kDa protein band and cannot be suppressed by 5 μM nonradioactive IP_4 (lanes marked "+"). Thus, no other proteins eluted from the CM-cellulose and the heparin-agarose column specifically bind IP_4.

Modified Purification Scheme

The following modification of the protocol for purification of the IP_4 receptor simplifies the procedure and gives a final preparation with a yield comparable to that described above. The membranes are solubilized, then dialyzed and applied to the CM-cellulose column (35 ml), as outlined above. The column is eluted with Tris buffer with stepwise-increased NaCl concentrations (50, 200, and 800 mM). IP_4 binding activity is detected only in the fraction obtained with 200 mM NaCl. This fraction ($\sim$70 ml) is dialyzed in 1 liter Tris buffer overnight and then subjected to heparin-agarose chromatography and hydroxylapatite chromatography (cf. Fig. 1). The second heparin-agarose chromatography is usually omitted because the increase in purity does not justify the loss in material. Analysis of samples obtained with the simplified purification protocol (Fig. 4) (29) shows that the final fraction (Fig. 4, lane 8) contains the IP_4 receptor as the predominant protein band. In some cases additional minor contaminating protein bands are observed.

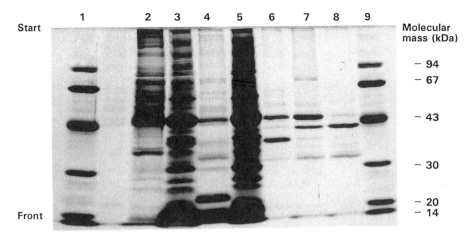

FIG. 4   Purification of the IP$_4$ receptor by a simplified scheme. Samples were subjected to SDS-PAGE analysis (cf. Fig. 2) with silver staining. Lanes 2, 3, and 4 contain fractions eluted from the CM-cellulose with buffer containing 50, 200, and 800 mM NaCl, respectively (18, 165, and 7 μg protein); lanes 5, 6, and 7, fractions eluted by 0.4, 0.5, and 0.8 M NaCl from the heparin-agarose column (85, 10, and 3 μg protein); lane 8, fraction eluted from the hydroxylapatite column by 1 M NaCl (3.5 μg protein); lanes 1 and 9, molecular mass markers. [Adapted from Hülser (29).]

Different Inositol 1,3,4,5-Tetrakisphosphate Receptors

A different protocol has been used to solubilize IP$_4$ binding activity from rat cerebellar membranes (17). Proteins were solubilized with buffer containing the detergent CHAPS (1%) and applied to heparin-agarose in buffer containing 250 mM NaCl. The eluate obtained with 750 mM NaCl showed IP$_4$ binding activity. Concanavalin A (Con A) chromatography was used to separate the glycosylated IP$_3$ receptor from the IP$_4$ binding activity, which does not adhere to the lectin column. The sample with the latter activity was applied to an IP$_4$ affinity resin and eluted with an NaCl concentration gradient. IP$_4$- and IP$_6$-binding proteins are obtained in different fractions. Two complexes of 182/123 kDa and 174/84 kDa show high-affinity IP$_4$ binding. The IP$_6$ receptor, comprising proteins of 115, 105, and 50 kDa, seems to be identical to the clathrin-associated assembly protein (18, 28).

Another inositol phosphate-binding protein has been isolated from bovine cerebellum by Chadwick *et al.* (21) with components of 111, 102, and 52 kDa. The receptor preparation has limited selectivity since it binds Ins(1,3,4,5)P$_4$, IP$_6$, and Ins(1,4,5)P$_3$ with similar affinities. The purified receptor preparation when reconstituted into planar bilayers displays ion channel activity, indicating that the protein complex could be an $Ins(1,3,4,5)P_4$-modulated K^+ channel.

Theibert *et al.* (30) have used a photoaffinity label similar to the one described by Reiser *et al.* (16). In the 182/123-kDa IP_4-binding protein complex the 182-kDa protein is specifically labeled, whereas in the 174/84-kDa complex both proteins are labeled by the photoaffinity analog. The relationship between these binding proteins and the IP_4 receptor described here still has to be established.

Summary

Membranes from pig cerebellum contain high-affinity binding sites for IP_4 (K_D 1 nM). IP_4 binding activity is solubilized using the nonionic detergent Brij 58 and purified by sequential chromatography with CM-cellulose, heparin-agarose, and hydroxylapatite. The IP_4 receptor is identified as a 42-kDa protein, and high-affinity binding of this protein is established by an IP_4 photoaffinity label (15, 16). From rat cerebellum various IP_4-binding proteins with molecular masses of 182 and 174/84 kDa have been isolated (18, 30).

The purified IP_4 receptor should provide us with the tools to localize this receptor in cells and to determine the actual functions of IP_4 in cellular Ca^{2+} homeostasis (24). Subcellular localization may give clues to help solve the problem of whether IP_4 induces resequestration of Ca^{2+} into internal stores, as suggested by Hill and co-workers (31), or whether IP_4 regulates Ca^{2+} entry into the cytoplasm through the plasma membrane (24).

Acknowledgments

Work carried out in the author's laboratory was supported by the Deutsche Forschungsgemeinschaft (Re 563/3-1). I thank Frédéric Donié, Eckehard Hülser, and Rolf Stricker for enthusiastic collaboration and valuable contributions.

References

1. M. J. Berridge and R. F. Irvine, *Nature (London)* **341,** 197 (1989).
2. S. Supattapone, P. F. Worley, J. M. Baraban, and S. H. Snyder, *J. Biol. Chem.* **263,** 1530 (1988).
3. C. D. Ferris, R. L. Huganir, S. Supattapone, and S. H. Snyder, *Nature (London)* **342,** 87 (1989).

4. T. Furuichi, S. Yoshikawa, A. Miyawaki, K. Wada, N. Maeda, and K. Mikoshiba, *Nature* (*London*) **342,** 32 (1989).

5. N. Maeda, T. Kawasaki, S. Nakade, N. Yokota, T. Taguchi, T. Kasai, and K. Mikoshiba, *J. Biol. Chem.* **266,** 1109 (1991).

6. R. F. Irvine, A. J. Letcher, J. P. Heslop, and M. J. Berridge, *Nature* (*London*) **320,** 631 (1986).

7. L. Changya, D. V. Gallacher, R. F. Irvine, B. V. L. Potter, and O. H. Petersen, *J. Membr. Biol.* **109,** 85 (1989).

8. P. Palade, C. Dettbarn, P. Volpe, B. Alderson, and A. Otero, *Mol. Pharmacol.* **36,** 664 (1989).

9. S. K. Josef, H. L. Rice, and J. R. Williamson, *Biochem. J.* **258,** 261 (1989).

10. P. J. Cullen, R. F. Irvine, and A. P. Dawson, *Biochem. J.* **271,** 549 (1990).

11. F. Donié and G. Reiser, *FEBS Lett.* **254,** 155 (1989).

12. G. Reiser and F. Donié, *Eur. J. Neurosci.* **2,** 769 (1990).

13. F. Donié and G. Reiser, *Biochem. Biophys. Res. Commun.* **181,** 997 (1991).

14. F. Donié, E. Hülser, and G. Reiser, *FEBS Lett.* **268,** 194 (1990).

15. F. Donié and G. Reiser, *Biochem. J.* **275,** 453 (1991).

16. G. Reiser, R. Schäfer, F. Donié, E. Hülser, M. Nehls-Sahabandu, and G. W. Mayr, *Biochem. J.* **280,** 533 (1991).

17. A. B. Theibert, S. Supattapone, C. D. Ferris, S. K. Danoff, R. K. Evans, and S. H. Snyder, *Biochem. J.* **267,** 441 (1990).

18. A. B. Theibert, V. A. Estevez, C. D. Ferris, S. K. Danoff, R. K. Barrow, G. D. Prestwich, and S. H. Snyder, *Proc. Natl. Acad. Sci. U.S.A.* **88,** 3165 (1991).

19. H. S. Penefsky, *J. Biol. Chem.* **252,** 2891 (1977).

20. B. Buchberger, Ph.D. Thesis, Universität Tübingen, Tübingen, Germany (1990).

21. C. C. Chadwick, A. P. Timerman, A. Saito, M. Mayrleitner, H. Schindler, and S. Fleischer, *J. Biol. Chem.* **267,** 3473 (1992).

22. S. R. Hingorani and W. S. Agnew, *Anal. Biochem.* **194,** 204 (1991).

23. J. M. Neugebauer, *in* "Methods in Enzymology" (M. P. Deutscher, ed.), Vol. 182, p. 239. Academic Press, San Diego, 1990.

24. T. Balla, L. Hunyady, A. J. Baukal, and K. J. Catt, *J. Biol. Chem.* **264,** 9386 (1988).

25. R. F. Irvine, *FEBS Lett.* **263,** 5 (1990).

26. S. B. Shears, *Biochem. J.* **260,** 313 (1989).

27. S. K. Danoff, S. Supattapone, and S. H. Snyder, *Biochem. J.* **254,** 701 (1988).

28. C. D. Ferris and S. H. Snyder, *J. Neurosci.* **12,** 1567 (1992).

29. E. Hülser, Diploma Thesis, Universität Tübingen, Tübingen, Germany (1991).

30. A. B. Theibert, V. A. Estevez, R. J. Mourey, J. F. Marecek, R. K. Barrow, G. D. Prestwich, and S. H. Snyder, *J. Biol. Chem.* **267,** 9071 (1992).

31. T. D. Hill, N. M. Dean, and A. L. Boynton, *Science* **242,** 1176 (1988).

[25] Inositol 1,4,5-Trisphosphate-Binding Proteins in Rat Brain Cytosol

Masato Hirata and Takashi Kanematsu

Introduction

myo-Inositol 1,4,5-trisphosphate [Ins(1,4,5)P$_3$], a product of the receptor-activated hydrolysis of phosphatidylinositol 4,5-bisphosphate (PIP$_2$), plays an important role as an intracellular second messenger by mobilizing Ca^{2+} from nonmitochondrial store sites (1). Ins(1,4,5)P$_3$ is metabolized by two known routes; one is dephosphorylation, catalyzed by Ins(1,4,5)P$_3$-5-phosphatase present in both cytosol and membrane fractions of cells, the result being formation of Ins(1,4)P$_2$ which is subsequently degraded to free inositol by other phosphatase activities (2). Alternatively, phosphorylation of the 3-hydroxyl group of Ins(1,4,5)P$_3$ by an ATP-dependent kinase present in the cell cytosol produces Ins(1,3,4,5)P$_4$ (3). The three types of proteins heretofore identified are Ins(1,4,5)P$_3$-interacting macromolecules: Ins(1,4,5)P$_3$ receptors on the endoplasmic reticulum are involved in Ca^{2+} release (4, 5) and two types of enzymes are related to Ins(1,4,5)P$_3$ metabolism.

In 1985, we described for the first time the chemical modification of Ins(1,4,5)P$_3$ (6). The analog has the azidobenzoyl group at the C-2 position for photoaffinity labeling and causes irreversible inactivation of the receptor protein for Ca^{2+} release, following photolysis. On the basis of these findings and the report (7) that biological activities of Ins(1,4,5)P$_3$ are related to two adjacent phosphates at C-4 and C-5 and the phosphate at C-1 increases the affinity for its recognition by the receptor site, we attempted further chemical modifications of Ins(1,4,5)P$_3$ at the C-2 position and examined the effects on the above-mentioned Ins(1,4,5)P$_3$-recognizable protein (8, 9). The Ins(1,4,5)P$_3$ analogs attach to other molecules through substituents at the C-2 position. We, therefore, prepared Ins(1,4,5)P$_3$ affinity matrices which proved to be useful for purifying the known Ins(1,4,5)P$_3$-interacting proteins (10). In this chapter, we describe the purification of novel Ins(1,4,5)P$_3$-binding proteins from rat brain cytosol, using the Ins(1,4,5)P$_3$ affinity matrices (11).

Methods in Neurosciences, Volume 18

Binding Assay

The specific radioactivity of [^{3}H]Ins(1,4,5)P$_3$ employed should be greater than 185 GBq/mmol to achieve significant specific over nonspecific binding, assayed in the presence of 1 μM unlabeled Ins(1,4,5)P$_3$. We regularly use [^{3}H]Ins(1,4,5)P$_3$ with a specific radioactivity of 629 GBq/mmol. The binding of [^{3}H]Ins(1,4,5)P$_3$ to soluble proteins is assayed by the polyethylene glycol precipitation method as follows.

The assay mixture in a microcentrifuge tube (0.45 ml) contains 50 mM Tris-HCl buffer (pH 8.3), 0.2% Triton X-100, 1 mM EDTA, 1.3 nM carrier-free [^{3}H]Ins(1,4,5)P$_3$ (370 Bq), and the protein sample. After incubation on ice for 15 min, 50 μl of 10 mg/ml bovine γ-globulin and 0.5 ml of 30% (w/v) polyethylene glycol 6000 are added to the mixture, then a further incubation on ice is conducted for 5 min. Following centrifugation at 15,000 rpm for 5 min at room temperature, the precipitates are dissolved in 1 ml of 0.1 N NaOH and then counted for ^{3}H radioactivity after mixing with 10 ml of a scintillation cocktail consisting of 0.4% (w/v) 2,5-diphenyloxazole (DPO) and 0.02% (w/v) 1,4-bis(5-phenyloxazol-2-yl)benzene (POPOP) in 666 ml of toluene and 334 ml of Triton X-100.

In routine assays, the specific binding varies from about 500 to 6000 disintegrations/min (dpm)/assay tube, depending on the protein sample, whereas the nonspecific binding is relatively constant at 150 to 250 dpm/tube. Incubation on ice in the presence of EDTA is required to prevent the hydrolysis of [^{3}H]Ins(1,4,5)P$_3$ by the 5-phosphatase present in the protein sample. If 0.25 mg of brain homogenate is incubated in the absence of EDTA or in the presence of 0.3 mM MgCl$_2$ without EDTA, about 10 or 48%, respectively, of the [^{3}H]Ins(1,4,5)P$_3$ is hydrolyzed, even on ice. The presence of 0.2% (v/v) Triton X-100 is required for precipitate formation by polyethylene glycol 6000, for reasons unknown.

Purification

Preaffinity Chromatography Step

Brains minus cerebellum from Wistar rats of either sex weighing 200–250 g are homogenized in an ice bath in a glass homogenizer with a Teflon pestle in 3 volumes of solution containing 50 mM NaCl, 10 mM HEPES buffer (pH 7.2), 1 mM EDTA, 2 mM NaN$_3$, and 10 mM 2-mercaptoethanol (designated as buffer A) supplemented with a mixture of protease inhibitors (1 μg/ml aprotinin, 1.25 μg/ml pepstatin A, 0.1 mM p-amidinophenylmethylsulfonyl fluoride, and 10 μM leupeptin). The following procedures are performed

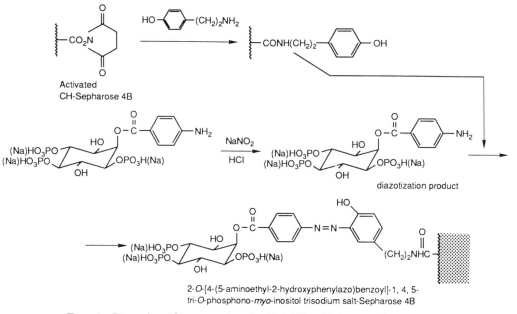

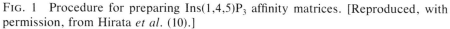

2-*O*-[4-(5-aminoethyl-2-hydroxyphenylazo)benzoyl]-1, 4, 5-
tri-*O*-phosphono-*myo*-inositol trisodium salt-Sepharose 4B

FIG. 1   Procedure for preparing Ins(1,4,5)P$_3$ affinity matrices. [Reproduced, with permission, from Hirata *et al.* (10).]

in a cold room (temperature 4–6°C). The cytosol fraction is obtained by centrifuging the homogenates at 130,000 *g* for 1 hr at 4°C.

Affinity Chromatography

Preparation of Inositol 1,4,5-Trisphosphate Affinity Gels

[(5-Aminoethyl-2-hydroxyphenylazo)benzoyl]-1,4,5-tri-*O*-phosphono-*myo*-inositol-Sepharose 4B is prepared in three steps, as follows (see Fig. 1).

1. After washing the activated CH-Sepharose 4B (1 g, Pharmacia, Uppsala, Sweden) with 1 m*M* HCl and subsequently with 0.1 *M* NaHCO$_3$ (pH 8.0), the resins are mixed with 2 μmol tyramine at room temperature, collected by suction filtration, washed with 0.5 *M* NaCl plus 50 m*M* Tris-HCl (pH 8.0) and 0.5 *M* NaCl plus 50 m*M* formic acid (pH 4.0), alternatively, and finally suspended in 0.1 *M* NaHCO$_3$ (pH 8.0).
2. Twenty microliters of 12 *N* HCl and 5 μmol NaNO$_2$ are mixed with 2 μmol of an Ins(1,4,5)P$_3$ analog, 2-(4-aminobenzoyl)-*myo*-inositol 1,4,5-trisphosphate, which is prepared according to the method by Ozaki and

Watanabe (12) in water cooled to 0°C, and the mixture is incubated at 0°C for 30 min for diazotization.

3. The diazotization product from Step 2 is mixed with the product at Step 1, and the mixture is incubated at room temperature for 1 hr. The resins coupled with the analog through tyramine are collected by passing the mixture through a sintered glass funnel, following by washing as described above.

While neither the analog nor the Ins(1,4,5)P$_3$ affinity gel are commercially available at the present time; however, both can be obtained from our laboratory or that of Professor Shoichiro Ozaki (Department of Applied Chemistry, Faculty of Engineering, Ehime University, Matsuyama, 790, Japan).

Properties of Affinity Gels

Although structures of the functionalized resins have not been fully characterized, the analogous reactions occur in solution, as mentioned above, and there is no recovery of the analog in immobilization procedures. Furthermore, when the analog-immobilized resins, but not control resins, are included in the reaction mixture for [^{3}H]Ins(1,4,5)P$_3$-5-phosphatase, the 3-kinase, or the binding protein, the activities are inhibited, as seen with the free analog (8, 9). These results indicate that the products are formed as illustrated in Fig. 1.

Preliminary Experiments with Affinity Column

The Ins(1,4,5)P$_3$ affinity column thus prepared has been examined for applicability for purifying the known Ins(1,4,5)P$_3$-metabolizing enzymes present in the cytosol fraction of rat brain. The cytosol fraction of two rat brains is applied to the Ins(1,4,5)P$_3$ affinity column (0.8 × 1 cm), and the adsorbed proteins are eluted by a stepwise increase in sodium concentrations (Fig. 2). All the media used contain 2 mM EDTA to protect the columns from attack by Ins(1,4,5)P$_3$-5-phosphatase activity present in the cytosol. Activation of the phosphatase, which is capable of hydrolyzing the analogs as substrate (8), requires the presence of Mg^{2+}, and thus inclusion of EDTA to chelate Mg^{2+} in the solution prevents activation of the enzyme. The cytosolic Ins(1,4,5)P$_3$-5-phosphatase (specific activity 51 nmol/mg of protein/min) that is retained on the column is eluted with 0.5 M NaCl, with a 7- to 8-fold increase in the specific activity. The cytosolic Ins(1,4,5)P$_3$-3-kinase activity (specific activity 0.23 nmol/mg of protein/min), mainly present in the cytosol fraction, is also determined in each fraction. The enzyme activities are eluted from the column by 2 M NaCl. Purification over the column increases the specific activity by 50- to 70-fold. These results indicate that the affinity

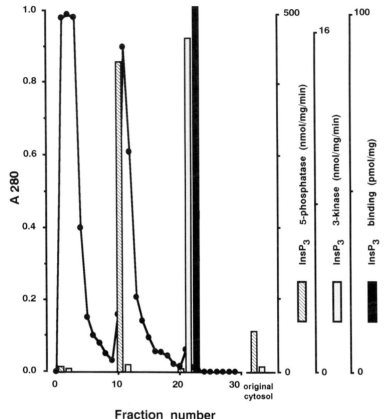

Fraction number

FIG. 2   Ins(1,4,5)P$_3$ affinity chromatography of the cytosol fraction of rat brain. The cytosol fraction was applied to an Ins(1,4,5)P$_3$ affinity column, and the adsorbed fraction was eluted by a stepwise increase in NaCl concentration. At fractions 11 or 21, a 0.5 or 2 M NaCl solution was applied, respectively. Fractions 2, 12, and 22 were assayed for [³H]Ins(1,4,5)P$_3$-metabolizing as well as binding activities. [³H]Ins(1,4,5)P$_3$-5-phosphate activity, hatched bar; [³H]Ins(1,4,5)P$_3$-3-kinase activity, dotted bar; [³H]Ins(1,4,5)P$_3$-binding activity, filled bar. [Adapted, with permission, from Hirata *et al.* (10).]

column is useful for purifying proteins capable of being recognized by Ins(1,4,5)P$_3$.

When we measured the [³H]Ins(1,4,5)P$_3$-binding activity as well as [³H]Ins(1,4,5)P$_3$-metabolizing activities in each fraction obtained with Ins(1,4,5)P$_3$ affinity chromatography, as shown in Fig. 2, we became aware of the presence of remarkable [³H]Ins(1,4,5)P$_3$-binding activity in the 2 M NaCl fraction. The specific binding of 110 pmol/mg protein at 1.3 nM

[^{3}H]Ins(1,4,5)P$_3$ is obtained with the 2 M NaCl eluate, whereas that with the cytosol fraction is 0.01 pmol/mg protein, the purification being 11,000-fold. Thus [^{3}H]Ins(1,4,5)P$_3$-binding activities are present in eluates with 2 M NaCl solution, along with that of Ins(1,4,5)P$_3$-3-kinase. This finding prompted us to purify the molecules responsible for the [^{3}H]Ins(1,4,5)P$_3$ binding in the 2 M NaCl eluate.

Reusability of Column

The affinity column could be used several times following regeneration by washing with a solution of 6 M urea and 2 M NaCl, followed by requilibration with an initial buffer. EDTA to chelate Mg^{2+} is included in the medium, thereby preventing the activation of Ins(1,4,5)P$_3$-5-phosphatase present in the sample. By including EDTA in the medium, the life span of the affinity resins is prolonged. Nevertheless, the resins do deteriorate with use; after the column had been exposed to detergent extracts or soluble fractions from 70–100 rat brains, the Ins(1,4,5)P$_3$-recognizable proteins such as the metabolic enzymes and Ins(1,4,5)P$_3$ receptor failed to be adsorbed, as assessed by measurement of the activities. One explanation for the deterioration may be the liberation of the Ins(1,4,5)P$_3$ moiety at the carboxyester bond on the second carbon of the inositol ring from its supporting medium (see Fig. 1) by activities of carboxyesterases present in various species of cells. However, this notion seems unlikely because the Ins(1,4,5)P$_3$ affinity matrices remained active even after having been extensively treated with commercially available carboxyesterase prepared from porcine liver (250 units at 25°C for 12 hr).

Purification with Affinity Column

For purification of the cytosolic [^{3}H]Ins(1,4,5)P$_3$-binding proteins, the cytosol fraction (~60 ml) obtained from 10 brains (minus cerebellum) is applied to the affinity column (0.8 × 3 cm), followed by washing of the column with 100 ml of buffer A containing 0.5 M NaCl. The column is gravity driven. The more extensive the wash with 0.5 M NaCl solution, the less the contamination in the following eluates. Buffer A containing 2 M NaCl is then applied to the column and fractions of 2 ml collected. When each fraction is assayed for [^{3}H]Ins(1,4,5)P$_3$-binding activity, fractions 2 to 5 have high binding activities.

Postaffinity Chromatography Step

Samples from the affinity column with high [^{3}H]Ins(1,4,5)P$_3$-binding activity are collected and further fractionated, without dialysis, by application to a HiLoad 26/60 Superdex 200 (Pharmacia) column (2.6 × 60 cm) equili-brated with solution containing 0.3 M NaCl, 20 mM HEPES/NaOH (pH 7.2), 2 mM NaN$_3$, and 10 mM 2-mercaptoethanol. As shown in Fig. 3A, the binding activity is eluted between molecular mass markers of 200K and 66K, giving two peaks. Ins(1,4,5)P$_3$-3-kinase activity, however, is eluted around 110 min of the elution time, thereby indicating that the [^{3}H]Ins(1,4,5)P$_3$-binding activities observed are not due to Ins(1,4,5)P$_3$-3-kinase. As shown in Fig. 3B, analyses of the fractions by sodium dodecyl sulfate (SDS)–polyacrylamide gel electrophoresis suggest that the protein with an apparent molecular mass of 130 or 85 kDa is likely to be responsible for the [^{3}H]Ins(1,4,5)P$_3$-binding activity. When there is little contamination of the purified sample with lower molecular weight proteins, further purification is most efficiently achieved by applying each sample to a TSK-DEAE-5PW (Tosoh, Tokyo, Japan) column (0.75 × 7.5 cm) mounted in a high-performance liquid chromatography (HPLC) system, as shown in Figs. 4 and 5, respectively.

Summary of Purification

Table I summarizes the purification procedures for the [^{3}H]Ins(1,4,5)P$_3$-bind-ing proteins. The purification was most satisfactory with Ins(1,4,5)P$_3$ affinity chromatography, and the subsequent gel-filtration chromatography separated the two binding activities with moderate purification. When an Ins(1,4,5)P$_3$ affinity column was used, the total binding activity in a 2 M NaCl eluate from the column was 20- to 30-fold over that obtained using the cytosol. These findings suggest that the crude cytosol fraction may have contained inhibitory factor(s) removable by application to an affinity column. Subse-quent anion-exchange chromatography led to further purification, as assessed by SDS–polyacrylamide gel electrophoresis; however, the specific binding was little improved.

The same Ins(1,4,5)P$_3$-binding proteins as purified from the brain cytosol were also isolated from Triton extracts of the brain membranes, using the affinity column (M. Hirata et al., manuscript in preparation). In this case, however, the Ins(1,4,5)P$_3$ receptor responsible for Ca^{2+} release present in the extract bound to the column, thereby reducing the binding of the Ins(1,4,5)P$_3$-binding proteins described here. Therefore, the conca-navalin A (Con A) affinity chromatography was required as a preaffinity chromatography step, because the well-known Ins(1,4,5)P$_3$ receptor is a glycoprotein, whereas the Ins(1,4,5)P$_3$-binding proteins passed through the column.

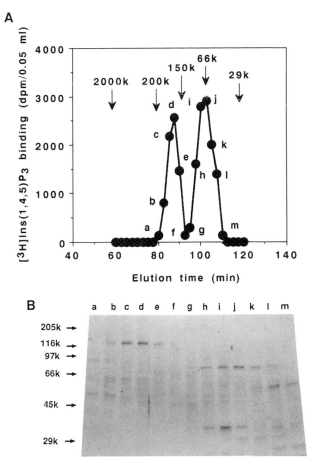

FIG. 3 Gel-filtration chromatography of active fractions eluted from the Ins(1,4,5)P₃ affinity column. (A) The second to fifth tubes eluted from an Ins(1,4,5)P₃ column with 2 M NaCl contained [³H]Ins(1,4,5)P₃-binding activities, and the mixture (~8 ml) was applied to a HiLoad 26/60 Superdex 200 column, equilibrated with a solution containing 0.3 M NaCl, 10 mM HEPES/NaOH (pH 7.2), 2 mM NaN₃, and 10 mM 2-mercaptoethanol. The flow rate was 120 ml/hr, and each fraction was collected over a 2.5-min period. Fifty microliters of each fraction was assayed for [³H]Ins(1,4,5)P₃-binding activity. Each value is the mean of duplicate determinations. Molecular weight markers used were blue dextran (2000K), β-amylase (200K), alcohol dehydrogenase (150K), bovine serum albumin (66K), and carbonate dehydratase (29K). (B) SDS–polyacrylamide gel electrophoresis of each fraction designated in A. Twenty microliters of each fraction was boiled with 5 μl of a 5× concentrated sample buffer containing SDS and 2-mercaptoethanol. Electrophoresis was carried out on an 8% (w/v) polyacrylamide gel, and kits were used to silver stain the gel. [Adapted, with permission, from Kanematsu et al. (11).]

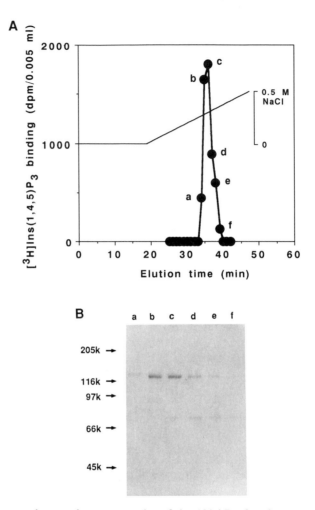

FIG. 4   Anion-exchange chromatography of the 130-kDa fraction separated by gel-filtration chromatography. (A) Fractions designated in Fig. 3 as b–e were collected and applied to a TSK-DEAE-5PW column (0.75 × 7.5 cm) equilibrated with a solution containing 10 mM HEPES/NaOH (pH 7.2), 2 mM NaN$_3$, 10 mM 2-mercaptoethanol, and 1 mM EDTA. A gradient with 0.5 M NaCl was made. Five microliters of each fraction was assayed for binding of [^{3}H]Ins(1,4,5)P$_3$. (B) SDS–polyacrylamide gel electrophoresis of each fraction designated in A. Electrophoresis was performed as described for Fig. 3.

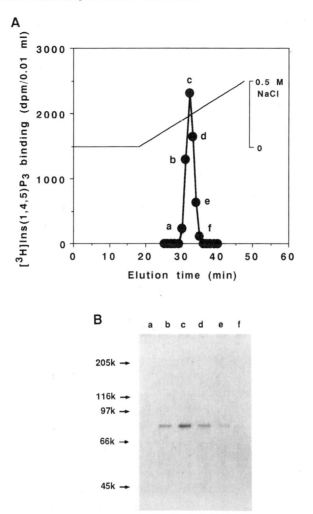

FIG. 5   Anion-exchange chromatography of the 85-kDa fraction separated by gel-filtration chromatography. (A) Fractions designated in Fig. 3 as i–k were collected and applied to a TSK-DEAE-5PW column (0.75 × 7.5 cm) equilibrated with a solution containing 10 mM HEPES/NaOH (pH 7.2), 2 mM NaN₃, 10 mM 2-mercaptoethanol, and 1 mM EDTA. A gradient with 0.5 M NaCl was made. Ten microliters of each fraction was assayed for binding of [³H]Ins(1,4,5)P₃. (B) SDS–polyacrylamide gel electrophoresis of each fraction designated in A. Electrophoresis was performed as described for Fig. 3.

TABLE I   Purification of [³H]Inositol 1,4,5-Trisphosphate-Binding Proteins from Rat Brain Cytosol[a]

Fraction	Protein (mg)	Specific binding (pmol/mg)	Total binding (pmol)	Purification (-fold)	Yield
Cytosol	188	0.011	2.1	1	1
Affinity chromatography	0.2	313	66.5	28,000	32
Gel filtration chromatography					
130-kDa protein	0.019	784	14.9	71,000	7.1
85-kDa protein	0.020	1530	30.6	139,000	14.6
DEAE chromatography					
130-kDa protein	0.013	750	9.8	68,000	4.7
85-kDa protein	0.015	1500	22.5	136,000	10.7

[a] Cytosol fraction obtained from 10 rat brains was used as starting material. Adapted, with permission, from Kanematsu *et al.* (11).

Properties of Cytosolic Inositol 1,4,5-Trisphosphate-Binding Proteins

Identification of Cytosolic Inositol 1,4,5-Trisphosphate-Binding Proteins

The possibility that the cytosolic Ins(1,4,5)P₃-binding proteins purified here are the proteolytic products of the well-characterized membranous Ins(1,4,5)P₃ receptor should be addressed. For this purpose, several peptides have been isolated after lysylendopeptidase digestion and then sequenced. Three peptides derived from the 130 kDa protein were sequenced (XPLXFMEGNQNTPXF, IVYFMAIIDIXTPYG, and NTETFXNNGLAD-QITEDXAF), and the sequences showed no similarity to those of the rat membrane Ins(1,4,5)P₃ receptor. Sequence similarity was examined using the SWISS-PROT protein database and NBRF protein database, but no similar proteins were found.

Three lysylendopeptidase peptides derived from the 85-kDa protein were also sequenced (TIWQESRK, IIHHSGSMDQRQK, and QGYRHV-HLLSK). The peptide sequences were the same as those of the δ isozyme of phospholipase C (PLC-δ), namely residues 50–57, 128–140, and 728–738, respectively. Thus, the 130-kDa protein is likely to be a newly identified Ins(1,4,5)P₃-binding protein, whereas the 85-kDa protein capable of binding Ins(1,4,5)P₃ is PLC-δ. PLC activity in each fraction obtained by gel-filtration chromatography and anion-exchange chromatography was assayed using [³H]phosphatidylinositol 4,5-bisphosphate as a substrate. The high PLC activities corresponded with the [³H]Ins(1,4,5)P₃-binding activities attributed

TABLE II   Binding Specificity of Inositol
1,4,5-Trisphosphate-Binding Proteins[a]

Inositol phosphate	IC$_{50}$ (nM)		
	130-kDa protein	85-kDa protein	Ins(1,4,5)P₃ receptor
Ins(1,4,5)P₃	2.4	5.9	6.3
Ins(3,4,5,6)P₄	4.8	32	600
Ins(1:2cyc,4,5)P₃	8.6	24	30
Ins(1,3,4,5)P₄	21	25	43
Ins(2,4,5)P₃	30	230	100
Ins(1,3,4,5,6)P₅	55	150	1000
Ins(1,3,4,6)P₄	180	90	170

[a] Various concentrations of inositol phosphates were incubated with purified samples of the 130- or 85-kDa proteins. The well-known Ins(1,4,5)P₃ receptor was also examined for comparison. Inositol phosphates used were chemically synthesized (12) and were racemic mixtures, except for Ins(1,4,5)P₃ and Ins(1:2-cyclic,4,5)P₃. Data for the 130-kDa protein were modified, with permission, from Kanematsu *et al.* (11).

to the 85-kDa protein, thereby confirming that the 85kDa protein is indeed PLC-δ (11).

Properties of Cytosolic Inositol 1,4,5-Trisphosphate-Binding Proteins

A wide variety of synthesized inositol phosphates have been examined for potency in inhibiting the binding of [³H]Ins(1,4,5)P₃. In the 130-kDa protein, noteworthy was the finding that Ins(3,4,5,6)P₄ was as potent as Ins(1,4,5)P₃, the order of potency being Ins(1,4,5)P₃ = Ins(3,4,5,6)P₄ > Ins(1:2cyc,4,5)P₃ > Ins(1,3,4,5)P₄ = Ins(2,4,5)P₃ > Ins(1,3,4,6)P₄ = Ins(1,3,4,5,6)P₅ > Ins(1,3,4)P₃. Ins(1,2,4,5)P₄ was equipotent to Ins(1,4,5)P₃ and Ins(3,4,5,6)P₄ (data not shown). On the other hand, in the 85-kDa protein, Ins(3,4,5,6)P₄ was not so potent as Ins(1,4,5)P₃ but was equipotent to Ins(1,3,4,5)P₄. Another difference from that seen with the 130-kDa protein was the potency of Ins(2,4,5)P₃, which was less potent. Table II summarizes the IC$_{50}$ values of a wide variety of inositol phosphates examined for the potential to inhibit the binding of [³H]Ins(1,4,5)P₃. These values were also determined for comparison with the well-known Ins(1,4,5)P₃ receptor.

The pH profiles for [³H]Ins(1,4,5)P₃ binding to the three Ins(1,4,5)P₃-binding proteins were determined (Fig. 6). Binding to the Ins(1,4,5)P₃ receptor increased as the pH value increased, whereas that to the 130- or 85-kDa protein was maximal at pH 8.3 and then declined at a more alkaline pH.

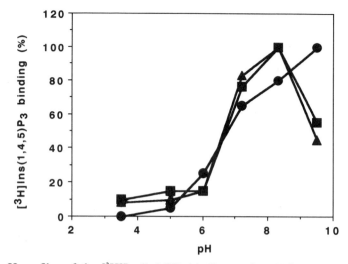

FIG. 6   pH profiles of the [^{3}H]Ins(1,4,5)P$_3$ binding to the 130-kDa protein, 85-kDa protein, or Ins(1,4,5)P$_3$ receptor. The pH values were changed during the assay of [^{3}H]Ins(1,4,5)P$_3$ binding to the 130-kDa (■) and 85-kDa proteins (▲). The Ins(1,4,5)P$_3$ receptor was also examined for comparison (●). The pH values of 3.5, 5.0, and 6.0, of 7.2, and of 8.3 and 9.5 were achieved with MES/NaOH, HEPES/NaOH, and Tris-HCl, respectively. Each point is the mean of three determinations.

Conclusion

We have prepared Ins(1,4,5)P$_3$ affinity matrices; two Ins(1,4,5)P$_3$-binding proteins in rat brain cytosolic fractions were purified. The apparent molecular masses, as estimated on SDS–polyacrylamide gel electrophoresis, were 130- and 85-kDa, respectively. Partial amino acid sequence determinations following proteolysis and reversed-phase HPLC revealed that the 85-kDa protein is the δ isozyme of PLC, and the 130-kDa protein appears to be a newly identified Ins(1,4,5)P$_3$-binding protein. Biological functions and structural features of the 130-kDa protein are the subjects of ongoing studies.

Acknowledgments

This work was supported by funding from The Kato Memorial Bioscience Foundation, The Ichiro Kanehara Foundation, and from a Grant-in-Aid for Scientific Research from the Ministry of Education, Science, and Culture of Japan.

References

1. M. J. Berridge and R. F. Irvine, *Nature* (*London*) **312,** 315 (1984).
2. S. B. Shears, *Biochem. J.* **260,** 313 (1989).
3. R. F. Irvine, A. J. Letcher, J. P. Heslop, and M. J. Berridge, *Nature* (*London*) **320,** 631 (1986).
4. S. Supattapone, P. F. Worley, J. M. Baraban, and S. H. Snyder, *J. Biol. Chem.* **263,** 1530 (1988).
5. T. Furuichi, S. Yoshikawa, A. Miyawaki, K. Wada, N. Maeda, and K. Mikoshiba, *Nature* (*London*) **342,** 32 (1989).
6. M. Hirata, T. Sasaguri, T. Hamachi, T. Hashimoto, M. Kukita, and T. Koga, *Nature* (*London*) **317,** 723 (1985).
7. R. F. Irvine, R. O. Brown, and M. J. Berridge, *Biochem. J.* **221,** 269 (1984).
8. M. Hirata, Y. Watanabe, T. Ishimatsu, T. Ikebe, Y. Kimura, K. Yamaguchi, S. Ozaki, and T. Koga, *J. Biol. Chem.* **264,** 20303 (1989).
9. M. Hirata, F. Yanaga, T. Koga, T. Ogasawara, Y. Watanabe, and S. Ozaki, *J. Biol. Chem.* **265,** 8404 (1990).
10. M. Hirata, Y. Watanabe, T. Ishimatsu, F. Yanaga, T. Koga, and S. Ozaki, *Biochem. Biophys. Res. Commun.* **168,** 379 (1990).
11. T. Kanematsu, H. Takeya, Y. Watanabe, S. Ozaki, M. Yoshida, T. Koga, S. Iwanaga, and M. Hirata, *J. Biol. Chem.* **267,** 6518 (1992).
12. S. Ozaki and Y. Watanabe, *in* "Inositol Phosphates and Derivatives" (A. B. Reitz, ed.), ACS Symp. Ser. No. 463, p. 43. American Chemical Society, Washington, D.C., 1991.

[26] Inositol 1,4,5-Trisphosphate Phosphatase and Kinase from Brain

Christophe Erneux, Kazunaga Takazawa, and Benoît Verjans

Introduction

Inositol 1,4,5-trisphosphate [Ins(1,4,5)P_3; IP_3] is metabolized by two routes, namely, IP_3-5-phosphatase (5-phosphatase) and IP_3-3-kinase (3-kinase), the products of which are inositol 1,4-bisphosphate [Ins(1,4)P_2] and inositol 1,3,4,5-tetrakisphosphate [Ins(1,3,4,5)P_4; IP_4], respectively (reviewed in Ref. 1). Both enzymes are possible candidates for physiological or pharmacological control of IP_3/IP_4 levels. The approaches that we have used to understanding these complex systems are to obtain specific cDNA clones for the proteins (2), to compare their sequences with other kinase(s) or phosphatase(s), and to study their expression by *in situ* hybridization (3). Because 5-phosphatase and 3-kinase are more active in brain than in any other tissue, brain was chosen as starting material for purification. Our strategy was to purify the protein in high yield and then prepare antibodies and/or microsequences to screen cDNA libraries from brain. To demonstrate that 5-phosphatase or 3-kinase is associated with a given protein band on sodium dodecyl sulfate (SDS) gels, regeneration of activities was performed after SDS-polyacrylamide gel electrophoresis (4–6). We propose the existence of three distinct 5-phosphatases: types I and II are present in rat or bovine brain (7), and type III has been purified in platelets ($M_r = 75,000$) and cloned (8). 3-Kinase appears to exist in two forms: 3-kinase A is present in rat (2), bovine, and human brain, and 3-kinase B has been isolated as a cDNA clone from a human hippocampus cDNA library (9). 3-Kinases A and B are associated with different genes on different chromosomes.

Assay of Enzymatic Activities

5-Phosphatase is incubated in 50 mM HEPES (pH 7.4), 2 mM $MgCl_2$, 48 mM mercaptoethanol, 1 mg/ml bovine serum albumin (BSA, >92% pure, Serva, Heidelberg, Germany), 30 μM cold IP_3, and [^{3}H]IP_3 (specific activity 17 Ci/mmol from NEN, Boston, MA) in a final volume of 0.1 ml. IP_3 is provided by Sigma (St. Louis, MO) and is checked to be 86% pure. Crude soluble enzymatic preparations of bovine brain are diluted 50-fold in 50 mM HEPES

Methods in Neurosciences, Volume 18

(pH 7.4), 2 mM MgCl$_2$, 48 mM mercaptoethanol, and 1 mg/ml BSA; 10 μl of this dilution is used for each assay per tube. Each sample is incubated at 37°C for 8 min, stopped by the addition of 1 ml of 0.1 M HCOOH, 0.4 M NH$_4$COOH, and then loaded on a 0.2-ml column of AG 1-X8 resin (200–400 mesh), formate form (10). Hydrolyzed inositol phosphates are eluted in 4 ml of 0.1 M HCOOH, 0.4 M NH$_4$COOH; the remaining [^{3}H]IP$_3$ is eluted in 5 ml of 0.1 M HCOOH, 0.8 M NH$_4$COOH. Ten milliliters of Instagel (Packard, Groningen, The Netherlands) is added to estimate radioactivity.

No 3-kinase activity is detected under these conditions. In crude samples, Ins(1,4)P$_2$ formed by 5-phosphatase is partially hydrolyzed to inositol 4-phosphate [Ins(4)P]. This is why we do not separate [^{3}H]Ins(4)P and [^{3}H]Ins(1,4)P$_2$ after incubation. 5-Phosphatase activity is linear for up to 10 min of incubation. [5-^{32}P]Ins(1,4,5)P$_3$ can also be used as substrate; in this case, a buffer containing 0.1 M HCOOH, 0.2 M NH$_4$COOH is used to stop the reaction and elute the reaction product, radiolabeled inorganic phosphate (^{32}P$_i$). The column separation technique is tested with standards of [^{3}H]Ins(1,4)P$_2$ and [^{3}H]Ins(1,4,5)P$_3$; blank values of 5-phosphatase assay usually range between 3 and 7% of the total radioactivity present in each tube.

3-Kinase is assayed by measuring the production of IP$_4$ from IP$_3$. The incubation mixture (0.1 ml) contains 84 mM HEPES/NaOH (pH 7.5), 1 mg/ml BSA, 1 mM ATP, 20 mM MgCl$_2$, 2.5–12.5 mM 2,3-bisphosphoglycerate, 1 mM EGTA, 1 μM calmodulin (CaM) (or water), and 10 μM IP$_3$ and [^{3}H]IP$_3$ (11). Ca^{2+} is added to adjust the free Ca^{2+} concentration to 10 μM when CaM is added to the incubation mixture. Each assay tube also contains 2-mercaptoethanol (0.84 μl/ml). The reaction is initiated by adding the enzyme, followed by an incubation of 8–10 min at 37°C. The rat brain crude enzyme in homogenates is diluted 100-fold (final dilution) in 84 mM HEPES/NaOH (pH 7.5), 0.1% Triton X-100, 2-mercaptoethanol (0.84 μl/ml). Each sample reaction is stopped by adding 1 ml of ice-cold 0.1 M HCOOH, 0.4 M NH$_4$COOH and loaded on a 0.6-ml AG 1-X8 column. Each column is washed with 3 ml of the same buffer, then 20 ml of 0.1 M HCOOH, 0.7 M NH$_4$COOH, and [^{3}H]IP$_4$ is eluted in 5 ml of 0.1 M HCOOH, 1.2 M NH$_4$COOH. The incubation mixture is sometimes supplemented with 0.1% Triton X-100 to stabilize the enzyme. We verify by three dilutions the linearity of the assay with respect to protein concentration. Blank values are of 3–4% of the radioactivity present in each tube. 2,3-Bisphosphoglycerate is added to block 5-phosphatase activity.

Assay in Sodium Dodecyl Sulfate Solutions

Purified 5-phosphatase and crude rat brain 3-kinase retain some activity even after denaturation by SDS (4, 5). We have studied the effect of various concentrations of SDS 5-phosphatase or 3-kinase activities in an incubation mixture containing Triton X-100 (1%) for 30–60 min of incubation at 37°C. The experiments are done by mixing enzyme with SDS (up to 2%, v/v), followed by dilution of the mixture in buffer with 0.1% Triton X-100. Triton (0.5–1%) by itself has no effect on enzymatic activity. In the presence of SDS, however, activity rapidly decreases; this effect is partly reversed by the addition of Triton X-100. Under these conditions, SDS gel electrophoresis identifies 5-phosphatase as a 43-kDa polypeptide (4) and 3-kinase as a 50-kDa polypeptide (5). Stimulation by Ca^{2+}-calmodulin is still maintained provided that the final SDS concentration is below 0.01% in an incubation mixture containing 1% Triton. Triton by itself does not prevent the interaction of 3-kinase with calmodulin.

Preparation of Resins for Assay and Purification

Dowex AG 1-X8

After swelling in water, the Dowex resin (Bio-Rad, Richmond, CA) is washed with 1 M NaOH (50–100 times the total gel volume) until a silver nitrate test for chloride is negative. The resin is then washed with 2 volumes of water followed by 4 volumes of 1 M HCOOH so that the pH of the eluate is below 2. Finally, the resin is washed with water until the pH reaches 4 to 5. The resin is recovered after assay, pooled, stirred for 1 hr in 0.1 M HCOOH, 1.5 M NH$_4$COOH, and reprepared as before. In this case, 1 volume of NaOH is generally sufficient to remove traces of chloride.

DEAE-Sephacel

DEAE-Sephacel resin (Pharmacia, Piscataway, NJ) is placed in a glass funnel (20 × 20 cm), washed with 2 volumes of water, and then washed with 5 volumes of 10 mM Tris-HCl, pH 8. Before use, the resin is equilibrated in DEAE buffer (see below). After use, it is washed with 4 volumes of 0.1 M NaOH, 2 volumes of water, and 10 mM Tris/HCl, pH 8, until the eluate reaches a pH of 8 to 8.5.

Blue-Sepharose

Blue-Sepharose resin (Pharmacia) is equilibrated by an overnight run of Blue Sepharose buffer (see below) at 100 ml/hr. After use, the column is washed with 150 ml of 2 M NaCl solution in the same buffer and reequilibrated for 6 hr in low-salt buffer.

Phosphocellulose

Phosphocellulose (Whatman, Clifton, NJ) is swollen in water, then washed in 25 volumes of 0.5 *N* NaOH for 5 min. This is followed by water to decrease the pH (<11). The resin is then washed in 25 volumes of 0.5 *N* HCl for 5 min, filtered, and washed with water to increase the pH (>3).

Purification of Type I Inositol 1,4,5-Trisphosphate-5-Phosphatase

The six purification steps are described in Verjans *et al.* (12). All operations are carried out at 4°C. Three fresh bovine brains are homogenized in a Teflon/ glass homogenizer in 1 liter of 20 m*M* Tris-HCl, pH 8.3, 0.25 *M* sucrose, 24 m*M* 2-mercaptoethanol, and protease inhibitors 5 μ*M* leupeptin (Sigma) and 50 mg/liter phenylmethylsulfonyl fluoride (Sigma) or Pefabloc (Pentapharm, Basle, Switzerland). After a 20,000 *g* centrifugation for 60 min (GSA rotor, 11,000 rpm), the supernatant is removed and kept; the pellet is resuspended in 1 liter of the same buffer and recentrifuged. Supernatants are pooled and diluted 2-fold in DEAE buffer (20 m*M* Tris-HCl, pH 8.3, 0.1 m*M* EDTA, 12 m*M* 2-mercaptoethanol, 10% glycerol, and protease inhibitors). It is important to achieve a pH of 8.3; otherwise, type I 5-phosphatase will not bind to the DEAE-Sephacel. If the pH is too low, it is adjusted with a saturated solution of Tris. DEAE resin (1 liter) must also be well equilibrated in buffer before mixing with crude enzyme. After 90 min of gentle stirring, the resin is filtered on a glass funnel (20 × 20 cm) and washed with 5 liters of DEAE buffer. For efficient protein binding, the resin must have a strong pink color. After resuspension, the resin is packed by gravity into the column (60 × 50 cm). A 2.4-liter (total volume) linear gradient from 0 to 0.5 *M* NaCl at a flow rate of 175 ml/hr is used to elute the enzyme. The volume of each fraction is about 20 to 25 ml (500 drops). Elution is performed overnight; the column can run dry. Fractions are assayed at a 1:600 dilution, and the protein content (absorbance at 280 nm) is measured on samples diluted 1:10. Type I enzyme activity is eluted with 60.1 ± 8.1% (mean ± S.D., *n* = 20) of total recovery.

The pooled fractions from the first step are made up to 2 liters in BD buffer (20 m*M* Tris-HCl, pH 7.5, 0.1 m*M* EGTA, 2 m*M* MgCl₂ 10% glycerol, and protease inhibitors) to decrease the salt concentration. This solution is loaded overnight onto a Blue-Sepharose column (26 × 2.5 cm). The column is washed with 150 ml of buffer. The enzyme is eluted with a linear 0–0.8 *M* NaCl gradient (400 ml) at a flow rate of 150 ml/hr. Fractions (10–12 ml) are assayed at a 1:600 dilution; activity comigrates with the major eluted peak as measured by optical density at 280 nm. Pooled peak fractions are concentrated to 15 ml in a 200-ml Amicon (Danvers, MA) ultrafiltration cell with a PM10 membrane. The concentrate is applied onto two Sephacryl S-200 columns in series (75 × 2.5 cm each), equilibrated with 20 mM Tris-HCl, pH 7.5, 1 mM EDTA, 100 mM NaCl, 10% (v/v) glycerol, and protease inhibitors. Some batches of Sephacryl can be used for several runs without an apparent decrease in efficiency, but others give broader protein peaks after a few runs. The enzyme is eluted at a flow rate of 50 ml/hr. Fractions (5 ml) are assayed after 1 : 750 dilution, and the pooled activity is concentrated to 7.5 ml in a 50-ml Amicon ultrafiltration cell. The resulting solution is diluted 1 : 2 in 10 mM Tris-HCl, pH 7.5, 10 mM KCl, 3 mM 2-mercaptoethanol, 10% glycerol, and protease inhibitors and applied to a phosphocellulose column (15 × 0.9 cm) at a flow rate of 15 ml/hr. The resin is washed with 10 ml of the last buffer and the enzyme eluted with a 80-ml linear gradient of 0–0.25 M sodium phosphate, pH 7.6. Phosphocellulose chromatography is performed at pH 7.5, owing to the fact that enzyme does not bind to the column at higher pH. The flow rate has to be very low (10 to 15 ml/hr maximum) in order to avoid compression of column resulting in a deceased flow rate.

At this step, total activity is approximately 20–30 μmol/min at 37°C and 30 μM IP$_3$ (3–5 mg of protein). Two or three preparations, depending on total activity (>40 μmol/min), are pooled, concentrated to 5 ml, and dialyzed overnight against 1 liter BD buffer without MgCl$_2$ to avoid proteolysis. The enzymes is diluted 1 : 6 in BD buffer, and [MgCl$_2$] is adjusted to 2 mM. The sample is applied to a Blue-Sepharose column (5 × 0.7 cm). The resin is washed with 10 ml of BD buffer and the enzyme eluted with a 44 ml (total volume) linear gradient of 0–10 mM 2,3-bisphosphoglycerate (flow rate 15 ml/hr). With fresh resin, the enzyme elutes at about 3 mM 2,3-bisphosphoglycerate. In this last step, we avoid using EGTA to prevent precipitation in the presence of acetonitrile/trifluoroacetic acid (see below). The resulting preparation generally contains a 2000-fold purified IP$_3$-5-phosphatase with 5 to 10% recovery and a total activity (at 30 μM IP$_3$) between 10 and 40 μmol/min/mg of protein. Kinetic constants are determined; a typical purified preparation has a K_m for IP$_3$ of 10.5 ± 1.8 μM and a V_{max} for IP$_3$ of 27.6 ± 4.2 μmol/min/mg of protein (means ± S.D., $n = 4$).

The last purification step is performed by high-performance liquid chromatography (HPLC) using a C$_{18}$ reversed-phase column (8P300 RP column from Chrompack, Antwerp, Belgium, 15 × 0.46 cm). We use an acetonitrile gradient to elute the activity with two solutions. The first contains 5% acetonitrile and 0.9% trifluoroacetic acid, the second 95% acetonitrile and a concentration of trifluoroacetic acid that allows suppression of the difference in absorbance at 214 nm between both solutions [~0.8% (v/v) trifluoroacetic acid]. After loading of the sample, the absorbance must be allowed to return to basal levels before the gradient is started. After an elution time of 1 min, the acetonitrile concentration is approximately 35%, this step is followed by a second one involving a 0.5% acetonitrile increase per minute from 35 to 55% acetonitrile (during 40 min). The 5-phosphatase is eluted at 46% acetonitrile and its identity checked by SDS–polyacrylamide gel electrophoresis and 5-phosphatase assay. The protein content of the HPLC peaks can be estimated either by calibration of the column with BSA or by determination of the protein percentage corresponding to each peak. The final yield is 50–100 μg of pure 5-phosphatase with an estimated V_{max} between 300 and 500 μmol/min/mg of 5-phosphatase. This material is sufficient for microsequence determination.

Purification of Rat Brain Inositol 1,4,5-Trisphosphate-3-Kinase

Purification of rat brain IP$_3$-3-kinase is described in Takazawa et al. (13). A typical procedure is given below.

Rat brain (80 g) is homogenized at 4°C in 240 ml (3 volumes) of 20 mM Tris-HCl (pH 7.5), 1 mM EDTA, 0.25 M sucrose, 24 mM 2-mercaptoethanol containing protease inhibitors (0.4 mM phenylmethylsulfonyl fluoride and 5 μM leupeptin). The homogenate is centrifuged at 35,000 g (SA 600 rotor, 15,000 rpm) for 60 min at 4°C, and the supernatants are pooled. The particulate fraction is resuspended in the same buffer, homogenized, and centrifuged for 60 min as before. The supernatants are removed and combined with the supernatants of the first centrifugation (total volume 400 ml; OD$_{280}$ 8.37). Twenty-six milliliters of 5 M NaCl is added to reach a final salt concentration of 0.3 M. The crude soluble fraction is applied to a Blue-Sepharose column (5 × 10 cm, ~215 ml resin) equilibrated with 20 mM Tris-HCl (pH 7.5), 1 mM EDTA, 0.02% Triton X-100, 24 mM 2-mercaptoethanol, and protease inhibitors (buffer A). The column is washed with buffer A made 0.8 M in NaCl and 0.03% in Triton X-100. The 3-kinase is eluted with 2.5 M NaCl and 1% Triton X-100. Recovery is 50% or 6.6 μmol/min as measured in the presence of Ca^{2+}/CaM and 10 μM InsP$_3$. The elution of the enzyme is largely influenced by both salt and detergent concentrations.

The enzyme, in a volume of approximately 275 ml, is dialyzed overnight against 1.5 liters of 10 mM Tris-HCl (pH 7.5), 10 mM KCl, 0.01% Triton X-100, 12 mM 2-mercaptoethanol, and protease inhibitors (buffer B), with two changes of buffer, and applied to a phosphocellulose column (20 ml of resin) equilibrated in buffer B. The column is washed with buffer B containing 150 mM potassium phosphate until no protein is further eluted (i.e., with 75 ml). The IP$_3$-3-kinase is eluted with 500 mM potassium phosphate in buffer B.

Two fractions of 32 and 10 ml are recovered. The 32-ml fraction has 2.8 μmol/min 3-kinase activity (49% recovery). It is adjusted to 0.1% Triton X-100 with a 20% stock solution of detergent and to 0.5 mM CaCl$_2$ with a

10 mM stock solution. The sample is applied to a CaM-Sepharose column (20 ml of resin) equilibrated with 20 mM Tris-HCl (pH 7.5), 0.2 mM CaCl$_2$, 0.1% Triton X-100, 0.4 M NaCl, 12 mM 2-mercaptoethanol, and protease inhibitors (buffer C). The column is first washed with 50 ml of buffer C made 0.5% in Triton X-100, then with 75 ml of buffer C without detergent, and subsequently eluted with 100 ml of 20 mM Tris-HCl (pH 7.5), 2 mM EGTA, 0.1 M NaCl, 12 mM 2-mercaptoethanol, and protease inhibitors (buffer D). The IP$_3$-3-kinase is eluted in buffer D containing 0.2% SDS and no NaCl. The yield of the last step is 598 nmol/min (29% of activity applied on the column). Pooled peak fractions are immediately concentrated to approximately 1 ml using an Amicon PM10 ultrafiltration membrane and verified to be pure by SDS–polyacrylamide gel electrophoresis.

Acknowledgments

This work was supported by grants from Boehringer Ingelheim (Bender and Co., Vienna, Austria), the Ministère de la Politique Scientifique (PAI), and Sciences de la Vie. We thank R. Lecocq and C. Moreau for cooperation and many helpful discussions. B. Verjans is supported by the Fonds National de la Recherche Scientifique (FNRS).

References

1. C. Erneux and K. Takazawa, *Trends Pharmacol. Sci.* **12,** 174 (1991).
2. K. Takazawa, J. Vandekerckhove, J. E. Dumont, and C. Erneux, *Biochem J.* **272,** 107 (1990).
3. P. Mailleux, K. Takazawa, C. Erneux, and J. J. Vanderhaeghen, *J. Neurochem.* **56,** 345 (1991).
4. M. Lemos, J. E. Dumont, and C. Erneux, *FEBS Lett.* **249,** 321 (1989).
5. K. Takazawa, H. Passareiro, J. E. Dumont, and C. Erneux, *Biochem. J.* **261,** 483 (1989).
6. O. Gabriel and D. M. Gersten, *Anal. Biochem.* **203,** 1 (1992).
7. C. Erneux, M. Lemos, B. Verjans, P. Vanderhaeghen, A. Delvaux, and J. E. Dumont, *Eur. J. Biochem.* **181,** 317 (1989).
8. T. S. Ross, A. Bennett-Jefferson, C. A. Mitchell, and P. W. Majerus, *J. Biol. Chem.* **266,** 20283 (1991).
9. K. Takazawa, J. Perret, J. E. Dumont, and C. Erneux, *Biochem. J.* **278,** 883 (1991).
10. C. Erneux, A. Delvaux, C. Moreau, and J. E. Dumont, *Biochem. Biophys. Res. Commun.* **134,** 351 (1986).

11. K. Takazawa, H. Passareiro, J. E. Dumont, and C. Erneux, *Biochem. Biophys. Res. Commun.* **153,** 632 (1988).

12. B. Verjans, R. Lecocq, C. Moreau, and C. Erneux, *Eur. J. Biochem.* **204,** 1083 (1992).

13. K. Takazawa, M. Lemos, A. Delvaux, C. Lejeune, J. E. Dumont, and C. Erneux, *Biochem. J.* **268,** 213 (1990).

[27]   Synthesis of ^{32}P-Labeled Phosphoinositides
and Inositol Phosphates: Characterization
and Purification of Inositol
1,3,4,5-Tetrakisphosphate-3-phosphatase
from Brain

Ariane Höer and Eckard Oberdisse

Introduction

Inositol 1,3,4,5-tetrakisphosphate-3-phosphatase [Ins(1,3,4,5)P$_4$-3-phosphatase] is one of the numerous inositol polyphosphate phosphatases that dephosphorylates inositol 1,3,4,5-tetrakisphosphate [Ins(1,3,4,5)P$_4$] to inositol 1,4,5-trisphosphate [Ins(1,4,5)P$_3$].* Ins(1,4,5)P$_3$ is well established as an intracellular second messenger which releases Ca^{2+} from intracellular stores (1). It is mainly a product of phosphatidylinositol 4,5-bisphosphate [PtdIns(4,5)P$_2$] degradation by phospholipase C enzymes that are activated by hormones, neurotransmitters, or growth factors via guanine nucleotide-binding proteins (G proteins) or receptor-coupled tyrosine kinases (2, 3). Ins(1,4,5)P$_3$ is dephosphorylated by a specific Ins(1,4,5)P$_3$/Ins(1,3,4,5)P$_4$-5-phosphatase, or it is phosphorylated by a 3-kinase to Ins(1,3,4,5)P$_4$ (4) which is then dephosphorylated by the same Ins(1,4,5)P$_3$/Ins(1,3,4,5)P$_4$-5-phosphatase, yielding Ins(1,4,5)P$_3$. This was long thought to be the only way of Ins(1,3,4,5)P$_4$ degradation. The existence of a 3-dephosphorylation of Ins(1,3,4,5)P$_4$ was discovered in the following cells and tissues: erythrocytes, platelets, lymphatic cells, brain, liver, parotic gland, and kidney (5–12). As yet the enzyme has only been detected in cytosol after ion-exchange chromatography, in permeabilized cells, or in membranes. The reason for this is that the Ins(1,3,4,5)P$_4$-3-phosphatase is inhibited by very low concentrations of inositol 1,3,4,5,6-pentakisphosphate [Ins(1,3,4,5,6)P$_5$] and inositol hexakisphosphate (IP$_6$) (12, 13), and these inositol polyphosphates are present in high concentrations in the cytosol (4, 14). Recent investigations have shown that Ins(1,3,4,5,6)P$_5$ and IP$_6$ are also substrates of the Ins(1,3,4,5)P$_4$-3-phosphatase (15).

---

* Inositol phosphates are designated according to IUPAC nomenclature, with reference to the 1-D-phosphate [*Biochem. J.* **258**, 1 (1989)].

Methods in Neurosciences, Volume 18

In this chapter we describe the preparation of the substrate [5-^{32}P]Ins(1,3,4,5)P$_4$ for the Ins(1,3,4,5)P$_4$-3-phosphatase and a standard assay to determine Ins(1,3,4,5)P$_4$-3-phosphatase activity. We also describe the enrichment of the enzyme from porcine brain as well as the removal of inositol polyphosphates by anion-exchange chromatography.

Preparation of Substrates

The easiest way to measure the 3-phosphatase activity is via incubation with [5-^{32}P]Ins(1,3,4,5)P$_4$. The synthesis of the compound starts with the preparation of [γ-^{32}P]ATP, which is used for the phosphorylation of phosphatidylinositol 4-phosphate [PtdIns(4)P] by a PtdIns(4)P 5-kinase to get [5-^{32}P]PtdIns(4,5)P$_2$. In the next step [5-^{32}P]Ins(1,4,5)P$_3$ is prepared from [5-^{32}P]PtdIns(4,5)P$_2$, and finally [5-^{32}P]Ins(1,3,4,5)P$_4$ is synthesized from [5-^{32}P]Ins(1,4,5)P$_3$ by an Ins(1,4,5)P$_3$ 3-kinase.

Preparation of [γ-^{32}P]ATP

The synthesis of [γ-^{32}P]ATP is a slight modification of the method described by Johnson and Walseth (16). The advantage of our modification is that the [γ-^{32}P]ATP will be in a small volume. The following solutions are necessary.

100 mM Tris-HCl, pH 9.0
0.5 M dithiothreitol (DTT)
Reaction mixture A (Table I)
    These solutions can be stored at −20°C for several months
1 mM ADP
10 mM Pyruvate
    Each of these compounds is dissolved in 100 mM Tris-HCl, pH 9.0, and must be prepared freshly
Enzyme mixture: The enzyme mixture is prepared exactly as described by Johnson and Walseth (16). From this mixture 24 μl is centrifuged at 13,000 g at 4°C in a bench-top centrifuge for 10 min. The supernatant is discarded and the pellet suspended in 80 μl of 100 mM Tris-HCl, pH 9.0, and stored on ice until use.
^{32}P$_i$: 5 mCi of phosphorus-32 as orthophosphoric acid (NEX-053C) from NEN/Dupont de Nemours (Boston, MA) is used. The concentration of radioactivity is 500 mCi/2 ml, and 5 mCi will be delivered in a volume of about 3 μl. The vial is centrifuged for 5–10 min to remove

TABLE I   Reaction Mixtures for Synthesis of Radiolabeled Substances

| Reaction mixture[a] | Substance | Concentration in (mM) | |
		In reaction mixture	Resulting final
A	MgCl$_2$	60.0	12.0
	L-α-Glycerol phosphate	4.0	0.8
	β-NAD[b]	2.5	0.5
	DTT	30.0	6.0
	EDTA, pH 8.0	0.5	0.1
	Tris-HCl, pH 9.0	100.0	20.0
B	MgCl$_2$	135.6	22.6
	Spermine	2.4	0.4
	DTT	22.8	3.8
	EGTA	3.0	0.5
	Tris-HCl, pH 7	120.0	20.0
C	KCl	40.0	20.0
	MgCl$_2$	20.0	10.0
	CaCl$_2$	2.4	1.2
	2,3-DPG[c]	6.0	3.0
	EDTA	1.2	0.6
	EGTA	2.0	1.0
	ATP[d]	52.0	26.0
	2-Mercaptoethanol	0.2%	0.1%

[a] All reaction mixtures can be prepared in larger amounts and stored in aliquots of 1 ml at −20°C.

[b] β-Nicotinamide adenine dinucleotide.

[c] 2,3-Diphosphoglyceric acid.

[d] ATP should be added from a stock solution of 100 mM. It is absolutely necessary to adjust the stock solution to pH 7 with NaOH.

radioactive material from the screw cap, and water is added to achieve a final volume of 13.8 μl.

A mixture of the above solutions is prepared as follows:

    6 μl of the ADP solution
    6 μl of the pyruvate solution
    12 μl of reaction mixture A
    2.4 μl of 0.5 mM DTT
    6 μl of the centrifuged enzyme mix

From this mixture, 16.2 μl is added to 13.8 μl of the ^{32}P$_i$ which had been transferred into a 1.5-ml polypropylene tube with screw cap (Sarstedt, 72.692, Nümbrecht-Rommelsdorf, Germany). The tube is briefly vortexed and incubated at 37°C. After 5 min, a pipette tip is dipped into the mixture without suction, and the tip is then dipped into 1 ml of water. The transferred radioactivity will be enough for the charcoal check, which is performed as described by Johnson and Walseth (16). Regularly, the reaction is finished after 10 min when about 99% of the $^{32}P_i$ has been incorporated into [γ-^{32}P]ATP. The reaction is terminated by incubating the closed reaction vial at 96°C for 5 min. After brief centrifugation to remove radioactive material from the cap, the [γ-^{32}P]ATP can be stored at −80°C until use.

Synthesis of [5-^{32}P]Phosphatidylinositol 4,5-Bisphosphate

The following reagents are needed.

>Reaction mixture B (see Table I)
>2 mM ADP (freshly prepared)
>Lipids: L-α-phosphatidylinositol 4-monophosphate [PtdIns(4)P] from Sigma (St. Louis, MO, P 9738) should be purchased in vials containing 1 mg; this amount is dissolved in 1 ml of chloroform/methanol (2 : 1, v/v). The solution can be stored at −20°C. DL-α-Phosphatidyl-L-serine, dipalmitoyl (PtdSer), is from Sigma (P 1902); 5 mg is dissolved in 500 μl of chloroform/methanol (2 : 1, v/v). The PtdSer solution can be stored for 1–2 weeks at −20°C, older solutions should not be used. Before withdrawal of lipids from the vials, these should be brought to room temperature
>For the enrichment of the PtdIns(4)P 5-kinase from rat brain, a Bio-Gel TSK-DEAE-5-PW HPLC column (Bio-Rad, Richmond, CA) and one rat brain are necessary. Rat brains can be frozen in liquid nitrogen and stored at −80°C in a suitable vial without any buffer for at least 1 year. For PtdIns(4)P 5-kinase preparation, a frozen brain is thawed during the homogenization procedure.

Enrichment of Phosphatidylinositol-4-Phosphate 5-Kinase from Rat Brain
PtdIns(4)P 5-kinase is enriched from rat brain exactly as described by Divecha and Irvine (17), using a DEAE high-performance liquid chromatography (HPLC) column. Fractions of 1 ml are collected and assayed for PtdIns(4)P 5-kinase. If a new column is used, check every other fraction from fraction 10 to fraction 60 for kinase activity. After a few runs, you will know when the enzyme will elute, and the number of tested fractions can be reduced. In our hands, it was sufficient to test every other fraction between fractions 30 and 60. After several runs (about 10), the column separation may become

impaired. The column can then be cleaned with pepsin and NaOH as described by Wregett *et al.* (18).

The PtdIns(4)P 5-kinase activity is assayed as follows. In each test tube, 18.75 μl of PtdSer (10 mg/ml) and 50 μl PtdIns(4)P (1 mg/ml) are dried under a stream of nitrogen. To the dried lipids, 21 μl of reaction mixture B, 6.25 μl of 2 mM ADP, and 32.75 μl of water are added, and the mixture is sonicated for 5 min to suspend the lipids. Then 1,000,000 counts/min (cpm) of [γ-^{32}P]ATP in 15 μl of reaction mixture A, which was diluted 1:5 with water, and 50 μl from each fraction to be tested are added to start the reaction. The incubation is carried out for 3 hr at 30°C. Terminating the reaction and phase separation are achieved by the addition of 300 μl of chloroform, 100 μl of 100 mM HCl, 50 μl of methanol, and 25 μl of water. The samples are vigorously vortexed and centrifuged for 10 min at 13,000 g in a bench-top centrifuge. From the upper phase 20 μl is removed for liquid scintillation counting. The rest of the upper phase and the protein pellet between the two phases is discarded, and the organic phase is washed twice with 50 μl of water/methanol (4:1, v/v). Two 20-μl aliquots are drawn from each organic phase for liquid scintillation counting. The radioactivity in the lower phase corresponds to the generated [5-^{32}P]PtdIns(4,5)P$_2$. The fraction with the highest PtdIns(4)P 5-kinase activity is used for the preparative synthesis of [5-^{32}P]PtdIns(4,5)P$_2$. The kinase should be enriched 1 or 2 days prior to a [5-^{32}P]PtdIns(4,5)P$_2$ preparation, because the kinase activity of the preparation described decreases rapidly. The half-time of PtdIns(4)P 5-kinase activity was estimated to be about 2 weeks at 4°C.

Preparative Synthesis of [5-^{32}P]Phosphatidylinositol 4,5-Bisphosphate

The preparative synthesis of [5-^{32}P]PtdIns(4,5)P$_2$ is carried out exactly as described above for the assay of PtdIns(4)P 5-kinase with 15 μl of [γ-^{32}P]ATP (2.5 mCi) instead of tracer amounts and 50 μl of the fraction with the highest PtdIns(4)P 5-kinase activity. It is recommended to use polypropylene tubes with screw caps as for the [γ-^{32}P]ATP synthesis. This will reduce to a minimum radioactive contamination of centrifuges, gloves, and vortex mixers during handling of the tube. Two 1-μl aliquots of the organic phase are sufficient to determine the radioactivity. Up to 30% of the employed radioactivity will be incorporated into the [5-^{32}P]PtdIns(4,5)P$_2$. The specific activity is about 3000 Ci/mmol.

Preparation of [5-^{32}P]Inositol 1,4,5-Trisphosphate

If a purified mammalian phospholipase C enzyme is available, it can be used for the enzymatic cleavage of [5-^{32}P]PtdIns(4,5)P$_2$ as described (13). Additionally, there are two methods for the chemical cleavage of

PtdIns(4,5)P_2. The method described by Wregett *et al.* (18) follows the deacylation protocol of Clarke and Dawson (19) with subsequent removal of the glycerol moiety with sodium periodate (20). This is probably the safest method of chemical degradation of PtdIns(4,5)P_2. We have successfully degraded [5-^{32}P]PtdIns(4,5)P_2 by alkaline hydrolysis, which can be performed easily and fast. The disadvantage is that two IP_3 isomers will be formed. Typically about 65% of the total radioactivity is Ins(1,4,5)P_3 and about 20% corresponds to another IP_3 isomer, probably Ins(2,4,5)P_3. Because the synthesis of [5-^{32}P]Ins(1,3,4,5)P_4 is not affected by the second IP_3 isomer, a purification step is not necessary. A shift of the radioactive label to other than the phosphate moiety in the 5-position of the inositol molecule does not occur; when we incubated [5-^{32}P]Ins(1,4,5)P_3 or [5-^{32}P]Ins(1,3,4,5)P_4 with a purified Ins(1,4,5)P_3/Ins(1,3,4,5)P_4-5-phosphatase, only $^{32}P_i$ was released, indicating that the radioactive label remains at the 5-position (A. Höer and E. Oberdisse, unpublished results).

The following reagents are needed for alkaline hydrolysis:

1 *M* KOH
1 *M* HCl
1 *M* HEPES/NaOH, pH 7.0
200 μM Cholic acid in chloroform/methanol (2 : 1, v/v): 4 mg cholic acid is dissolved in 1 ml of chloroform/methanol and diluted 1 : 50 in chloroform/methanol

For alkaline hydrolysis, 10 μl of a 200 μM cholic acid solution is dried in a polypropylene tube with screw cap under nitrogene. To the cholic acid [5-^{32}P]PtdInsP$_2$ is added repetitively in volumes of 25 μl and dried. Warming the tube to 40°C in a dry block hastens this procedure. The cholic acid will facilitate the suspension of the lipid. When all the lipids are dried, 30 μl of 1 *M* KOH is added, and the mixture is incubated for 45 min at 96°C. A brief centrifugation will pellet the small volume, and the solution must be neutralized immediately by addition of 25 μl of 1 *M* HCl, 100 μl of water, and 15 μl of 1 *M* HEPES, pH 7.0. The pH is checked with pH-indicator strips, and the final neutralization is achieved by adding 1-μl amounts of 1 *M* HCl and subsequent testing of pH with pH-indicator strips. When the pH is about 7, water is added to a final volume of 200 μl. Normally 50% of the employed radioactivity will be recovered. The other 50% is probably lost by unspecific binding to the vial. This "disappearance" of radioactivity is a typical problem which occurs in handling [5-^{32}P]PtdIns(4,5)P_2. Addition of unlabeled PtdIns(4,5)P_2 as a carrier would probably reduce the unspecific binding, but it would also reduce the specific activity of the radiolabeled substances.

The [5-^{32}P]Ins(1,3,4,5)P$_4$ synthesis is performed in the same vial without further purification of the [5-^{32}P]Ins(1,4,5)P$_3$. If it is desired to use [5-^{32}P]Ins(1,4,5)P$_3$ as a substrate for other enzymes of inositol polyphosphate metabolism, the [5-^{32}P]Ins(1,4,5)P$_3$ has to be purified by HPLC, using a gradient which allows the separation of Ins(1,4,5)P$_3$ from Ins(2,4,5)P$_3$ (see below).

Synthesis of [5-^{32}P]Inositol 1,3,4,5-Tetrakisphosphate

Preparation of Rat Brain Cytosol

Rat brain cytosol serves as a source for Ins(1,4,5)P$_3$ 3-kinase. One rat brain is homogenized at 4°C in 10 ml of homogenization buffer containing 250 mM sucrose, 1 mM DTT, and 20 mM HEPES/NaOH, pH 7.0, and subsequently centrifuged for 60 min at 100,000 g (4°C). The supernatant is stored in aliquots of 100 μl at -80°C until use. The Ins(1,4,5)P$_3$ 3-kinase present in the cytosol is very stable. We have used one preparation for 3 years without significant loss of activity. Typically, the final concentration of protein, which is employed for the synthesis of [5-^{32}P]Ins(1,3,4,5)P$_4$, is 100 μg/ml. The optimal amount of protein can be found by incubation of different cytosol concentrations and 0.5 μM [5-^{32}P]Ins(1,4,5)P$_3$ (20,000 cpm) under the conditions described for the preparative synthesis (see below).

Practical Procedure of [5-^{32}P]Inositol 1,3,4,5-Tetrakisphosphate Synthesis

Reaction mixture C is prepared as shown in Table I. Note that some KCl and HEPES/NaOH, pH 7.0, are derived from the neutralization carried out to terminate the alkaline hydrolysis. Thus, the final concentrations of KCl and HEPES/NaOH, pH 7.0, for the [5-^{32}P]Ins(1,3,4,5)P$_4$ synthesis will be 80 and 30 mM, respectively. To inhibit the Ins(1,4,5)P$_3$/Ins(1,3,4,5)P$_4$-5-phosphatase, 2,3-diphosphoglyceric acid (3 mM) is added; otherwise the reaction product [5-^{32}P]Ins(1,3,4,5)P$_4$ would be degraded to some extent during the synthesis.

The reaction is performed in a final volume of 500 μl. To the 200 μl of [5-^{32}P]Ins(1,4,5)P$_3$ is added 180 μl of reaction mixture C. Rat brain cytosol is supplemented to give a final concentration of 100 μg protein/ml, and water is added to 500 μl before the addition of cytosol. The synthesis is carried out at 37°C, and after 10 min an aliquot of about 1 μl should be taken and

TABLE II   Chromatography Gradients[a]

Gradient	Time (min)	B (%)[b]	Flow (ml/min)
A	0.0	0	1.75
	2.0	0	1.75
	2.5	5	1.75
	12.0	30	1.75
	17.0	60	1.75
	20.0	100	1.75
	30.0	100	1.75
B	0.0	0	1.25
	4.0	25	1.25
	27.0	33	1.25
	28.0	100	1.25
	33.0	100	2.00
C	0.0	0	1.25
	6.0	0	1.25
	31.0	30	1.25
	41.0	50	1.25
	55.0	50	1.25
	56.0	100	1.25
	65.0	100	1.25
D[c]	0.0	0	1.25
	6.0	6	1.25
	18.0	20	1.25
	59.0	20[d]	1.25
	60.0	100	1.25
	70.0	100	1.25

[a] For all gradients a Partisil 10 SAX column (4.5 × 200 mm; Whatman) is used. It is necessary to wash the column with water for at least 10 min at a flow rate of 1.25 ml/min after each gradient.

[b] Eluent B is 3.4 M ammonium formate adjusted to pH 3.7 with o-phosphoric acid (85%).

[c] L. R. Stephens, P. T. Hawkins, A. F. Stanley, T. Moore, D. R. Poyner, P. J. Morris, M. R. Hanley, R. R. Kay, and R. F. Irvine, *Biochem. J.* **275,** 485 (1991).

[d] With a new packed column, it may be necessary to increase eluent B from 20 to 25% between 18 and 59 min, because the IP$_3$ isomers elute in some cases at 100% and will not be separated.

analyzed by HPLC with gradient A (Table II) to check whether the reaction has started. The reaction is stopped after 45–60 min by the addition of 500 μl of methanol. The protein is pelleted by centrifugation at 13,000 g for 10 min, and the formed [5-^{32}P]Ins(1,3,4,5)P$_4$ is purified by HPLC (see below). Normally about 70% of the employed radioactivity is incorporated into

[5-^{32}P]Ins(1,3,4,5)P$_4$. The specific activity is estimated to be 1000–3000 Ci/mmol.

Purification of ^{32}P-Labeled Inositol Phosphates

Purification of the [5-^{32}P]Ins(1,4,5)P$_3$ and [5-^{32}P]Ins(1,3,4,5)P$_4$ is achieved by anion-exchange chromatography on a Partisil 10 SAX column (4.5 × 200 mm, Whatman, Clifton, NJ). The purification procedure, which is described here, is principally the same for each of the inositol phosphates except that different gradients are used. The column should be of high quality and should not used for analytical runs, as considerable amounts of radioactivity will be retained on the column.

The practical procedure is as follows. The inositol phosphate to be purified is loaded on the column by a 1–1.5 ml sample loop. For the purification of [5-^{32}P]Ins(1,3,4,5)P$_4$, gradient C is used, and for the purification of [5-^{32}P]Ins(1,4,5)P$_3$ gradient D is necessary (see Table II). When [5-^{32}P]Ins(1,3,4,5)P$_4$ is purified, fractions are collected at intervals of 20–30 sec from 40 to 55 min. [5-^{32}P]Ins(1,3,4,5)P$_4$ will elute at 45–48 min, but the retention time shortens when the column has been used several times. For the purification of [5-^{32}P]Ins(1,4,5)P$_3$ fractions should be collected at intervals of 20–30 sec from 40 to 65 min. [5-^{32}P]Ins(1,4,5)P$_3$ elutes as the first IP$_3$ isomer at about 55 min from a freshly packed column, but every run shortens the retention time of [5-^{32}P]Ins(1,4,5)P$_3$ significantly. Therefore, it is recommended to check the retention time with a small amount of [5-^{32}P]Ins(1,4,5)P$_3$ before the purification.

The following procedures are the same for [5-^{32}P]Ins(1,3,4,5)P$_4$ and [5-^{32}P]Ins(1,4,5)P$_3$. When all fractions have been collected, the peaks of radioactivity are localized. This can be done simply with a hand-held radioactivity monitor. It may be necessary to put a β shield (1–1.5 cm plexiglass) between the monitor and the vial when the radioactivity in the vial is above the range of the monitor.

The peak fractions are pooled and desalted using any method described for desalting of inositol phosphates (21). We exchange the salt of the eluent for KCl. For this purpose the pooled peak fractions are diluted 1:10 with water and transferred to a centrifugation tube which can be properly closed by a cap. Subsequently, for each 1 ml of the diluted inositol phosphates 5 μl of a Partisil 10 SAX suspension is added, which is prepared as follows: 100 mg of Partisil 10 SAX is filled in a suitable centrifugation tube, and 1 ml of 3.4 M ammonium formate adjusted to pH 3.7 with H$_3$PO$_4$ is added. After vortexing and centrifugation, the supernatant is discarded, and the anion exchanger is washed at least 5 times with 1 ml of water to remove the salt.

The Partisil mixed with the inositol phosphate is shaken for at least 24 hr at 4°C, then pelleted by centrifugation; the supernatant is carefully removed by aspiration. The bound $[5-^{32}P]Ins(1,3,4,5)P_4$ or $[5-^{32}P]Ins(1,4,5)P_3$ is eluted with 5×100 μl of 1 M HCl from the anion exchanger by vigorous mixing and subsequent centrifugation. The supernatants are pooled, and neutralization is achieved with 10 M KOH and buffer: 50 μl of 1 M HEPES/NaOH, pH 7.0, and 40 μl of 10 M KOH are added and the pH is checked with pH-indicator strips. The pH is then adjusted to about 7 by adding small volumes (1–2 μl) of 10 M KOH. The final concentration of KCl will be about 830 mM. The inositol phosphates are stored at -20°C until use.

Assay for Inositol-1,3,4,5-Tetrakisphosphate-3-Phosphatase

$[5-^{32}P]Ins(1,3,4,5)P_4$ is dephosphorylated by the 3-phosphatase, and the reaction products are $[5-^{32}P]Ins(1,4,5)P_3$ and unlabeled inorganic phosphate (P_i). If $Ins(1,4,5)P_3/Ins(1,3,4,5)P_4$-5-phosphatase activity is also present, the substrate $[5-^{32}P]Ins(1,3,4,5)P_4$ is degraded to unlabeled $Ins(1,3,4)P_3$ and $^{32}P_i$. As $[5-^{32}P]Ins(1,4,5)P_3$ is a substrate of the $Ins(1,4,5)P_3/Ins(1,3,4,5)P_4$-5-phosphatase, $^{32}P_i$ will also accumulate as a degradation product of this reaction (Fig. 1). Tritiated $Ins(1,3,4,5)P_4$ may also be used as substrate (NEN/Dupont de Nemours or Amersham Buchler). With tritiated $Ins(1,3,4,5)P_4$ as the substrate, $[^3H]Ins(1,4,5)P_3$ and $[^3H]Ins(1,3,4)P_3$ will accumulate as the reaction products of 3-phosphatase and 5-phosphatase, respectively. The advantage of tritiated substrate is the long half-life; the disadvantage is the necessity of scintillation liquid additive, as well as the disposal of the radioactive waste. After separation of the radioactive reaction products by HPLC, radiation can be detected using an on-line radioactivity detector or a liquid scintillation counter.

Assay Procedure

All stock solutions, radioactive compounds and protein are diluted in 1 mM DTT and 30 mM HEPES/NaOH, pH 7.0. The final concentrations in the assay are as follows:

140 mM KCl
30 $\mu$$M$ EDTA
1 mM DTT
500 nM $Ins(1,3,4,5)P_4$ (from Boehringer Mannheim, Mannheim, Ger-

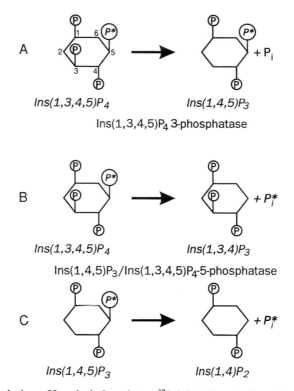

A   Ins(1,3,4,5)P$_4$ → Ins(1,4,5)P$_3$ + P$_i$

Ins(1,3,4,5)P$_4$ 3-phosphatase

B   Ins(1,3,4,5)P$_4$ → Ins(1,3,4)P$_3$ + P$_i^*$

Ins(1,4,5)P$_3$/Ins(1,3,4,5)P$_4$-5-phosphatase

C   Ins(1,4,5)P$_3$ → Ins(1,4)P$_2$ + P$_i^*$

FIG. 1   Degradation of Inositol phosphates ^{32}P-labeled at the 5-position of the inositol molecule by the Ins(1,3,4,5)P$_4$-3-phosphatase and the Ins(1,4,5)P$_3$/Ins(1,3,4,5)P$_4$-5-phosphatase. *P marks the position of the radioactive label. (A) Degradation of [5-^{32}P]Ins(1,3,4,5)P$_4$ by Ins(1,3,4,5)P$_4$-3-phosphatase. (B) Degradation of [5-^{32}P]Ins(1,3,4,5)P$_4$ by Ins(1,4,5)P$_3$/Ins(1,3,4,5)P$_4$-5-phosphatase. (C) Degradation of [5-^{32}P]Ins(1,4,5)P$_3$ by Ins(1,4,5)P$_3$/Ins(1,3,4,5)P$_4$-5-phosphatase.

many, or Calbiochem, La Jolla, CA), stock solution of 1 mM in water stored at $-20°C$

30 mM HEPES/NaOH, pH 7.0

10,000–20,000 cpm (0.01 μCi) of [5-^{32}P]Ins(1,3,4,5)P$_4$ or 0.05 μCi of [^{3}H]Ins(1,3,4,5)P$_4$

10–100 μg of protein/ml

The final assay volume is 100 μl. The reaction is started by the addition of substrate or, if kinetic parameters of the enzyme are tested, by the addition of protein. The incubation is performed for 30 min at 37°C. For termination of the reaction 400 μl of the stopping solution is added, and the samples are centrifuged for 10 min at 13,000 g in a bench-top centrifuge to pellet the protein. The stopping solution is prepared as follows: 180 mg of phytic acid is dissolved in 125 ml of water, then 170 μl of phosphoric acid (85%), 625 μl of 0.4 M EDTA, pH 7.4, and 125 ml of methanol are added.

Analysis of Reaction Products

From the centrifuged sample 450 μl of the supernatant is removed and loaded on a Partisil 10 SAX column. For the separation of ^{32}P-labeled substances, gradient A (see Table II) is run. The retention times are about 8, 17–18, and 20–22 min for P_i, $Ins(1,4,5)P_3$, and $Ins(1,3,4,5)P_4$, respectively, depending on the quality and the age of the column. Radioactivity can be detected by Cerenkov radiation using an on-line radioactivity monitor or by collecting the eluate in intervals of 0.5–1 min and counting each fraction in a liquid scintillation counter.

Gradient A described above does not allow separation of $Ins(1,3,4)P_3$ from $Ins(1,4,5)P_3$. For the analysis of tritiated reaction products, gradient B is run (see Table II). The retention times for a freshly packed column are as follows: $PtdIns(1,4)P_2$, 12 min; $Ins(1,3,4)P_3$, 22 min; $Ins(1,4,5)P_3$, 25 min; $Ins(1,3,4,5)P_4$, 34 min. With an on-line radioactivity detector, a scintillation cocktail that is miscible with high salt solutions has to be mixed to the eluate (e.g., 6.25 ml/min Flow-scint VI, Canberra-Packard, Meriden, CT). If fractions of the eluate are collected, they are diluted with water, and any suitable scintillation cocktail can be added for liquid scintillation counting.

If $[5-^{32}P]Ins(1,3,4,5)P_4$ is used as a substrate for the $Ins(1,3,4,5)P_4$-3-phosphatase separation of the released $[5-^{32}P]Ins(1,4,5)P_3$ from $[5-^{32}P]Ins(1,3,4,5)P_4$ can be attempted by anion-exchange chromatography with Bio-Rad AG 1.8 anion-exchange columns, which are batch eluted with HCl as described elsewhere (22). The problem with this method is that $InsP_3$ and $InsP_4$ may not be separated properly. Therefore, this approach is not appropriate for kinetic studies of the 3-phosphatase.

Assay for Inositol-1,4,5-Trisphosphate/Inositol-1,3,4,5-Tetrakisphosphate-5-Phosphatase

Investigation of $Ins(1,3,4,5)P_4$ degradation by the $Ins(1,3,4,5)P_4$-3-phosphatase from membranes or enriched from porcine brain cytosol as described below is disturbed by the $Ins(1,4,5)P_3/Ins(1,3,4,5)P_4$-5-phosphatase, which dephosphorylates the substrate Ins(1,3,4,5)P_4 and Ins(1,4,5)P_3. If the 3-phosphatase should be purified, it is necessary to measure 5-phosphatase activity until a separation of enzymes is achieved. There are two types of 5-phosphatase: the type I enzyme degrades Ins(1,3,4,5)P_4 and Ins(1,4,5)P_3, and the type II enzyme has a very high K_m value for Ins(1,3,4,5)P_4 and therefore mainly dephosphorylates Ins(1,4,5)P_3 (23).

The 5-phosphatases can be measured with [5-^{32}P]Ins(1,4,5)P_3 as substrate, following the same protocol as for the 3-phosphatase, except that the incubation buffer is supplemented with 1 mM MgCl$_2$ and 1000–2000 cpm of [5-^{32}P]Ins(1,4,5)P_3 is added. Unlabeled Ins(1,3,4,5)P_4 is exchanged for 500 nM Ins(1,4,5)P_3. The released ^{32}P$_i$ can easily be separated from the reaction mixture, using Dowex 1-X8 columns as described (24). For this purpose, 5-ml pipette tips [about 4 × 100 mm; there are also complete packages with columns and closures commercially available (Pierce, Rockford, IL)], which have been prepared with glass wool or another suitable material to retain the anion-exchange material, are filled with 1 ml of Dowex 1-X8 in the formate form and washed with two 5-ml volumes of water. The sample is loaded in 5 ml of water, and P$_i$ is eluted with two 5-ml portions of 0.2 M ammonium formate/0.1 M formic acid. The eluate is collected and the Cerenkov radiation detected in a liquid scintillation counter.

Enrichment of Inositol-1,3,4,5-Tetrakisphosphate-3-Phosphatase from Porcine Brain

Preparation of Cytosol

All steps are carried out at 4°C. From 25 fresh porcine brains, which can be obtained from a slaughterhouse, the arachnoideae, cerebelli, and medullae oblongatae are removed, and the brains are washed in 0.9% (w/v) NaCl. About 25 brain hemispheres are homogenized using a 4 liter Waring blendor in 2.5 liter of a buffer containing 250 mM sucrose, 20 mM 2-mercaptoethanol, 4 mM EDTA, and 20 mM HEPES–NaOH, pH 8.0. The homogenate is filtered through gauze or a kitchen sieve to remove large particles, diluted with 2.5 liter of homogenization buffer, and then centrifuged at 300 g for 30 min. The supernatant is carefully removed and diluted 2-fold with buffer containing 20 mM 2-mercaptoethanol, 1 mM EDTA, and 20 mM HEPES/ NaOH, pH 8.0.

The pellet obtained by a second centrifugation at 14,000 g for 30 min corresponds to a crude membrane preparation, and the supernatant is centrifuged at 100,000 g for 1 hr. The supernatant is collected, and 430 ml of ethylene glycol is added per each liter of supernatant, resulting in a final content of 30% ethylene glycol (v/v). This cytosolic fraction contains about 10 g of protein and will be used for column chromatography.

Materials for Ion-Exchange Chromatography

DEAE-Sephacel (Pharmacia, Piscataway, NJ) is prepared and filled in a column (5 × 100 cm) as recommended by the manufacturer. For a column of the above size, 2 liters of ion-exchange material is needed. The following buffers are prepared.

Buffer A: 20 mM 2-mercaptoethanol, 1 mM EDTA, 30% ethylene glycol (v/v), 20 mM HEPES/NaOH, pH 8.0
Buffer B: 0.6 M NaCl, 20 mM 2-mercaptoethanol, 1 mM EDTA, 30% ethylene glycol (v/v), 20 mM HEPES/NaOH, pH 8.0

Anion-Exchange Chromatography of Inositol-1,3,4,5-Tetrakisphosphate-3-Phosphatase

The column is equilibrated with buffer A. All steps are performed with a flow rate of 120 ml/hr. The cytosol preparation (~10 g protein) is loaded, and the column is washed with 5 liters of buffer A. Washing is followed by a linear 6-liter gradient from 0 to 100% buffer B. Fractions of 10–15 ml are collected and assayed for 3-phosphatase activity (Fig. 2). For this purpose, 10 μl of each fraction diluted 1 : 10 to 1 : 30 is employed. The 3-phosphatase elutes at a NaCl concentration of about 200 mM. This procedure removes the inhibitors of the 3-phosphatase, Ins(1,3,4,5,6)P$_5$ and IP$_6$. Peak fractions containing 3-phosphatase activity are pooled and used for further purification or stored in aliquots at −80°C for the investigation of enzyme properties. At −80°C, the enzyme is stable for several months; after 1 year, some loss of activity will occur. After this purification step, the 3-phosphatase still contains 5-phosphatase activity. The large-scale preparation described can be adapted for smaller amounts of material. A purification procedure for the Ins(1,3,4,5)P$_4$-3-phosphatase from rat liver has been described (15).

Properties of Inositol-1,3,4,5-Tetrakisphosphate-3-Phosphatase

Influence of MgCl$_2$

The Ins(1,4,5)P$_3$/Ins(1,3,4,5)P$_4$-5-phosphatase is dependent on MgCl$_2$ (25), whereas the 3-phosphatase is independent of Mg^{2+} (26). Therefore, the addition of EDTA to the incubation buffer will completely inhibit the

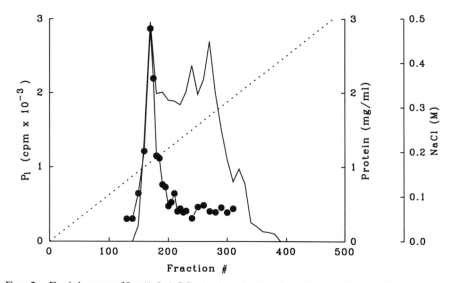

FIG. 2   Enrichment of Ins(1,3,4,5)P$_4$-3-phosphatase by anion-exchange chromatography on DEAE-Sephacel. Porcine brain cytosol was loaded on and eluted from the column as described in the text. Circles show the 3-phosphatase activity measured as [5-^{32}P]Ins(1,4,5)P$_3$ released from [5-^{32}P]Ins(1,3,4,5)P$_4$. The eluted protein and the NaCl concentration are indicated by the solid and the dotted line, respectively.

5-phosphatase activity that may interfere with kinetic investigations of the 3-phosphatase. The incubation buffer for the 3-phosphatase can be supplemented with EDTA of concentrations up to 1 mM to avoid 5-phosphatase activity.

Influence of Monovalent Cations

The standard assay contains 140 mM KCl. We have studied the influence of varying concentrations of KCl, NaCl, and LiCl on the activity of the 3-phosphatase (7). The enzyme is activated by increasing concentrations of all salts tested; KCl is most effective. An activation by KCl was also described for the Ins(1,3,4,5)P$_4$-3-phosphatase from permeabilized platelets (9) and erythrocyte membranes (27).

Other Properties

The Ins(1,3,4,5)P$_4$-3-phosphatase from porcine brain cytosol has been well characterized using the methods described. The K_m for the substrate Ins(1,3,4,5)P$_4$ is about 400 nM (26). Several inositol polyphosphates were found to inhibit the enzyme activity. For Ins(1,4,5)P_3, Ins(1,3,4)P_3, and Ins(3,4,5,6)P_4, we determined K_i values of 2, 1.75, and 0.5 μM, respectively (26). The most potent inhibitors of the enzyme are Ins(1,3,4,5,6)P_5 and IP$_6$ with K_i values of 60 and 3 nM, respectively (13). Other inhibitors of the 3-phosphatase activity are GTP, UTP, and CTP (13), acting in the range of 10–100 μM. The molecular mass of the 3-phosphatase from pig brain cytosol was estimated by gel filtration and was found to be 36 kDa (13).

Acknowledgments

We thank D. Höer for practical and theoretical contributions to the methods, especially the synthesis of radiolabeled substances. The helpful discussion of G. Schultz is appreciated. This work was supported by the Deutsche Forschungsgemeinschaft.

References

1. M. J. Berridge and R. F. Irvine, *Nature (London)* **341,** 197 (1989).
2. S. J. Taylor, H. Z. Chae, S. G. Rhee, and J. H. Exton, *Nature (London)* **350,** 516 (1991).
3. S. G. Rhee, *Trends Biochem. Sci.* **16,** 297 (1991).
4. S. B. Shears, *Biochem. J.* **260,** 313 (1989).
5. J. R. Cunha-Melo, N. M. Dean, H. Ali, and M. A. Beaven, *J. Biol. Chem.* **268,** 14245 (1988).
6. C. Doughney, M. A. McPherson, and R. L. Dormer, *Biochem. J.* **251,** 927 (1988).
7. D. Höer, A. Kwiatkowski, C. Seib, W. Rosenthal, G. Schultz, and E. Oberdisse, *Biochem. Biophys. Res. Commun.* **154,** 668 (1988).
8. P. J. Cullen, R. F. Irvine, B. K. Drobak, and A. P. Dawson, *Biochem. J.* **259,** 931 (1989).
9. E. Oberdisse, R. D. Nolan, and E. G. Lapetina, *J. Biol. Chem.* **265,** 726 (1989).
10. E. R. Lazarowski, D. A. Winegar, R. D. Nolan, E. Oberdisse, and E. G. Lapetina, *J. Biol. Chem.* **265,** 13118 (1990).
11. P. J. Hughes and S. B. Shears, *J. Biol. Chem.* **265,** 9869 (1990).
12. M. E. Hodgson and S. B. Shears, *J. Biol. Chem.* **267,** 831 (1991).
13. A. Höer and E. Oberdisse, *Biochem. J.* **278,** 219 (1991).
14. D. Pittet, W. Schlegel, D. P. Lew, A. Monod, and G. W. Mayr, *J. Biol. Chem.* **264,** 18489 (1989).
15. K. Nogimori, P. J. Hughes, M. C. Glennon, M. E. Hodgson, J. W. Putney, Jr., and S. B. Shears, *J. Biol. Chem.* **266,** 16499 (1991).
16. R. A. Johnson and T. F. Walseth, *Adv. Cyclic Nucleotide Res.* **10,** 135 (1979).
17. N. Divecha and R. F. Irvine, *in* "Methods in Inositide Research" (R. F. Irvine, ed.), p. 179. Raven, New York, 1990.
18. K. A. Wregett, D. J. Lander, and R. F. Irvine, *in* "Methods in Enzymology" (S. Fleischer and B. Fleischer, eds.), Vol. 191, p. 707. Academic Press, San Diego, 1990.

19. N. Clarke and R. M. C. Dawson, *Biochem. J.* **195,** 301 (1981).
20. D. M. Brown and J. C. Stewart, *Biochim. Biophys. Acta* **124,** 413 (1966).
21. L. R. Stephens, *in* ''Methods in Inositide Research'' (R. F. Irvine, ed.), p. 9. Raven, New York, 1990.
22. C. E. L. Spencer, L. R. Stephens, and R. F. Irvine, *in* ''Methods in Inositide Research'' (R. F. Irvine, ed.), p. 39. Raven, New York, 1990.
23. C. A. Hansen, R. A. Johanson, M. T. Williamson, and J. R. Williamson, *J. Biol. Chem.* **262,** 17319 (1987).
24. M. J. Berridge, R. M. C. Dawson, C. P. Downes, J. P. Heslop, and R. F. Irvine, *Biochem. J.* **212,** 473 (1982).
25. T. M. Conolly, T. E. Bross, and P. W. Majerus, *J. Biol. Chem.* **260,** 7868 (1985).
26. A. Höer, D. Höer, and E. Oberdisse, *Biochem. J.* **270,** 715 (1990).
27. T. Estrada-Garcia, A. Craxton, C. J. Kirk, and R. H. Michell, *Proc. R. Soc. London* **244,** 63 (1991).

[28] Species Differences in the Response of Second Messenger Inositol 1,4,5-Trisphosphate to Lithium

Lowell E. Hokin and John F. Dixon

Introduction

Receptor activation of phosphodiesteratic cleavage of phosphoinositides generates intracellular second messenger molecules, such as inositol 1,4,5-trisphosphate [$Ins(1,4,5)P_3$; IP_3], which mobilizes intracellular Ca^{2+}, and diacylglycerol, which activates protein kinase C (for recent reviews, see Refs. 1–5). The $Ins(1,4,5)P_3$ formed on agonist stimulation is rapidly metabolized by a kinase, which is specific for the 3′-position of inositol, or by a phosphatase, which is specific for the 5′-position. The 3′-kinase generates inositol 1,3,4,5-tetrakisphosphate [$Ins(1,3,4,5)P_4$; IP_4], which has been suggested, but not proved, to act as another second messenger involving Ca^{2+} movements (6).

Li$^+$ is effective in the treatment of manic-depressive psychosis or bipolar disorder (7). The mechanism of its therapeutic action is not clear, although several hypotheses have been advanced. The most well-known hypothesis, put forward by Berridge (8), is based on the fact that in agonist-stimulated brain preparations, therapeutic concentrations of Li$^+$ cause accumulation of certain inositol phosphates, primarily inositol monophosphates but also inositol 1,3,4-trisphosphate [$Ins(1,3,4)P_3$] and inositol 1,4-bisphosphate. This is brought about by inhibition of inositol monophosphatases and inositol polyphosphate-1-phosphatase(s) (9, 10). The accumulation of inositol phosphates has been suggested to ultimately reduce the supply of phosphoinositides and thus attenuate agonist-induced $Ins(1,4,5)P_3$ formation and intracellular Ca^{2+} mobilization (8).

In apparent support of the Berridge hypothesis, Nahorski and co-workers (11) found that in cerebral cortex slices of rat Li$^+$ inhibited by 15–25% muscarinic receptor-stimulated $Ins(1,4,5)P_3$ and $Ins(1,3,4,5)P_4$ accumulation. However, Whitworth et $al.$ (12) reported that chronic Li$^+$ enhanced both stimulated and unstimulated levels of $Ins(1,4,5)P_3$ and $Ins(1,3,4,5)P_4$ in mouse brain in $vivo$, a result opposite to their findings on IP_4, but not IP_3, in $vitro$ (13).

Experimental Procedures

Guinea Pig, Rabbit, Rat, and Mouse

Preparation of Brain Slices, Labeling, and Drug Treatment

The following methods have been described by Lee *et al.* (14). Guinea pig and rodent cerebral cortex slices (0.5 × 0.35 × 0.35 mm) are prepared by a modification (15) of the method of Brown *et al.* (16). Slices from the brains of two 350–400 g guinea pigs (or, where indicated, four 250 g rats or nine 25 g mice) are placed in a 50-ml Erlenmeyer flask with 5 ml of oxygenated Krebs–Henseleit bicarbonate saline (KHBS) containing (in m*M*) 113 NaCl, 4.7 KCl, 2.5 CaCl$_2$, 1.2 KH$_2$PO$_4$, 1.0 MgSO$_4$, 25 NaHCO$_3$, and 11.5 glucose, pH 7.4. Slices are preincubated with vigorous shaking for 15 min at 37°C. Prior to all incubations, the flasks are oxygenated for 30 sec and tightly stoppered. Preincubation is repeated three times (for 15, 15, and 30 min). The slices are prelabeled with 0.25 mCi *myo*-[2-³H]inositol (specific activity 15–20 Ci/mmol) in fresh incubation medium for 1 hr. At the end of this period, the slices are rinsed four times with 30 ml of fresh KHBS to remove free labeled compound. The slices are suspended in approximately 15 ml of incubation medium, and 1-ml aliquots are pipetted into 25-ml Erlenmeyer flasks.

In the samples containing LiCl, the ionic strength is adjusted by reducing the concentration of NaCl. The slices are then incubated with and without Li$^+$ for 20 min. Finally, they are incubated with or without acetylcholine (ACh) (supplemented with 100 μM eserine) for various times at 37°C. At the end of the incubation, the samples are transferred to tubes containing 2 ml of ice-cold 4.5% perchloric acid and 20 μg sodium phytate to terminate the reaction. Phytate is found to increase recoveries of Ins(1,3,4,5)P$_4$ by up to 20%, but it had no significant effect on the recovery of Ins(1,4,5)P$_3$ (data not shown). Because phytate interferes in the binding assays for both Ins(1,4,5)P$_3$ and Ins(1,3,4,5)P$_4$, it is excluded from the quenching medium in those experiments in which the binding assay is used.

Extraction of [³H]Inositol Polyphosphates

The quenched samples are homogenized with a Polytron (Brinkmann Instruments, Westbury, NY) for 20 sec, followed by centrifugation at 10,000 rpm for 20 min. The supernatant is neutralized with KOH in the presence of 5 m*M* Na$_2$EDTA, 10 m*M* NaHCO$_3$, and 5 μl of pHydrion indicator solution (range, pH 1–11). The neutralized supernatant is centrifuged at 10,000 rpm for 20 min to remove KClO$_4$ and subsequently stored at −20°C. Before application to the high-performance liquid chromatography (HPLC) column, a further accumulation of $KClO_4$ is removed by centrifugation. The pellets containing the particulate matter from the perchloric acid-treated homogenate are homogenized with 3.8 ml of methanol/chloroform/water (2 : 1 : 0.6, v/v) and 20-μl aliquots are taken to determine the radioactivity in total phosphoinositides. A comparison of various extraction procedures is discussed elsewhere (14).

Chromatographic Analysis of Inositol Polyphosphates

Neutralized extracts (pH 6–7) are applied to a 25-cm analytical Whatman (Clifton, NJ) Partisil SAX column and eluted with a linear gradient of $NH_4H_2(PO_4)$, pH 3.8, as follows: 0 min, water; then 5 min, 0.5 M [in $NH_4H_2(PO_4)$]; 35 min, 0.7 M; 40 min, 1.7 M; 80 min, 1.7 M; 85 min, water; and 120 min, water. This elution program is based on the method of Dean and Moyer (17). An automated HPLC system and peak detection system, as previously described (18), are used. Continuous-flow counting is adequate for peak detection, but quantitative measurement requires collection of peaks for recounting in a liquid scintillation counter.

Binding Assays for Measurement of Mass of Inositol Polyphosphates

Ins(1,4,5)P₃ is assayed by the method of Chaliss et al. (19) with the following modifications: A final incubation volume of 0.4 ml is used. The pH of the 25 mM Tris-HCl buffer is increased to 9.0. The binding protein (from bovine adrenal cortex) is diluted in buffer, and 0.2 ml is added to the reaction mixture. The larger volume facilitates equal sampling of the particulate suspension. At the end of the binding period, the protein is separated from the reaction mixture by centrifugation through a 0.3-ml cushion of 5% sucrose in 25 mM sodium acetate, pH 5.0. The lower pH of the cushion is necessary for good pelleting of the binding protein. Ins(1,3,4,5)P₄ is assayed by the method of Donié and Reiser (20). At the conclusion of both assays, the binding protein (pellet) is dispersed in 0.35 ml of water and counted in 8-ml glass vials in 5 ml of Polyfluor, a biodegradable scintillation mixture.

Cerebral Cortex Slices from Rhesus Monkeys

The following methods have been described by Dixon et al. (21). Individual female rhesus monkeys, aged 12 to 15 years, which are being sacrificed at the Wisconsin Regional Primate Center (Madison, WI), are subjected to deep anesthesia with sodium pentobarbital, and the skull cap is removed after cutting with an electric saw. The brain is removed and placed cortex down on ice overlaid with aluminum foil. After a delay of under 5 min to allow dissection of subcortical structures, a cortical hemisphere is submerged in ice-cold KHBS, modified to be nominally Ca^{2+} free.

Preparation, prelabeling, and incubation of slices are as described by Lee *et al.* (14) with the following modifications. Nominally Ca^{2+}-free KHBS is always used during the 1 hr of restorative incubation prior to prelabeling and, where indicated, is used during some subsequent incubations. Omission of Ca^{2+} during slicing and restoration helps preserve tissue viability (22). Omission of Ca^{2+} also minimizes $Ins(1,4,5)P_3$ accumulation during preincubation with Li^+. The final slice dimensions are changed to $0.5 \times 0.8 \times 0.8$ mm. The concentration of Mg^{2+} is 1 mM. Prelabeling is omitted when the mass of $Ins(1,4,5)P_3$ is measured by the receptor binding assay.

Specific drug treatment and incubation conditions are described in figure legends. Quench, extraction, and separation of inositol phosphates by HPLC are carried out as previously described (14). The receptor binding assay is as previously described (14), except the $Ins(1,4,5)P_3$-binding protein is prepared from beef liver (20). This binding protein is found to be easier to prepare and to use than the binding protein from beef adrenal glands. All experiments are performed two or more times with at least triplicate slice incubations for all points.

Results

Chromatographic Separation of [^3H]Inositol-Labeled Inositol Phosphates
Figure 1 shows a typical HPLC separation of various [^{3}H]inositol phosphates present in a trichloroacetic acid extract of serotonin-stimulated cerebellar slices (23). It should be pointed out that the amounts of the various inositol phosphates varies with respect to different neural structures and with respect to stimulation with different agonists.

Effects of Lithium on Accumulation of Inositol Polyphosphates in Brain Cortex Slices of Guinea Pig
Quite by accident, we found that Li^+ increased $Ins(1,4,5)P_3$ and $Ins(1,3,4,5)P_4$ in guinea pig brain cortex slices incubated with ACh and therapeutic concentrations of Li^+ (14). There was a progressive increase in second messenger $Ins(1,4,5)P_3$, putative second messenger inositol 1,3,4,5-tetrakisphosphate [$Ins(1,3,4,5)P_4$], and nonmessenger inositol 1,3,4-trisphosphate [$Ins(1,3,4)P_3$] between 1 and 5 mM Li^+ (Fig. 2). In the presence of 1 mM inositol, there was a statistically significant increase in $Ins(1,4,5)P_3$ at 1 mM Li^+, which is the midpoint of the therapeutic range in man. [In more recent studies with improved incubation conditions, a statistically significant increase in

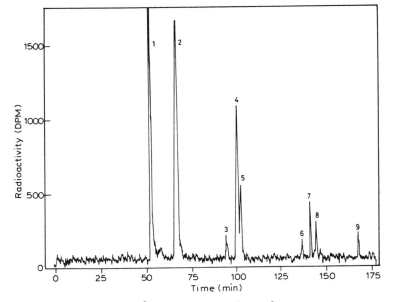

FIG. 1   HPLC separation of [^{3}H]inositol phosphates from an aqueous extract of serotonin-stimulated guinea pig cerebellar slices prelabeled with [^{3}H]inositol. Guinea pig cerebellar slices were prelabeled with [^{3}H]inositol for 1 hr. They were preincubated for 10 min in the absence of [^{3}H]inositol and further incubated with serotonin (1 mM) for 10 min. The reaction was quenched with trichloroacetic acid. Preparation of the extract and conditions for HPLC separation are described in Sastry *et al.* (23). Peaks are as follows: 1, inositol 1- and 3-monophosphates; 2, inositol 4-monophosphate; 3, inositol 1,3-bisphosphate; 4, inositol 1,4-bisphosphate; 5, inositol 3,4-bisphosphate; 6, glycerophosphoryl inositol bisphosphate; 7, inositol 1,3,4-trisphosphate; 8, inositol 1,4,5-trisphosphate; 9, inositol 1,3,4,5-tetrakisphosphate. [Reproduced from Sastry *et al.* (23) by permission of the *Journal of Neurochemistry*.]

Ins(1,4,5)P$_3$ in the absence of added inositol can be seen in guinea pig brain cortex slices at therapeutic concentrations of Li$^+$ (J. F. Dixon and L. E. Hokin, unpublished observations, 1992).]

Effect of Lithium on Accumulation of Inositol Polyphosphates in Cholinergically Stimulated Rat and Mouse Brain Cortex Slices in Presence and Absence of Inositol

Figure 3A,C shows that Li$^+$ suppressed the levels of Ins(1,4,5)P$_3$ and Ins(1,3,4,5)P$_4$ in cholinergically stimulated rat and mouse brain cortex slices incubated without inositol supplementation. This confirms previous observations in the rat (24). Whitworth and Kendall (13) did not find an inhibition

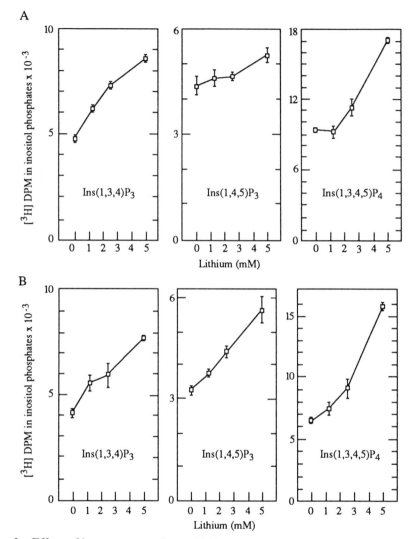

FIG. 2   Effect of low concentrations of Li$^+$, without and with inositol supplementation, on the accumulation of Ins(1,4,5)P$_3$, Ins(1,3,4,5)P$_4$, and Ins(1,3,4)P$_3$ in guinea pig brain cortex slices in the presence of ACh. Brain cortex slices, labeled with [^{3}H]inositol, were preincubated for 20 min with various concentrations of LiCl and then incubated in the same medium for 10 min with 0.1 mM ACh. (A) No inositol supplementation; (B) 1 mM inositol present during the 20-min preincubation and during stimulation. Quench, extraction, and separation of inositol phosphates were carried out as described by Lee *et al.* (14). [Reproduced from Lee *et al.* (14) by permission of the *Biochemical Journal.*]

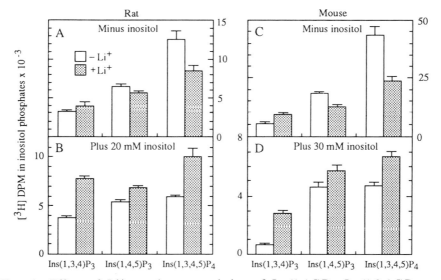

FIG. 3   Effect of Li$^+$ on the accumulation of Ins(1,4,5)P$_3$, Ins(1,3,4,5)P$_4$, and Ins(1,3,4)P$_3$ in rat and mouse brain cortex slices in the presence of ACh, without and with inositol supplementation. Brain cortex slices, labeled with [^{3}H]inositol, were preincubated for 20 min with or without 10 mM LiCl and, as indicated, without or with inositol. The slices were then incubated in the same medium with 0.1 mM ACh for 5 min (B) or for 10 min (A, C, and D). An inositol phosphate extract was analyzed by HPLC. Quench, extraction, and separation of inositol phosphates were carried out as described by Lee *et al.* (14). [Reproduced from Lee *et al.* (14) by permission of the *Biochemical Journal*.]

of IP$_3$ accumulation in mouse brain cortex slices, but Ins(1,4,5)P$_3$ and Ins(1,3,4)P$_3$ were not separated, and, as shown by others and ourselves (see, e.g., Fig. 2), Li$^+$ rather consistently stimulates accumulation of Ins(1,3,4)P$_3$. One possible explanation for the species differences between guinea pig, on the one hand, and rat and mouse, on the other hand, is that in the presence of Li$^+$ inositol may be more rate-limiting for resynthesis of phosphoinositides in the rat and mouse. Figure 3B,D shows that this was in fact the case. If sufficient inositol was added so it was not rate-limiting for phosphoinositide synthesis, a Li$^+$-induced increment in both Ins(1,4,5)P$_3$ and Ins(1,3,4,5)P$_4$ levels could be seen. There is a basis for the species differences. Rat and mouse brain cortices contain half the brain inositol concentration of that of guinea pig (25, 26), rat brain cortex slices are depleted of inositol by 80% on incubation (25), and they require 10 mM inositol supplementation to restore *in vivo* levels of inositol (25). Thus, the species differences appeared

TABLE I   Effects of Lithium on the Accumulation of [^{3}H]Inositol
1,4,5-Trisphosphate in Monkey Brain Cortex Slices[a]

Experiment	[Li$^+$] (mM)	Ins(1,4,5)P$_3$ ([^{3}H]dpm ± S.E.M.)	p	Increase (% ± S.E.M.)
Experiment 1	0	2565 ± 85		
($n = 8$)	0.325	2699 ± 97	0.315	5.2 ± 3.8
	2.5	3082 ± 118	0.003	20.2 ± 4.6
Experiment 2	0	2522 ± 48		
($n = 12$)	1	2881 ± 69	<0.001	16.0 ± 1.8

[a] Reproduced from Dixon *et al.* (21) by permission of the *Journal of Neurochemistry.*

to be due to rate-limiting concentrations of inositol in rat and mouse cerebral cortex slices.

Effects of Lithium on Inositol Polyphosphates Accumulation in Cerebral Cortex Slices of Rhesus Monkeys

With the exception of our recent studies in guinea pig and rabbit (14), studies of the effects of Li$^+$ on inositol phosphate metabolism in brain have been carried out in rat and, to a lesser extent, in mouse. Of greater relevance to the mechanism of the therapeutic action of Li$^+$ in man would be studies of the effects of Li$^+$ in brain structures in a primate. Rhesus monkeys share 94% gene identity with humans.

Effects of Therapeutic Concentrations of Lithium on Accumulation of Inositol 1,4,5-Trisphosphate in Monkey Brain Cortex Slices

As stated above, the therapeutic serum concentrations of Li$^+$ in the treatment of bipolar disorders range from 0.5 to 1.5 mM. Table I shows the effects of concentrations of Li$^+$ ranging from 0.325 to 2.5 mM on the accumulation of [^{3}H]Ins(1,4,5)P$_3$ in monkey brain cortex slices. There were highly significant stimulations of Ins(1,4,5)P$_3$ accumulation at 1 and 2.5 mM Li$^+$.

Effects of Lithium on Accumulation of Inositol Polyphosphates in Presence and Absence of Acetylcholine

Figure 4 shows the effects of 25 mM Li$^+$ on the accumulation of Ins(1,4,5)P$_3$ in monkey brain cortex slices incubated in the presence and absence of ACh. The high concentration of Li$^+$ was used to accentuate its effects on Ins(1,4,5)P$_3$ accumulation. Slices were washed to remove [^{3}H]inositol prior to addition of Li$^+$. At no time was nonradioactive inositol added to the incubation medium. Ins(1,4,5)P$_3$ accumulated more or less linearly over the 70-min period. There was a marked lithium-induced increase in accumulation

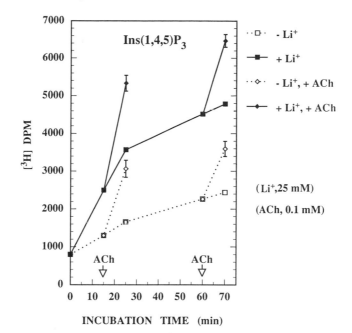

FIG. 4   Time-dependent formation of $[^3H]Ins(1,4,5)P_3$ in monkey cerebral cortex slices incubated with and without ACh in the presence and absence of Li⁺. Monkey cerebral cortex slices were prepared and prelabeled in Krebs–Henseleit bicarbonate saline with 2.5 mM Ca²⁺. The prelabeled slices were then incubated in the absence and presence of 25 mM LiCl before addition of 100 μM ACh and eserine to the indicated samples. Quench, extraction, and separation of inositol phosphates were carried out as described by Lee *et al.* (14), as modified by Dixon *et al.* (21). [Reproduced from Dixon *et al.* (21) by permission of the *Journal of Neurochemistry*.]

of $Ins(1,4,5)P_3$ up to 25 min, after which the elevation remained constant up to 70 min. In a previous study (14), the increase in $Ins(1,4,5)P_3$ in guinea pig brain cortex slices depended on the presence of ACh. This is clearly not the case here, although the species differences may not be fundamental, since with the newer methodology used here we have preliminary evidence that a Li⁺ effect can also be observed without agonist in the non-primate species (J. F. Dixon and L. E. Hokin, unpublished observations, 1992). On a percentage basis, the stimulation of $Ins(1,4,5)P_3$ accumulation by Li⁺ was the same in the presence or absence of ACh. However, the absolute increment of $[^3H]Ins(1,4,5)P_3$ was 57% higher in the presence of ACh. There was a concentration-dependent increase in $Ins(1,4,5)P_3$ with increasing concentrations of Li⁺ between 1 and 25 mM (data not shown).

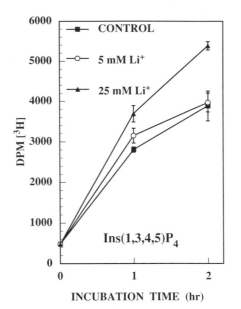

FIG. 5 Time-dependent formation of [³H]Ins(1,3,4,5)P₄ in monkey brain cerebral cortex slices incubated without agonists in the presence and absence of Li⁺. Monkey cerebral cortex slices were prepared and prelabeled as described by Lee *et al.* (14), as modified by Dixon *et al.* (21). The prelabeled slices were incubated for 1 and 2 hr in the presence of 0, 5, and 25 m*M* LiCl and quenched with perchloric acid. Quench, extraction, and separation of inositol phosphates were carried out as described previously (14). [Reproduced from Dixon *et al.* (21) by permission of the *Journal of Neurochemistry*.]

In a separate experiment, 5 m*M* Li⁺, a concentration well above the therapeutic range, did not increase Ins(1,3,4,5)P₄ over a 2-hr period, although there was an increase at 25 m*M* Li⁺ (21) (Fig. 5). It would thus appear that at least in rhesus monkey brain cortex slices, which are incubated in the absence of agonist, increases in Ins(1,3,4,5)P₄ at therapeutically relevant concentrations of Li⁺ do not occur, at least over a 2-hr period. As has been reported by ourselves and others, we observed increases in inositol monophosphates, inositol 1,4-bisphosphate, and inositol 1,3,4-trisphosphate in the presence of Li⁺ (data not shown).

Effects of Lithium on Inositol 1,4,5-Trisphosphate Mass

In a previous study (14), we showed that the enhancement of Ins(1,4,5)P₃ or Ins(1,3,4,5)P₄ by Li⁺ in guinea pig brain cortex slices was essentially the same whether measured by the [³H]inositol prelabeling technique or by mass determination. In monkey brain cortex slices, mass assay showed a 26%

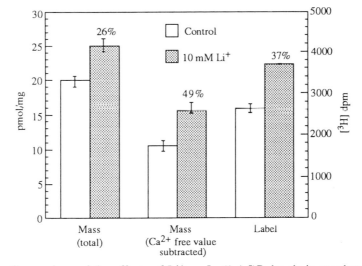

FIG. 6   Comparison of the effects of Li⁺ on Ins(1,4,5)P₃ levels in monkey cerebral cortex slices, as measured by the [³H]inositol prelabeling technique and by mass determinations. Brain cortex slices were prepared and restored (see text) in nominally Ca^{2+}-free KHBS and then incubated for 2 hr in fresh buffer with and without 10 mM LiCl. Calcium was then added (2.5 mM final concentration) and the incubation continued for 20 min before quench. The protein concentration in the suspension prior to quench was kept above 3 mg/ml. Quenching, extraction, and the receptor binding assay were as previously described (14). Mass (Ca^{2+} subtracted) was calculated by subtracting mass in the absence of Ca^{2+} from total mass. [Reproduced from Dixon *et al.* (21) by permission of the *Journal of Neurochemistry*.]

increase in Ins(1,4,5)P₃ with 10 mM Li⁺ (Fig. 6). The prelabeling technique showed a 37% increase. There is a possible explanation for this difference. There is a pool of Ins(1,4,5)P₃ seen by mass assay that is metabolically inactive. We could demonstrate this pool by incubating in the absence of Ca^{2+}. In the absence of Ca^{2+}, mass assay revealed Ins(1,4,5)P₃, but there was no label present, as measured by the prelabeling technique. If one subtracts this pool, the mass assay shows a 49% increase with Li⁺, which is greater than that seen with the prelabeling technique. Thus, the prelabeling results fall between those of the mass assay calculated by the two methods. In any event, it appears that the two assay methods give fairly similar results.

Discussion

We have shown here that therapeutic concentrations of Li⁺ increase accumulation of Ins(1,4,5)P₃ in cerebral cortex slices in species ranging from the mouse to rhesus monkey if inositol in the slice is not rate-limiting. In the monkey, but not in other species, $Ins(1,3,4,5)P_4$ is not increased with therapeutic concentrations of Li^+. In the monkey, neither agonist nor inositol supplementation was required to demonstrate the lithium effect. Our data in monkey and in other mammals (14) are at variance with the well-known hypothesis for the anti-manic-depressive action of Li^+, as put forward by Berridge (8), derived from earlier work of Allison and Stewart (26) and Hallcher and Sherman (27). According to this hypothesis, the trapping of inositol, primarily in the form of the inositol monophosphates, leaves less inositol available for resynthesis of phosphoinositides, and it is postulated that this results in a fall in second messengers. In support of the above hypothesis were the findings that Li^+ produced small inhibitions (13–25%) in accumulation of $Ins(1,4,5)P_3$ and a somewhat larger inhibition (50%) in accumulation of $Ins(1,3,4,5)P_4$ in rat brain cortex slices (28) and inhibitions in $Ins(1,3,4,5)P_4$, but not IP_3 (see above), in mouse brain cortex slices (13). These inhibitions were only seen when brain cortex slices were stimulated with high concentrations of cholinergic agents (0.1–1 mM), which produce massive breakdown of phosphoinositides, a condition which, in the presence of Li^+, is more likely to trap considerable inositol as inositol phosphates. In this connection, Whitworth and Kendall (13) showed that Li^+ did not decrease, and in fact increased, $Ins(1,3,4,5)P_4$ and IP_3 in mouse brain cortex slices stimulated with several other agonists.

The stimulatory effects of therapeutic concentrations of Li^+ on $Ins(1,4,5)P_3$ accumulation were not high but, statistically, were highly significant. It is not known whether this change in $Ins(1,4,5)P_3$ is large enough to affect release of Ca^{2+} from internal stores, but it is similar to the inhibition by Li^+ of $Ins(1,4,5)P_3$ accumulation shown by others and ourselves in rat brain cortex slices not supplemented with inositol—data marshaled in support of the Berridge hypothesis (24, 28). In studying the effects of Li^+ in a network of neurons in brain cortex slices, one is likely to be dealing with responsive and unresponsive neurons. The rise in $Ins(1,4,5)P_3$ in the lithium-sensitive neurons may be blunted by $Ins(1,4,5)P_3$ in the insensitive neurons, but in the therapeutic situation in man there may not be drastic changes in $Ins(1,4,5)P_3$ levels, even in the responsive neurons. This seems rather likely, since large changes in $Ins(1,4,5)P_3$, and thus Ca^{2+}, would be toxic. This may be responsible for the narrow margin of safety in the treatment of bipolar disorders with Li^+.

In the monkey, there was no effect of 1–10 mM inositol on the percentage stimulation of $Ins(1,4,5)P_3$ accumulation by Li^+ in the presence of 0.1 and 1.0 mM ACh and in the presence of 1.0, 10, and 25 mM Li^+ (21), but in the guinea pig 1 mM inositol increased the stimulation over the therapeutic range of Li^+ (14). At higher Li^+ concentrations inositol was not required in guinea pig brain cortex slices. Apparently, the "washout" of inositol which occurs in monkey brain cortex slices is insufficient to reduce the substrate to the point of making it rate-limiting, so as to reduce or reverse the Li$^+$ effect. The inhibitions of Ins(1,4,5)P$_3$ and Ins(1,3,4,5)P$_4$ by Li$^+$ in rat and mouse appear to be the result of artifactual *in vitro* "washout" of inositol, which is already at a low level as compared to guinea pig, for example, and this is supported by our restoration of Li$^+$ stimulations in these inositol polyphosphates in rat and mouse by supplementation with inositol (14).

Washout does not occur *in vivo*, and existing *in vivo* studies do not show inhibitions of resting Ins(1,4,5)P$_3$ by Li$^+$. Employing *in vivo* quench by microwave radiation, Whitworth *et al.* (12) found that chronic Li$^+$ treatment increased Ins(1,4,5)P$_3$ in mouse brain cortex *in vivo*. Jope *et al.* (29), using a similar protocol, found that the concentration of Ins(1,4,5)P$_3$ in rat brain cortex was unaltered by acute or chronic Li$^+$ treatment. With administration of pilocarpine, Ins(1,4,5)P$_3$ was substantially increased by Li$^+$ at 20 min but fell at 60 min. Again, a cholinergic agent, because of its powerful effect on phosphoinositide breakdown, would be expected to tie up substantial inositol in the presence of Li$^+$, and in rat brain cortex, which already contains low inositol levels as compared to other species that have been examined, resynthesis of phosphoinositides could be considerably impaired under these conditions. Studies that involve chronic Li$^+$ treatment, followed by decapitation and *ex vivo* slice incubation (30, 31), are difficult to interpret because of the method of sacrifice and because of alteration of the *in vivo* conditions by *ex vivo* incubation of slices. The effects of chronic treatment of monkeys with Li$^+$ on Ins(1,4,5)P$_3$ concentrations in brain cortex *in vivo* would be of considerable interest.

Because addition of agonist was not required to demonstrate the Li$^+$ effect, it was not unreasonable to assume that the Li$^+$ effect was under the control of an endogenous agonist or agonists, since brain cortex slices contain many intact neurons and synapses. To investigate this possibility we tested a variety of antagonists to various receptors in monkey brain cortex slices (32). Ketanserin, phentolamine, and chlorpheniramine, antagonists at 5-HT$_2$-serotoninergic, α_1-noradrenergic, and H$_1$-histaminergic receptors, respectively, had no significant effects on Ins(1,4,5)P$_3$ in the presence of Li$^+$, even though these receptors are coupled to phosphoinositidase C. Atropine, an antagonist to muscarinic cholinergic receptors, also coupled to phospholipase C, showed a marginal and statistically inconsistent inhibition of Ins(1,4,5)P$_3$ accumulation in the presence of Li$^+$. On the other hand, antagonists to the *N*-methyl-D-aspartate (NMDA) receptor, namely, ($\pm$)CPP [($\pm$)-3-(2-carboxypiperazine-4-yl)-propyl-1-phosphonic acid], ketamine, and MK801 (dizoclipine), abolished or reduced considerably the Li$^+$ effect, suggesting that the Li$^+$ effect in the absence of added agonist is rather specifically dependent on glutaminergic transmission via the NMDA receptor, presumably by regulation of intracellular Ca^{2+}. Antagonists to other glutamate receptors did not inhibit the Li^+ effect.

How do these studies relate to the therapeutic effects of Li^+ in manic-depressive disorders? It is not difficult to visualize that the elevating effect of Li^+ on $Ins(1,4,5)P_3$ and thus Ca^{2+} could lift the depressive phase of manic-depressive psychosis. But how could this explain the lessening of mania? In this connection, the therapeutic effect of Li^+ requires treatment for 1 week or longer to be established, even after therapeutic blood concentrations have been achieved, suggesting an adaptive mechanism. These adaptive changes might tend to reduce Ca^{2+} by down-regulating the $Ins(1,4,5)P_3$ receptor, although we do not know whether the increases in $Ins(1,4,5)P_3$ due to therapeutic concentrations of Li^+ would be sufficient to do this. If the $Ins(1,4,5)P_3$ receptor is down-regulated, however, and at the same time the $Ins(1,4,5)P_3$ remains elevated, a new set point for Ca^{2+} closer to normal from either the direction of depression or mania may be established. We have recently shown that chronic treatment of mice with Li^+ down-regulates the $Ins(1,4,5)P_3$ receptor in the forebrain of mice (G. V. Los, J. F. Dixon, and L. E. Hokin, unpublished observations, 1993).

The mechanism of the Li^+-induced accumulation of $Ins(1,4,5)P_3$ is not known. Direct inhibition of the $Ins(1,4,5)P_3$-5-phosphatase by Li^+ does not appear to occur (33). A possible enzymatic mechanism is suggested by the observation that low concentrations of Li^+ stimulate phospholipase C in PC12 cells in the presence of nerve growth factor (34). However, irrespective of the mechanism of the elevation of $Ins(1,4,5)P_3$ by Li^+, the $Ins(1,4,5)P_3$ receptors, which control release of intracellular microsomal Ca^{2+} stores, see the steady-state level of this messenger and respond accordingly.

Summary

The salient observations reviewed here are that, if inositol is not rate-limiting, there is a consistent stimulation of $Ins(1,4,5)P_3$ accumulation by Li^+ in brain cortex slices in species ranging from the mouse to the monkey, and of $Ins(1,3,4,5)P_4$ accumulation in all species except the monkey. In the monkey, addition of inositol to the incubation medium did not increase $Ins(1,4,5)P_3$ accumulation at therapeutic concentrations of Li^+. In the monkey, no neurotransmitter need be added, and antagonists to the NMDA (glutamate) receptor appear to selectively inhibit the lithium effect. These observations may have therapeutic implications for humans in the treatment of bipolar disorders with Li^+.

Acknowledgments

The authors thank Connie Bowes for technical assistance and Karen Wipperfurth for assistance in the preparation of the manuscript. We are also grateful to Dr. H. Uno of the Wisconsin Regional Primate Center for samples of monkey brain cortex. This work was supported by National Institutes of Health Grant HL16318.

References

1. M. J. Berridge and R. F. Irvine, *Nature* (*London*) **341**, 197 (1989).
2. R. S. Rana and L. E. Hokin, *Physiol. Rev.* **70**, 115 (1990).
3. A. Farago and Y. Nishizuka, *FEBS Lett* **268**, 350 (1990).
4. R. H. Michell, *Trends. Biochem. Sci.* **17**, 274 (1992).
5. P. W. Majerus, *Annu. Rev. Biochem.* **61**, 225 (1992).
6. A. P. Morris, D. V. Gallacher, R. F. Irvine, and O. H. Petersen, *Nature* (*London*) **330**, 653 (1987).
7. A. J. Wood and G. M. Goodwin, *Psychol. Med.* **17**, 579 (1987).
8. M. J. Berridge, C. P. Downes, and M. R. Hanley, *Cell* (*Cambridge, Mass.*) **59**, 411 (1989).
9. J. H. Allison, M. E. Blisner, W. H. Holland, P. P. Hippius, and W. R. Sherman, *Biochem. Biophys. Res. Commun.* **71**, 664 (1976).
10. W. R. Sherman, L. Y. Munsell, B. G. Gish, and M. P. Honchar, *J. Neurochem.* **44**, 798 (1985).
11. I. R. Batty and S. R. Nahorski, *Biochem. J.* **247**, 797 (1987).
12. P. Whitworth, D. J. Heal, and D. A. Kendall, *Br. J. Pharmacol.* **101**, 39 (1990).
13. P. Whitworth and D. A. Kendall, *J. Neurochem.* **51**, 258 (1988).
14. C. H. Lee, J. F. Dixon, M. Reichman, C. Moummi, G. Los, and L. E. Hokin, *Biochem. J.* **282**, 377 (1992).
15. M. Reichman, W. Nen, and L. E. Hokin, *Mol. Pharmacol.* **34**, 823 (1988).
16. E. Brown, D. A. Kendall, and S. R. Nahorski, *J. Neurochem.* **42**, 1379 (1984).
17. N. M. Dean and J. D. Moyer, *Biochem. J.* **242**, 361 (1987).
18. J. F. Dixon and L. E. Hokin, *J. Biol. Chem.* **264**, 11721 (1989).
19. J. Challiss, I. H. Batty, and S. R. Nahorski, *Biochem. Biophys. Res. Commun.* **157**, 683 (1988).
20. F. Donié and G. Reiser, *FEBS Lett.* **254**, 155 (1989).
21. J. F. Dixon, C. H. Lee, G. V. Los, and L. E. Hokin, *J. Neurochem.* **59**, 2332 (1992).
22. S. Feig and P. Lipton *J. Neurochem.* **55**, 473 (1990).
23. P. S. Sastry, J. F. Dixon, and L. E. Hokin, *J. Neurochem.* **58**, 1079 (1992).
24. E. G. Kennedy, R. I. Challiss, C. I. Ragan, and S. F. Nahorski, *Biochem. J.* **267**, 781 (1990).
25. W. R. Sherman, B. G. Gish, M. P. Honchar, and L. Y. Munsell, *Fed. Proc.* **46**, 2639 (1986).

26. J. H. Allison and M. A. Stewart, *Nature (London) New Biol.* **233,** 267 (1971).
27. L. M. Hallcher and W. R. Sherman, *J.Biol. Chem.* **255,** 10896 (1980).
28. E. D. Kennedy, R. A. J. Challiss, and S. R. Nahorski, *J. Neurochem.* **53,** 1652 (1989).
29. R. S. Jope, L. Song, and K. Kolassa, *Biol. Psychiatry* **31,** 505 (1992).
30. P. P. Godfrey, S. J. McClue, A. M. White, A. J. Wood, and D. G. Grahame-Smith, *J. Neurochem.* **52,** 498 (1989).
31. T. L. Casebolt and R. S. Jope, *Biol. Psychiatry* **25,** 329 (1989).
32. J. F. Dixon, G. V. Los, and L. E. Hokin, in preparation.
33. S. B. Shears, D. J. Storey, A. J. Morris, A. B. Cubitt, J. B. Parry, R. H. Michell, and C. J. Kirk, *Biochem. J.* **242,** 393 (1987).
34. C. Volonté and E. Racker, *J. Neurochem.* **51,** 1163 (1988).

Index